W9-AVI-544

REAL-WORLD NURSING SURVIVAL GUIDE:
ECGs & the HEART

REAL-WORLD NURSING SURVIVAL GUIDE SERIES

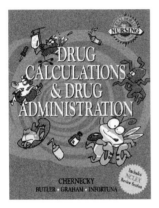

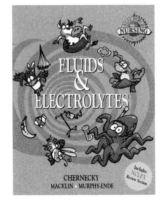

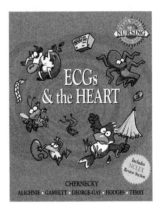

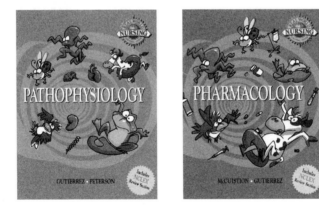

REAL-WORLD NURSING SURVIVAL GUIDE:

ECGs & the HEART

CYNTHIA CHERNECKY, PhD, RN, CNS, AOCN
Associate Professor, Department of Adult Health
Medical College of Georgia, School of Nursing
Augusta, Georgia

M. CHRISTINE ALICHNIE, PhD, RN
Chairperson and Professor
Department of Nursing
Assistant Dean
School of Health Sciences
College of Professional Studies
Bloomsburg University
Bloomsburg, Pennsylvania

KITTY GARRETT, MSN, RN, CCRN
Critical Care Nurse Clinician
St. Joseph Hospital
Augusta, Georgia

BEVERLY GEORGE-GAY, MSN, RN, CCRN
Medical College of Georgia
School of Nursing
Augusta, Georgia

REBECCA K. HODGES, RN, CCRN
Critical Care Nurse Clinician
St. Joseph Hospital
Augusta, Georgia

CYNTHIA TERRY, RN, CCRN
Assistant Professor, Nursing Program
Lehigh Carbon Community College
Schnecksville, Pennsylvania
Staff Nurse, Intensive Care Unit
Warren Hospital
Phillipsburg, New Jersey

W. B. SAUNDERS COMPANY
A Harcourt Health Sciences Company
Philadelphia London Montreal Sydney Tokyo Toronto

W.B. Saunders Company
A Harcourt Health Sciences Company

The Curtis Center
Independence Square West
Philadelphia, Pennsylvania 19106-3399

Library of Congress Cataloging-in-Publication Data

Real-world nursing survival guide. ECGs & the heart / Cynthia Chernecky ... [et al.].
    p. ; cm.
    Includes bibliographical references and index.
    ISBN 0-7216-9036-X
    1. Electrocardiography—Interpretation. 2. Arrhythmia—Nursing. 3. Heart—
Diseases—Nursing. I. Title: ECGs & the heart. II. Title ECGs and the heart.
III. Electrocardiograms and the heart. IV. Chernecky, Cynthia C.
    [DNLM: 1. Electrocardiography—methods—Nurses' Instruction. 2. Arrhythmia—
diagnosis—Nurses' Instruction. 3. Heart Diseases—diagnosis—Nurses' Instruction.
WG 140 R288 2001]
RC683.5.E5 R388 2001
616.1'207547—dc21   2001034811

Vice President and Publishing Director, Nursing: Sally Schrefer
Acquisitions Editor: Robin Carter
Developmental Editor: Gina Hopf
Project Manager: Catherine Jackson
Production Editor: Clay S. Broeker
Designer: Amy Buxton
Cover Designer and Illustrator: Chris Sharp, GraphCom Corporation

NOTICE

Nursing is an ever-changing field. Standard safety precautions must be followed, but as new research and clinical experience broaden our knowledge, changes in treatment and drug therapy may become necessary or appropriate. Readers are advised to check the most current product information provided by the manufacturer of each drug to be administered to verify the recommended dose, the method and duration of administration, and the contraindications. It is the responsibility of the licensed prescriber, relying on the experience and knowledge of the patient, to determine dosages and the best treatment for each individual patient. Neither the publisher nor the editor assumes any liability for any injury or damage to persons or property arising from this publication.

The Publisher

REAL-WORLD NURSING SURVIVAL GUIDE:
ECGs & THE HEART   ISBN 0-7216-9036-X

Copyright © 2002 by W.B. Saunders Company

All rights reserved. No part of this publication may be reproduced or transmitted in any form or by any means, electronic or mechanical, including photocopy, recording, or any information storage and retrieval system, without permission in writing from the publisher.

Printed in the United States of America

Last digit is the print number: 9 8 7 6 5 4 3 2 1

About the Authors

Dr. Cynthia Chernecky earned her degrees at the University of Connecticut (BSN), the University of Pittsburgh (MN), and Case Western Reserve University (PhD). She also earned an NCI fellowship at Yale University and a postdoctorate visiting scholarship at UCLA. Her clinical area of expertise is critical care oncology, with publications including *Laboratory Tests and Diagnostic Procedures* (third edition) and *Advanced and Critical Care Oncology Nursing: Managing Primary Complications*. She is a national speaker, researcher, and published scholar in cancer nursing. She is also active in the Orthodox Church and enjoys life with family, friends, colleagues, and two West Highland white terriers.

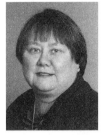

M. Christine (Chris) Alichnie earned a Bachelor's degree from the University of Pittsburgh, an MSN degree from the University of Pennsylvania, and a Master's degree of Science in Education from Wilkes College. She also holds a PhD in educational leadership from the University of Pennsylvania. Chris has worked as part of the nursing faculty at Northern Michigan University and at Wilkes College. Currently she is Chairperson and Professor of the Department of Nursing and Assistant Dean of the School of Health Sciences at Bloomsburg University. Chris is an appointed representative to the Pennsylvania State Board of Nursing and an appointed Program Evaluator for the National League of Nursing's Council of Baccalaureate and Higher Degree Programs. Her professional activities include membership in the Xi and Theta Zeta chapters of Sigma Theta Tau where she has held the positions of Finance Committee Chairperson and President and Eligibility Chairperson. She is also active in Phi Kappa Phi, Pi Lambda Theta (Eta chapter), the National Association of Female Executives, the National Council of State Boards of Nursing, and the American Nurses Association.

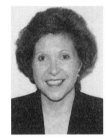

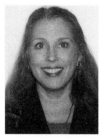

Kitty Garrett is a Critical Care Clinician at St. Joseph Hospital in Augusta, Georgia. She has 20 years of experience teaching basic dysrhythmias, 12-lead ECGs, and BCLS, ACLS, and CCRN Reviews at St. Joseph Hospital and is a consultant in the community. She is a national and local member and past program chair of the American Association of Critical Care Nurses and is certified through AACN as a CCRN. She pursued graduate studies in the Critical Care Clinical Nurse Specialist Program at the Medical College of Georgia and graduated in May 2001. She enjoys gardening, walking, playing tennis, and teaching Sunday school classes to teenagers.

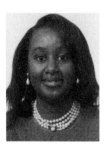

Beverly George-Gay started her nursing career in 1978, during which she completed a Practical Nursing Program at Clara Barton High School for Health Professions in Brooklyn, New York. After working in various areas of nursing and earning several degrees, she found herself at Shands Hospital at the University of Florida where she worked as a staff nurse and then as a charge nurse in the Surgical ICU. Beverly advanced to a Clinical Research Coordinator position for the Division of Critical Care Medicine, also at Shands Hospital. It was during this time that she completed her MSN degree at the University of Florida. Beverly then relocated to Augusta, Georgia, and began a career in academic nursing at the Medical College of Georgia, School of Nursing. She teaches Medical-Surgical Nursing, Critical Care Nursing, and Pathophysiology. Beverly also maintains a clinical practice and has served as a Clinical Nurse Intensivist for the Surgical Intensive Care Unit for the Division of Critical Care Nursing at the Medical College of Georgia Hospital and Clinics. Beverly is a wife and mother of three children, Reese, Joseph, and Dominique.

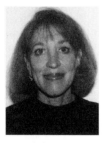

Rebecca (Becki) Hodges is a Critical Care Nurse Clinician with 24 years experience in an acute care setting. She has been actively involved in consulting and lecturing. Becki received her BSN from the Medical College of Georgia and is currently pursuing a graduate degree in nursing. She has maintained CCRN certification since 1982, was a charter member and past President of the CSRA chapter of AACN, and has been named to *Who's Who in Nursing*. In her spare time, she is also an avid gardener (specializing in topiary and herb gardening) and was a past President of the Azalea Garden Club.

Cynthia (Cindy) L. Terry earned her BSN from the Pennsylvania State University and completed her MSN at Villanova University. Since 1977 she has held various staff nurse positions in CCUs and ICUs. She obtained her CCRN in 1979 and has maintained it ever since. Cindy has served as a nurse manager of the CCU/Cardiac Catheterization Holding Area, but her primary work has been as a nurse educator in the hospital and academic settings for the last 22 years. Currently, she teaches at Lehigh Carbon Community College in Schnecksville, Pennsylvania, and also works in the CCU/ICU at Warren Hospital in Phillipsburg, New Jersey. She is a member of the American Association of Critical Care Nurses and Sigma Theta Tau (Rho Chapter). Cindy is also very active in the National Ski Patrol and serves as a Basic Patroller and Instructor at the Blue Mountain Ski Resort Area in Palmerton, Pennsylvania.

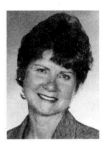

Contributors

Mary Ann Cegielsky, MSN, RN
Assistant Professor
Department of Nursing
Bloomsburg University
Bloomsburg, Pennsylvania

Sharon Kribbs, MN, RN
Assistant Chairperson and Assistant Professor
Department of Nursing
Bloomsburg University
Bloomsburg, Pennsylvania

Roseanne LeVan, MSN, RN
Former Instructor
Department of Nursing
Bloomsburg University
Bloomsburg, Pennsylvania

Dorette Sugg Welk, PhD, MSN, RN
Professor
Department of Nursing
Bloomsburg University
Bloomsburg, Pennsylvania

Faculty & Student Reviewers

FACULTY

Betty Nash Blevins, MSN, RN, CCRN, CS
Bluefield State College
Bluefield, West Virginia

Elizabeth M. Christensen, RN, MN, CCRN
Affiliate Faculty
University of Phoenix
New Orleans, Louisiana

Ronald Mitchell, PhD, RN
Idaho State University
Pocatello, Idaho

Jay K. Ober, RN, BS, CCRN, CEN
Cardiac Intensive Care Unit
Baystate Medical Center
Springfield, Massachusetts

Elizabeth A. O'Connor, MSN, RN, CS, FNP, CCRN
Bozeman College of Nursing
Montana State University, Great Falls Campus
Bozeman, Montana

Thena E. Parrott, PhD, RNCS
Associate Degree Nursing Program
Blinn College
Bryan, Texas

Jeffrey J. Paurus, RN, MS
Instructor
Minneapolis Community and Technical College
Staff Nurse
Fairview University Hospital
Minneapolis, Minnesota

Nancy L. Sarpy, RN, MS, CCRN
Assistant Professor of Nursing
School of Nursing
Loma Linda University
Loma Linda, California

STUDENTS

Edith Benham, LPN
WorWic Community College
Salisbury, Maryland

Kimberly A. Bloom
Bloomsburg University
Bloomsburg, Pennsylvania

Evelyn DeMoss
Austin Community College
Austin, Texas

Christine Griffin
Child Care Counselor
Lehigh Carbon Community College
Schnecksville, Pennsylvania

Elizabeth Hartzell, CNA
Lehigh Carbon Community College
Schnecksville, Pennsylvania

Carol A. Haverty, CAN
Lehigh Carbon Community College
Schnecksville, Pennsylvania

Sheila Holliday
Austin Community College
Austin, Texas

Mary Jo Lampart
Bloomsburg University
Bloomsburg, Pennsylvania

Nicole E. Landis
Lehigh Carbon Community College
Schnecksville, Pennsylvania

John Daniel Luchansky
Bloomsburg University
Bloomsburg, Pennsylvania

Maria E. Mulinos, LPN
Nanticoke Memorial Hospital
Seaford, Delaware

Melissa L. Normann
Bloomsburg University
Bloomsburg, Pennsylvania

Michelle Ratliff, CNA
Lehigh Carbon Community College
Schnecksville, Pennsylvania

Frederic W. Strohl, LPN
President, Phi Theta Kappa
Presidential Ambassador, SGA Senator
Lehigh Carbon Community College
Schnecksville, Pennsylvania

Dina M. Timko
Bloomsburg University
Bloomsburg, Pennsylvania

Deborah Warner, CNA
Lehigh Carbon Community College
Schnecksville, Pennsylvania

Beata F. Wirth
President, Student Nurse Program
College Senator, Phi Theta Kappa
Lehigh Carbon Community College
Schnecksville, Pennsylvania

Series Reviewers

FACULTY

Edwina A. McConnell, PhD, RN, FRCNA
Professor
School of Nursing
Texas Technical University Health Sciences Center
Lubbock, Texas
Consultant
Gorham, Maine

Judith L. Myers, MSN, RN
Health Sciences Center
St. Louis University
School of Nursing
St. Louis, Missouri

FEATURED STUDENTS

Shayne Michael Gray, RN, was born in Little Rock, Arkansas, and graduated with a BSN degree from the University of Arkansas for Medical Sciences (UAMS) in 1999. He has spent a year working at the University as an Intensive Care Nurse and has also applied for a medical commission in the Naval Reserve. Future plans include becoming a CRNA. Before nursing school, Shayne played drums in a band that eventually signed with a record label and was distributed by Polygram and Phillips Multimedia; this afforded him the opportunity to tour the United States and Canada for 3 years. Following that, he left the band and earned a leading role in an independent film that was shown at the prestigious Sundance Film Festival. It is the earnings from this movie role that Shayne credits with helping him finish his nursing school prerequisites at the University of Arkansas at Little Rock, and he married his wife Michelle in 1996, just as he was being accepted into the nursing program. He spent 2 years serving as a volunteer for the Arkansas Lung Association, speaking about the dangers of smoking to local school children, and has also been a volunteer for many of UAMS's fundraisers and community clean-up projects. A former Helicopter Flight Medic in the Army National Guard, Shayne is a certified scuba diver and loves the outdoors, playing guitar, and writing. He is also ACLS qualified and hopes to participate in nursing/medical research in the future.

For **Jill Hall,** attending nursing school has been the fulfillment of a childhood dream. Before that opportunity, she served an apprenticeship as a Mechanical and Production Engineer with British Aerospace. She then spent 2 years as a stay-at-home mother for her two children. When her husband accepted a job in California, the family moved from northern England to Huntington Beach, where Jill began taking prerequisite nursing classes at Golden West College. Once into the nursing program, she knew she had found what she was meant to do. She became involved in the Student Nurses' Association, and a trip to the mid-year NSNA convention in Dallas sparked her enthusiasm to run for national office. At the annual convention in Pittsburgh, she was elected to the Nominations and Elections Committee, and her year in office involved conventions in both Charlotte and Salt Lake City. In her own community, she is a member of the United Methodist Church and the high school PTO. She has been a Girl Scout leader, Sunday school teacher, soccer coach, and soccer camp coordinator, as well as a volunteer in the emergency room of a local hospital. She is currently employed in the Pediatric ICU at Miller Children's Hospital in Long Beach, California. She also plans to pursue both BSN and MSN degrees. She offers special thanks to two instructors who have served as mentors during her time in the nursing program at Golden West College, Nadine Davis and Marcia Swanson: "Their standards of excellence have inspired me to achieve more than I ever thought I could. Gracious thanks for all they have done for me."

Elizabeth J. Hoogmoed, RN, BSN, recently graduated from William Paterson University and is currently a neurological nurse at Valley Hospital in Ridgewood, New Jersey. She serves on the Executive Board of Sigma Theta Tau as Corresponding Secretary for the Iota Alpha chapter. She also served as Membership and Nominations Chair for New Jersey Nursing Students from 1998 to 1999 and continues to be a sustaining member of the organization. She has also been a volunteer for her local ambulance corps for 7 years. She has been accepted into the program at New York University, where she will complete her Masters degree to become a Nurse Practitioner. Her hope is to promote the profession of nursing and show its importance to the future of health care. In this era of computers and technology, she believes it is reassuring to know that a select number of individuals continue to follow the inner call to care for people and promote wellness in society: "These are the nurses."

Katie Scarlett McRae, BA, BSN, says that if you talk to her for more than a few minutes, you'll be sure to hear her say, "I love my job." She serves as a staff RN on the cardiovascular/telemetry floor at Oregon Health Sciences University (OHSU) in Portland, caring for patients who have had heart transplants or other cardiac/vascular surgeries or who suffer from congestive heart failure, diabetes, or arrhythmias. Working with many experienced nurses "great at sharing their insights and knowledge," Katie loves the teaching hospital environment and jokes that nursing is her "second career"; when she graduated from the OHSU nursing program in 1999, it was actually her second Bachelor's degree, but "the two degrees were 24 years apart!" Katie credits the rigorous OHSU program with giving her the confidence to know she could practice nursing safely. During nursing school, she was active in student government, and she is also a current member of the Oregon Nurses' Association, the ANA, and the AACN. She plans to return to OHSU soon to begin work on a Master's degree in Adult Health and Illness, with a focus on diabetes, and her ideal career would be to create and manage a comprehensive diabetes management for the state of Oregon.

STUDENTS

Angela M. Boyd, AS
University of Tennessee at Martin
Martin, Tennessee

Jennifer Hamilton
University of Virginia
Charlottesville, Virginia

Joy Kutlenios Amos, RN, BSN
Piedmont Medical Center
Rock Hill, South Carolina
Former student
Wheeling Jesuit University
Wheeling, West Virginia

Preface

The *Real-World Nursing Survival Guide* series was created with your input. Nursing students told us about certain topics they found difficult to master, such as dosage calculations, fluids and electrolytes, ECGs, pathophysiology, and pharmacology. Focus groups were held at the National Student Nurses Association meeting, and we asked you what would be the best way to learn this difficult material. Your responses were certainly interesting! You said we should keep the text to a minimum; use an engaging, fun approach; provide ample space to write on the pages; include a variety of activities to appeal to students with different learning styles; make the content visually appealing; and provide NCLEX review questions so you could check your understanding of key topics and perform any necessary review. The *Real-World Nursing Survival Guide* series is the result of your ideas.

An understanding of the heart and its electrical conduction system is necessary for excellence in nursing care, and an ability to apply knowledge related to the heart is also needed throughout the nursing process. Such knowledge provides an avenue for nursing assessment, leading to an increased quality and quantity of life for all those for whom nurses care.

Such knowledge is also the focus of *ECGs & the Heart*. To understand the diagnostic ECG test associated with the heart, you need to comprehend the electrophysiology of the heart muscle itself. You then need to incorporate knowledge of ECG leads to their specific cardiac areas and learn to interpret their output, which provides guidelines for care and intervention. We have made every effort to discuss similar principles of ECG interpretation as a related group of concepts to help you understand ECG interpretation and its relationship to cardiac electrophysiology. However, it is important to remember that ECG output is only one diagnostic test and one piece of assessment datum. You must examine the entire picture of a patient before interventions are implemented, and this book will help you understand the heart muscle, how this muscle works, and how to incorporate ECG data into your larger plan of care.

We include many features in the margins to help you focus on the vital information you'll need to succeed in the classroom and in the clinical setting. TAKE HOME POINTS are composed of both study tips for classroom tests and "pearls of wisdom" to assist you in caring for patients. Both are drawn from our many years of combined academic and clinical experience. Content marked with a caution icon is vital and usually involves nursing actions that may have life-threatening consequences or may significantly affect patient outcomes. The lifespan icon and the culture icon highlight variations in treatment that may be necessary for specific age or ethnic groups. A calculator icon will draw your eye to important equations and examples that will help you calculate proper medication dosages. Finally, a web links icon will direct you to sites on the Internet that will give more detailed information on a given topic. Each of these icons are designed to help you focus on real-world patient care, the nursing process, and positive patient outcomes.

We also use consistent headings that emphasize specific nursing actions. What It IS provides a definition of a topic. What You NEED TO KNOW provides the explanation of the topic. What You DO explains what you do as a practicing nurse. Finally, Do You UNDERSTAND? provides questions and exercises that are both entertaining and useful to reinforce the topic's concepts. This four-step approach provides you with information and helps you learn how to apply it to the clinical setting.

We have used our own real world clinical experiences, our memories of being nursing students, and the expert experiences of nursing faculty, clinicians, and current nursing students to bring you a text that will help you understand ECGs and therefore help you implement better patient care. We believe that understanding is the key to critical thinking, and critical thinking is the key to the art and science of nursing. We believe that this book and series will ultimately result in excellent nursing care. The race to acquire knowledge is never ending, so let the games begin!

Cynthia C. Chernecky, PhD, RN, CNS, AOCN
M. Christine Alichnie, PhD, RN
Kitty Garrett, RN, CCRN
Beverly George-Gay, MSN, RN, CCRN
Rebecca K. Hodges, RN, CCRN
Cynthia Terry, RN, CCRN

Acknowledgments

This book has been filled with expert clinical content from true colleagues whose goals are always to care for patients, students, and fellow nurses. The dedication, professionalism, and teamwork necessary to complete this project is nothing short of miraculous. My heartfelt thanks and admiration to all of the authors. I believe we have made a true difference and continue to model the excellence and caring that makes life truly worthwhile. I also could not continue in my professional career without mentors whose integrity is inspiring and reflects the best within the profession—thank you Dr. Ann Kolanowski and Dr. Linda Sarna.

Cynthia (Cinda) Chernecky

This book is dedicated to my family and professional colleagues who helped to make this book a reality; for their support and encouragement, I am eternally thankful. To my husband, Bill, and my children, William and Diana—your presence in my life means more than any professional award or accomplishment. To my professional colleagues and the departmental secretaries who assisted with the manuscript and supported this project—I am eternally grateful. To the senior nursing students, Mel, Dina, John, and Mary Jo, who critiqued parts of the book—my thanks for being the driving force to continue my pursuit of intellectual challenges. Last, to Cynthia Chernecky and Cynthia Terry and the excellent staff at Harcourt Health Sciences, whose guidance, encouragement, and support provided this opportunity—you have my sincere appreciation.

Christine Alichnie

Thanks to my husband Michael and to my three sons, Trey, Brian, and Michael, for their patience, understanding, and support during the preparation of this, my publishing debut. I would also like to thank Becki Hodges, my partner, co-author, and friend, who was always there to consult when the need arose. Special thanks to Cinda Chernecky, my faculty mentor, who has given me the opportunity to contribute to this book. Most importantly, thank you to my Creator for blessing me with the ability and motivation to share my knowledge with others in hopes that we may all make a difference in this world.

Kitty Garrett

To my husband Mont, who is my best friend and biggest fan and supporter. To my parents, Agnes and Joseph George, who always come to the rescue. Finally, to my children, Reese, Joseph, and Dominique, because they love me back.

Beverly George-Gay

It is with deep appreciation that I acknowledge those who have brought me endless joy and led me to the path of learning. Thanks to the contributors of this book, who shared their knowledge and made this a reality, and to Gina Hopf, Developmental Editor at Harcourt Health Sciences, who helped me keep the details straight. Thanks to Dr. Cinda Chernecky, my mentor, who got me involved in this project. A special thanks to my dad, Dr. Hubert King, and my mom, Betty, who have continually encouraged me and always provided love and support. To Drs. Hurley Jones and Wade Strickland, who first introduced me to the joys of cardiology. I am forever indebted to Kitty Garrett, a co-author and special friend who was always there for moral support. And finally, the most special thanks to my husband, Jack, my family, Stuart, Paige, Brad, Havird, Hodges, Phyllis, Rob, Riah, Blake, Jordan, and my sister, Debbie, for their limitless love.

Rebecca Hodges

I would like to thank the ADN faculty at LCCC for teaching me to go deeper than the surface and my family for giving me time to work on this book.

Cynthia Terry

Contents

1 Anatomy and Physiology

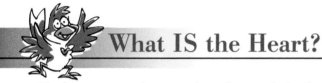 ## What IS the Heart?

The *heart* is a muscular organ about the size of a fist, located between the second and sixth left ribs and behind the sternum.

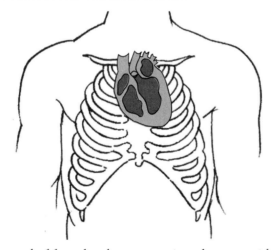

It is composed of four chambers: two *atria* and two *ventricles*. The main function of the atria, located at the top of the heart, is to act as reservoirs for incoming blood. However, the atria also contribute as much as 30% to the output of blood from the heart. This output of blood from the atria is known as *atrial kick*.

The ventricles are the heart's main pumping chambers. They are separated by valves that promote forward flow and allow synchrony between the filling and pumping of blood. The valves between the atria and ventricles are called the *atrioventricular* (AV) *valves*. These include the *tricuspid valve*

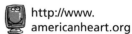 http://www.
americanheart.org

1

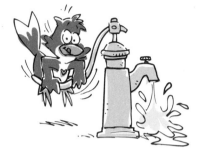

and the *mitral valve*. The tricuspid valve separates the right atrium from the right ventricle, and the mitral valve separates the left atrium from the left ventricle.

The valves leading away from the heart are called the *semilunar valves*. These include the *aortic valve* and the *pulmonic valve*. The aortic valve separates the left ventricle from the aorta, and the pulmonic valve separates the right ventricle from the pulmonary artery. To be competent, valves must open and close easily.

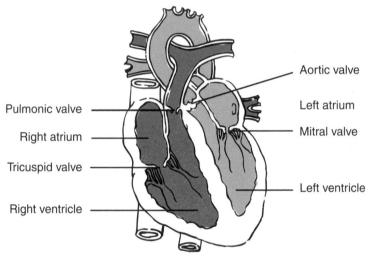

The heart has four layers: (1) the *myocardium*, (2) the *endocardium*, (3) the *epicardium*, and (4) the *pericardium*. The myocardium is the main muscular layer. This is the layer that is injured in a *myocardial infarction* (MI). The endocardium is the inner lining, which is continuous with the valves and the *endothelium* that lines the blood vessels. The epicardium is the outer surface from which the coronary arteries originate. The pericardium is a fibrous sac that surrounds and protects the heart.

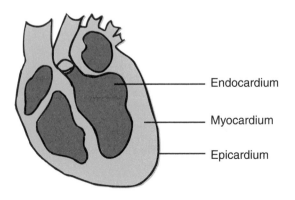

Heart sounds are caused by the closure of valves. The first heart sound (lub), or S1, is caused by closure of the AV valves. The second heart sound (dup), or S2, is caused by closure of the semilunar valves. A valve that does not close tightly allows backflow of blood (i.e., insufficiency or regurgitation). A valve that does not open wide enough causes turbulent flow secondary to obstruction or narrowing (i.e., stenosis). Both of these conditions may be detected clinically by auscultating for a murmur specific to the valve involved.

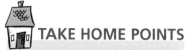

TAKE HOME POINTS

- Subendocardium is used to describe the portion of the myocardium that is closest to the heart's inner lining but does not go through the entire thickness of the heart muscle.
- *Transmural* means full thickness of the myocardium.

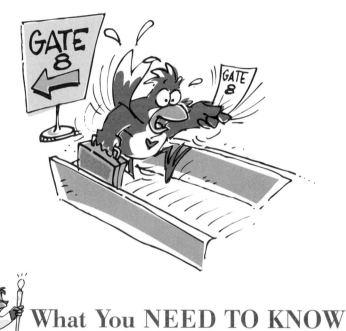

What You NEED TO KNOW

There are three systems that must work together for the heart to beat efficiently: (1) circulatory, (2) conduction, and (3) coronary. The circulatory system is the continuous network of vessels through which the heart mechanically pumps blood. The conduction system is the electrical wiring system that simulates the heart to pump. The coronary system is a system of arteries and veins that provide oxygenated blood to meet the metabolic needs of the heart muscle itself.

Circulatory System

The heart is actually two pumps in one. The left side pumps blood through the arterial system to deliver oxygenated blood to the tissues; the right side receives blood returning from the body and pumps it to the lungs to be reoxygenated. Although the left and right sides of the heart are separated by

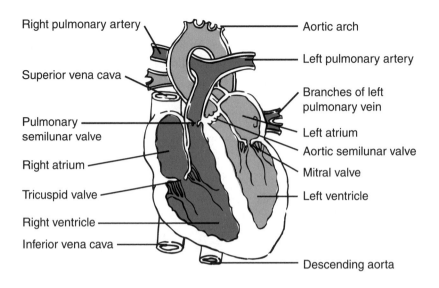

a septum, they pump in synchrony with each other. While the left ventricle is ejecting blood to the aorta, the right ventricle is ejecting blood to the pulmonary artery and out to the lungs.

The right heart receives venous blood from the systemic circulation through the *superior* and *inferior vena cavae,* which enter the right atrium. Blood leaves the right ventricle and enters the pulmonary circulation through the pulmonary artery. The pulmonary artery divides into right and left pulmonary arteries to transport nonoxygenated blood from the right heart to the right and left lungs.

The pulmonary arteries branch further into the pulmonary capillary bed, where oxygen and carbon dioxide exchange occurs. The four pulmonary veins, two from the right lung and two from the left lung, carry oxygenated blood from the lungs to the left side of the heart. The oxygenated blood moves through the left atrium and ventricle and out into the aorta, which delivers the blood to systemic arteries and arterioles that supply the body.

The left ventricular muscle is thicker than the right because it has to work harder to generate higher pressures to pump blood throughout the body. The right ventricle only has to pump from the heart to the lungs, and therefore does not have to work as hard.

The cardiac cycle is the pumping and resting (*systole* and *diastole*) action. In systole, the ventricles contract, the semilunar valves (pulmonic and aortic) open, and the AV valves (mitral and tricuspid) close. Then, during diastole, the ventricles refill again from the atria. The AV valves are open, and the semilunar valves are closed. One cycle of filling and contracting is equal to one heartbeat.

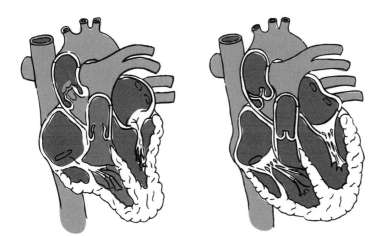

🏠 **TAKE HOME POINTS**

Ventricular filling occurs during diastole. There are four factors that affect how much blood is pumped from the heart (cardiac output) every minute:

1. Heart rate
2. Amount of blood
3. Volume of resistance
4. Squeezing ability of the ventricular myocardium

Heart rate should not be too fast or too slow, and the heart must have the right amount of blood to pump. There needs to be enough blood volume to fill and stretch the left ventricle to maximize its contraction, but not so much that the ventricle is over stretched and unable to keep up with the demand. The stretching caused by blood in the left ventricle is called *preload*. Remember the Frank-Starling curve: "The greater the stretch, the more forceful the contraction—up to a point.

The heart also needs to pump freely without meeting a lot of resistance. The main cause of resistance is constriction of the blood vessels *(arterioles)*. This constriction increases the aortic pressure and causes the heart to work harder to get the blood through the constricted vessels. This is called *afterload*.

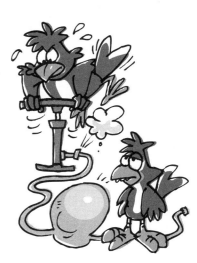

Finally, the squeezing ability of the ventricular myocardium affects the amount of blood pumped from the heart. The force of the contraction depends on the degree of fiber shortening (contractility). Two major factors determine the force of contraction: (1) preload and (2) sympathetic nervous system stimulation. Stimulation of the sympathetic nervous system increases myocardial contractility. If the muscle fibers are not well-oxygenated or if they have been damaged by past heart attacks, depressant effects of drugs, or electrolyte imbalances, myocardial fibers may not shorten maximally.

Conduction System

How is the heart stimulated to beat? The heart's own internal pacemaker, called the sinoatrial (SA) node, stimulates the heart. The SA node is a specialized bundle of nerve fibers located at the junction of the superior vena cava and right atrium, near the epicardial surface. The SA node fires and sends an electrical impulse down a group of three internodal tracts that connect the SA node to the *atrioventricular* (AV) *node*.

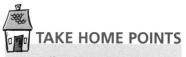

🏠 **TAKE HOME POINTS**

Factors affecting contractility are called *inotropic agents.* Positive inotropic drugs (e.g., digitalis, dobutamine) increase myocardial contractility. Negative inotropic drugs (e.g., beta blockers, calcium channel blockers) decrease myocardial contractility.

The AV node, also known as the *AV junction*, is located in the inferior portion of the right atrial wall, directly above the right ventricle. Once the impulse has reached the AV node, it is delayed for a short time to allow the ventricles to fill. It then continues from the AV node down a common pathway called the *bundle of His* and splits into two branches (the left and right bundle branches). These lead to the left and right ventricles, respectively.

The left bundle branch further divides into an anterior and posterior branch. The terminal portions of the bundle branches are called *Purkinje fibers*. The Purkinje fibers are like small fingers that reach throughout the myocardium to stimulate the muscle to contract. This electrical activation of the muscle cells is called *depolarization*. After depolarization, the cells are then deactivated, a process called *repolarization* (see Chapter 5).

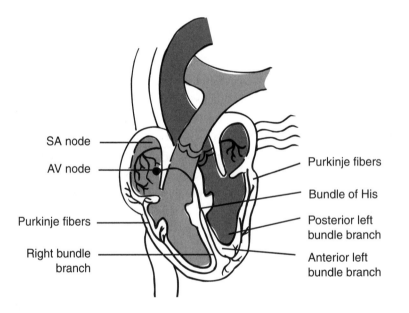

How does the heart know how fast to beat? The average heart rate is 60 to 100 beats per minute (bpm). Heart rate is determined by a balance of sympathetic and parasympathetic innervation. The normal physiologic response is for the heart rate to change to meet the demands of the body. For example, during exercise the skeletal muscles need more oxygen, so heart rate increases to send more blood to the muscles. However, during sleep metabolic needs are decreased, so heart rate is also decreased. (As a health care provider, you should be prepared to see some of your patients' heart rates drop into the 50s during the night.) In most cases the sympathetic and parasympathetic nervous systems are balanced to keep the heart rate within normal limits. However, one can override the other when it becomes necessary.

If the heart beats too slowly, tissue oxygenation is affected. Also, if the heart beats too rapidly, there is less time between beats for the ventricles to fill. This can cause a decrease in the amount of blood pumped from the heart, which can also decrease tissue perfusion.

Should the SA node fail to fire or fire too slowly, or if the impulse does not make it through to the AV node, the AV node can initiate impulses. The inherent rate of the AV node as the pacemaker is 40 to 60 bpm. If the SA node and the AV node fail to fire, fire too slowly, or the impulse fails to reach the ventricles, the ventricles can also stimulate themselves from the Purkinje fibers. However, this is the least efficient "pacemaker," because the ventricles can only initiate impulses at a rate of 20 to 40 bpm. This rate is too slow to meet the body's oxygenation needs, and the patient will require an artificial pacemaker to maintain good health.

Circulatory Circulation

The heart beats an average of 70 times a minute, 24 hours a day, 7 days a week for a lifetime. Unlike other body organs, it never gets a break. The heart has its own circulatory system to supply the myocardium with the necessary blood and oxygen. The heart "feeds itself first." It pumps an average of 5 to 6 L of blood every minute. The system of blood vessels supplying the heart is called the *coronary system*. The left and right coronary arteries branch off of the aorta just past the aortic valve. Most coronary filling occurs during diastole.

The left coronary artery descends in a common branch called the *left main* and then divides into the *left anterior descending* (LAD) and *circumflex arteries*. The LAD feeds the interventricular septum and anterior left ventricle. The circumflex feeds the left atrium and the lateral portion of the left ventricle.

The right coronary artery descends and winds around the back of the heart. It feeds the right atrium, the SA and AV nodes, the right ventricle, and the inferior and posterior surfaces of the left ventricle.

 TAKE HOME POINTS

It is imperative to be familiar with the conduction system to understand normal and abnormal heart rhythms (*dysrhythmias*).

 TAKE HOME POINTS

Ectopic beats
Although the SA node is the *normal pacemaker* of the heart, every cell in the heart has the ability to initiate an electrical impulse. This property is called *excitability,* and it explains how ectopic beats and rhythms can form. Common triggers for ectopic beats are ischemia, hypoxemia, electrolyte imbalances, caffeine, nicotine, and emotional stress.

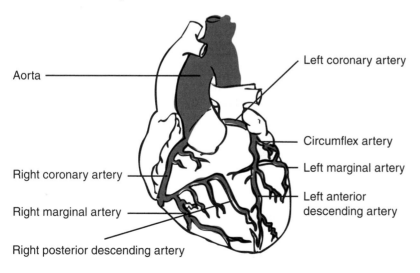

Aorta

Right coronary artery

Right marginal artery

Right posterior descending artery

Left coronary artery

Circumflex artery

Left marginal artery

Left anterior descending artery

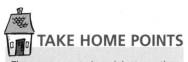

TAKE HOME POINTS

The coronary arteries originate on the epicardial surface of the myocardium and terminate on the endocardial surface, which explains why sub-endocardial ischemia, or ST depression, is the earliest ECG sign of ischemia. A strong knowledge of coronary artery anatomy is needed to interpret ECG results and to locate MI.

The coronary arteries may develop *atherosclerosis*. Atherosclerotic plaque narrows the lumen of the blood vessels, thereby compromising the blood flow to the myocardium. This can lead to ischemia, causing angina and, ultimately, MI.

Do You UNDERSTAND?

DIRECTIONS: **Complete the crossword puzzle.**

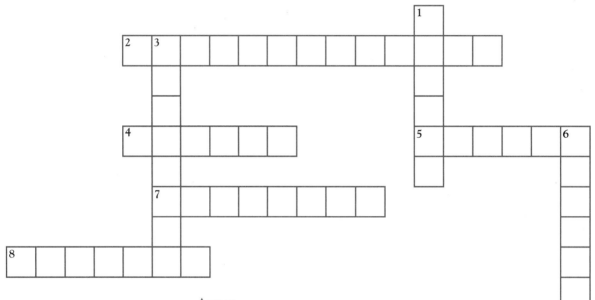

Across

2. The major gaseous waste product from heart circulation.
4. Blood is collected back to the heart by the _____ system.
5. This valve is located between the left ventricle and aorta, and it produces the S2 sound when closing.
7. The bottom of the heart is called the _____ surface.
8. Ventricular contraction.

Down

1. This valve is located between the left atrium and left ventricle and produces the S1 sound when closing.
3. Blood is pumped to the body through the _____ system.
6. These arteries supply the heart with oxygenated blood.

Answers:

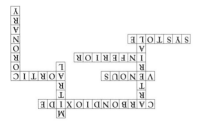

DIRECTIONS: **Match Column A with the terms listed in Column B.**

Column A

1. _____ Resistance the heart pumps against
2. _____ Number of heartbeats per minute
3. _____ Volume and stretch of the heart
4. _____ Squeezing ability of the heart

Column B

a. Preload
b. Afterload
c. Contractility
d. Heart rate

Principles of Rhythm Interpretation Waveform Analysis

To interpret a rhythm strip accurately, you must be able to identify waveforms correctly. This chapter discusses waveform identification and the electrical events of depolarization and repolarization. The relationship of waveforms and intervals to the cardiac cycle are also covered.

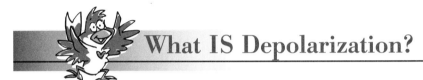

What IS Depolarization?

Depolarization is an electrical event that can be recorded on the electrocardiographic (ECG) or rhythm strip. It is a process in which the positive ions (mainly potassium) move from inside the cell to an area of less concentration outside the cell. This loss of positively charged ions causes the inside of the myocardial cell to become more negative. Once the cell becomes stimulated, the cell membrane allows sodium to rush from the extracellular space to the intracellular space. This process results in a sudden change in electrical charge within the cell that can be recorded on the ECG as indicated by the P wave and QRS complex.

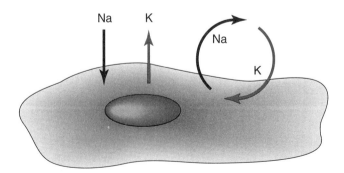

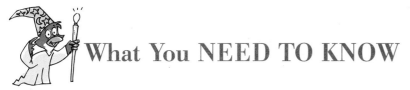

What You NEED TO KNOW

The movement of electrolytes stimulates cardiac cells. The ECG machine records the movement of sodium inside a cardiac cell at the same time that potassium moves out of the cell. Cardiac cells have the ability to conduct this current of energy from one cell to the next.

Electrodes placed on the chest and limbs pick up the electrical energy from this wave of depolarization. Depolarization normally begins in the sinoatrial (SA) node and moves through the atrium to the atrioventricular (AV) node, where there is a slight pause to allow both atria to contract. Then the wave travels to the bundle of His, through the right and left bundle branches to the Purkinje fibers, and finally to the ventricular cells. The mechanical process of contraction usually follows the electrical process of depolarization within a few milliseconds (ms). (See Chapter 1 for a review of the conduction system.)

Rule of Electrical Flow

The waveforms on the ECG created by the process of depolarization may be positive, negative, or *isoelectric* (flat). One of the basic principles of electrocardiography explains the reason for positive, negative, or isoelectric waveforms. This principle states that if the energy from the depolarization process flows toward a positive recording electrode, the waveform will appear upright or positive.

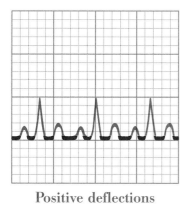

Positive deflections   Negative deflections

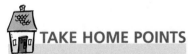

TAKE HOME POINTS

- The heart is three dimensional. Therefore when the process of depolarization occurs, it travels in several directions at one time.
- Depending on the lead being monitored, the recording electrode in that lead will view the majority of electrical current as either traveling toward or away from the electrode. It will then write the waveform as positive, negative, or isoelectric.

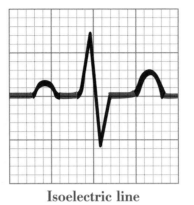

Isoelectric line

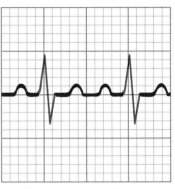

Biphasic waveforms

If the energy from the depolarization process flows toward a negative recording electrode or away from a positive electrode, the waveform will appear as a negative deflection. If the energy is directed away from the positive and the negative electrode, there will be an isoelectric line recorded. A *biphasic waveform* (a two-phased waveform that goes up and down) occurs when the flow of energy is first directed toward a positive electrode and then toward a negative electrode (or vice versa).

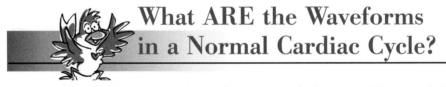

What ARE the Waveforms in a Normal Cardiac Cycle?

On the ECG, one cardiac cycle is composed of a P wave, PR interval, QRS complex, ST segment, and T wave. These waveforms electrically represent one heart beat.

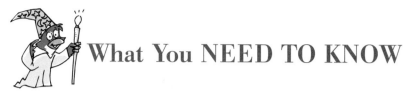

What You NEED TO KNOW

P Wave

The *P wave* represents the firing of the SA node and atrial depolarization. It should be the first waveform in the cardiac cycle. Normally, P waves are upright, particularly in lead II. Both atria depolarize simultaneously, resulting in one P wave.

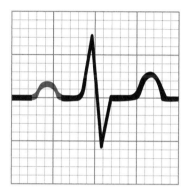

Normally, the P wave indicates the SA node started the impulse that depolarized the atrium. If a P wave changes in shape, it may indicate the impulse was initiated somewhere else in the atria or possibly in the junctional tissue, but outside the SA node.

In some abnormal rhythms, the atria may be stimulated more than once before the ventricles contract. In this case there may be two or more P waves for each QRS complex.

TAKE HOME POINTS

If conduction is normal, there should always be one P wave before every QRS complex.

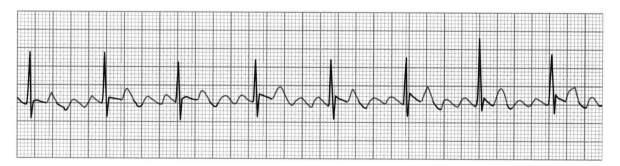

In some abnormal rhythms or beats, the P wave may be completely absent.

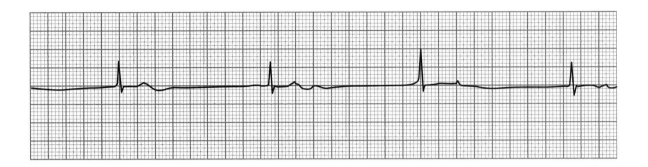

Inverted P Wave

If a P wave is upside down (particularly in lead II where they are expected to be upright), it is considered inverted. *Inverted P waves* in lead II indicate that conduction through the atria occurred in an opposite, backward (retrograde) manner.

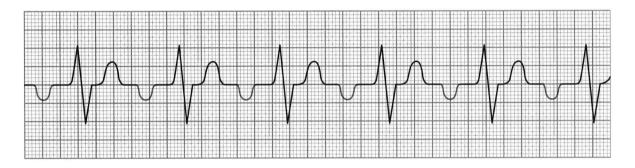

When this happens, the impulse originates in the AV junctional tissue, rather than in the SA node. In the normal heart, the SA node should always initiate the impulse and cause atrial depolarization, resulting in an upright P wave. Absent P waves, too many P waves, or inverted P waves compromise normal atrial contraction (atrial kick). The loss of synchronized, regular atrial contraction decreases the atrial contribution to ventricular filling and stretch, which reduces cardiac output.

PR Segment

The *PR segment* is an isoelectric (straight) line that occurs from the end of the P wave to the beginning of the QRS complex. The PR segment represents the delay of the electrical impulse at the AV node to allow for atrial contraction.

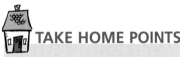

TAKE HOME POINTS

- A normal P wave is upright, rounded, and symmetrical.
- There should be one P wave for every QRS complex.
- Whenever the P wave changes, note whether the change occurs with one beat or whether the entire rhythm has changed.

PR Interval

The *PR interval* represents atrial depolarization and AV delay. It is measured from the beginning of the P wave to the end of the PR segment, which is the beginning of the QRS complex.

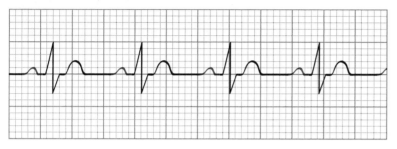

QRS Complex

The *QRS complex* represents ventricular depolarization. It may have a Q, R, or S wave, or it may have any combination of these waves.

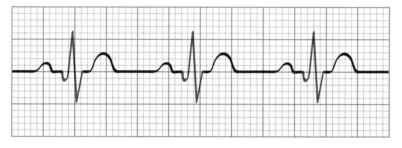

Q Wave. The *Q wave* is defined as the first negative deflection in the QRS complex. Not every QRS complex has a Q wave. Q waves may be considered a normal part of the QRS complex, or they may be considered significant, indicating that a myocardial infarction (MI) has occurred. The diagnosis of MI is based on many factors, including signs or symptoms, cardiac enzymes or markers, 12-lead ECG, and other tests (both invasive and noninvasive).

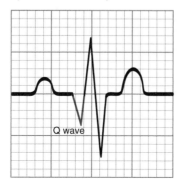

R Wave. An *R wave* is the first positive deflection after the P wave. R waves may differ in size, ranging from tall to small to absent. QRS complexes may or may not have an R wave.

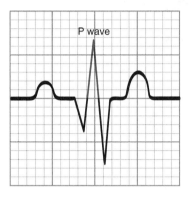

TAKE HOME POINTS

- The QRS complex represents ventricular depolarization.
- Although a QRS complex may contain a Q, R, or S wave (or some combination of these waves), it is still called a QRS complex.
- The Q wave is the negative deflection before the R, or it is the first negative deflection.
- The S wave is the negative deflection after the R, or it is the second negative deflection.
- The R wave is always a positive deflection.

S Wave. The *S wave* is also a negative wave. It is defined as the negative wave that follows the R wave or the second negative wave. As with other waves in the QRS complex, the S wave can be small, tall, or not there at all.

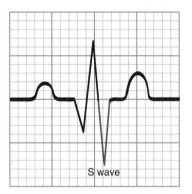

ST Segment

The *ST segment* is the line that follows the QRS complex and connects it to the T wave. It represents part of the ventricular repolarization process and, under normal circumstances, should be isoelectric.

In conditions where oxygen delivery to the myocardium is compromised, such as in myocardial ischemia, injury, or MI, the ST segment may be depressed or elevated.

T Wave

The *T wave* follows the QRS complex and represents ventricular repolarization. Changes in T wave amplitude can occur with electrolyte imbalances or ischemic processes to the myocardium. If you have difficulty finding P waves in heart rhythms that are very fast, look on top of the T wave.

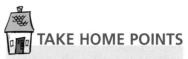

TAKE HOME POINTS

- T waves follow the QRS complex. Often they are greater in amplitude than the P wave.
- P waves should occur before the QRS complex.
- In most cases the QRS complex is the easiest waveform to identify on the ECG. You should look for P waves where they are supposed to be (i.e., before the QRS complex), and look for T waves following the QRS complex.
- If you have difficulty finding P waves in heart rhythms that are very fast, look on top of the T wave.

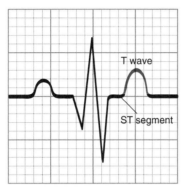

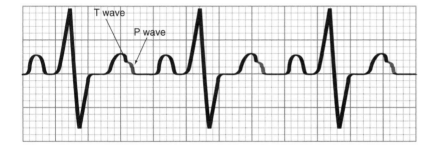

There is a time during the resting state of the ventricle (during ventricular repolarization when the T wave occurs) when the cardiac cell is regaining a negative charge. This is called the *relative refractory period.*

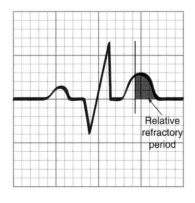

Any abnormal stimulus that occurs during the relative refractory period (e.g., an abnormal beat from the ventricles) could send the heart into electrical chaos.

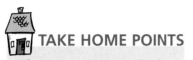

TAKE HOME POINTS

- If present, U waves immediately follow T waves.
- U waves are similar in appearance to P waves. When in doubt, look in additional leads to confirm the waveform.

U Wave

A *U wave* is a small waveform of unknown origin that may follow the T wave. If a U wave is present, it may have the same deflection as the T wave. U waves can be associated with electrolyte imbalances, particularly hypokalemia. (See *Real-World Nursing Survival Guide: Fluids & Electrolytes*, Chapter 5.)

QT Interval

The *QT interval* is measured from the beginning of the QRS complex to the end of the T wave. It represents the amount of time that it takes for ventricular depolarization and repolarization to occur. QT intervals vary with heart rate. Faster heart rates have shorter QT intervals, whereas slower heart rates have longer QT intervals.

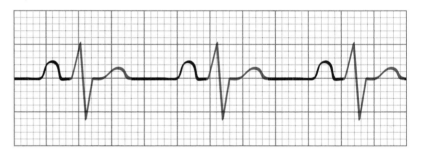

⚠ **Prolonged QT intervals have been associated with the life-threatening dysrhythmia, known as Torsade de pointes, a unique, polymorphic type of ventricular tachycardia.**

Certain antidysrhythmic drugs that prolong ventricular repolarization result in lengthened QT intervals. Treatment for this unique, polymorphic type of ventricular tachycardia, known as *torsade de pointes*, is aimed at shortening the refractory period (thus the QT interval) by interventions such as artificial overdrive pacing or the administration of intravenous (IV) isoproterenol, phenytoin, or Lidocaine. Administration of magnesium has also shown beneficial results in terminating torsade de pointes.

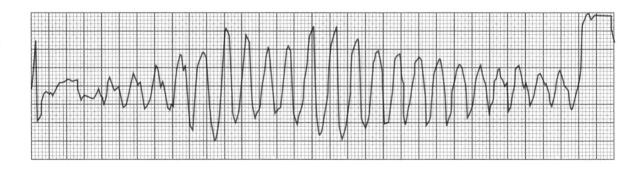

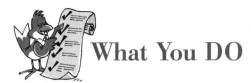

What You DO

- Assess your patient for any signs and symptoms (e.g., chest pain, shortness of breath, changes in consciousness level, changes in blood pressure) when a rhythm change occurs.
- Record a rhythm strip, and place it in the patient's chart for documentation.
- Note any antidysrhythmic medication the patient may be taking, and notify the prescribing professional.
- Follow accepted institution or ACLS protocols for emergency interventions in patients with life-threatening dysrhythmias.

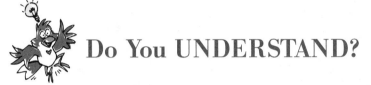

Do You UNDERSTAND?

DIRECTIONS: **What wave would each type of deflection produce?**

1. _____ Positive
2. _____ Negative
3. _____ Biphasic
4. _____ Isoelectric

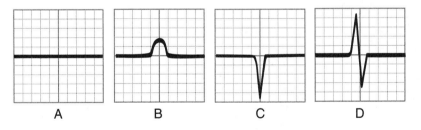

| A | B | C | D |

DIRECTIONS: **Write the normal and abnormal characteristics of a P wave.**

5. Normal: _____

_____

_____

6. Abnormal: _____

_____

_____

DIRECTIONS: Describe the normal Q, R, and S waves. What does the QRS complex indicate?

7. Q wave: _____

8. R wave: _____

9. S wave: _____

10. QRS complex: _____

Reference Points for Rhythm Strip Measurements

Electrocardiograms (ECGs) provide information about time and voltage of electrical events in the heart. To obtain these measurements, you need to understand important reference points on the ECG recording paper. This chapter discusses how to measure *time and voltage* on ECG paper.

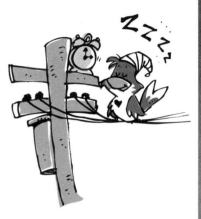

What IS Measuring Time and Voltage?

The ECG is printed on ruled paper with vertical and horizontal lines. These lines make up small boxes with thin lines, inside large boxes with heavy lines. Each small box is 1 mm in height and 1 mm in length. Each large box contains 25 small boxes. Height indicates voltage on the vertical axis, measured in millimeters (mm) or millivolts (mV). Width indicates time on the horizontal axis, measured in milliseconds (ms).

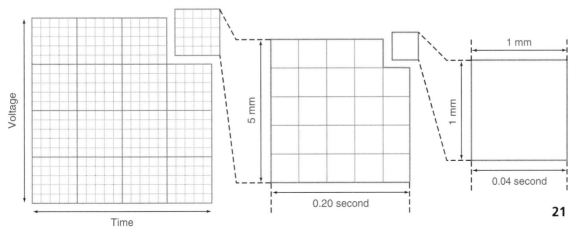

Both time and voltage are measured from the baseline. It is important to view this as an imaginary line drawn through the ECG complex, starting from the beginning of the complex and continuing on the paper to the end of the waveform. When you record a strip, the ECG tracing must be flat (not moving up and down) across the page as in the following example. If the tracing is not flat, you will need to troubleshoot the equipment and check your patient. (See Chapter 6 for more information about troubleshooting ECG waveforms.)

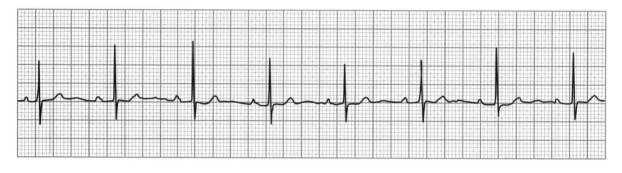

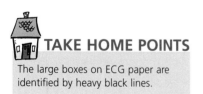

What You NEED TO KNOW

Measuring Time

One of the main goals of obtaining an ECG is to determine the patient's heart rate and its regularity. Therefore the ECG recording paper must be able to measure time. Time can be measured by counting the small and large boxes on the horizontal axis of the ECG paper, or it can be measured by the *second markers* (small, regularly spaced marks at the top or bottom of the ECG paper). As a health care provider, you should be familiar with both of these time-measurement methods.

Measuring time by counting boxes. Time can be measured by counting the number of boxes that encompass each waveform along the horizontal axis of the ECG paper.

Each small box on a horizontal line is equal to 0.04 seconds (or 40 milliseconds [ms]), and five small boxes on a horizontal line equal one large box. Five times 0.04 equals 0.20 seconds. Therefore one large box (measured horizontally) equals 0.20 seconds or 200 ms.

TAKE HOME POINTS

The large boxes on ECG paper are identified by heavy black lines.

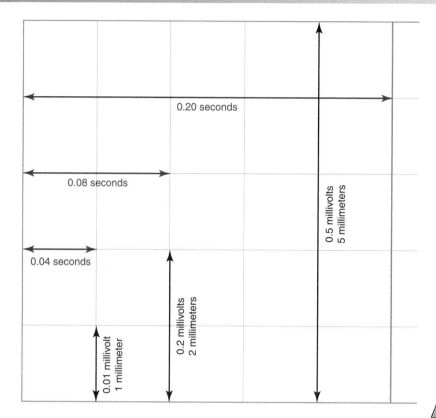

Five large boxes equal 1 second. The time duration of each wave of the ECG can be measured by counting the small boxes within a wave on the horizontal line.

Measuring time by second markers. *Second markers* can appear on ECG paper as vertical lines, triangles, or dots (depending on the paper manufacturer). These markers may also be called tics or hatch marks, and they can occur every 1, 3, or 6 seconds. Second markers are most common in the form of vertical lines.

TAKE HOME POINTS

- To measure time, count the number of small boxes across the horizontal line.
- Multiply the number of small boxes by 0.04 seconds (5 × 0.04 = 0.20 seconds); five large boxes (or 25 small boxes) on the horizontal line equals 1 second.

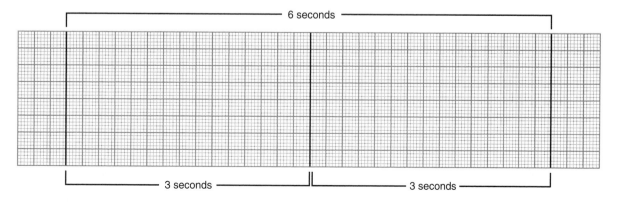

Remember, five large boxes equals 1 second. This means the marker occurring after every fifth large box indicates a 1-second interval (1 marker per second), a marker after every fifteenth large box indicates a 3-second interval, and a marker after each thirtieth large box indicates a 6-second interval.

Most ECG paper has 3- or 6-second markers or both. Since you will analyze and document 6-second strips, it is important to recognize when these markers appear on the ECG paper.

Measuring Voltage

Voltage is measured on the vertical axis. Therefore the height, or depth, of a wave represents a measure of voltage. Voltage is measured either upward or downward from the *isoelectric line*.

Each small vertical box is equal to 0.1 mV. Therefore 10 small vertical boxes or 2 large vertical boxes equal 1 mV. If the heart contracts forcefully or if the patient is experiencing enlargement of the heart muscle (hypertrophy) voltage will be increased. This can be observed as increased height (number of vertical boxes) of the waveforms.

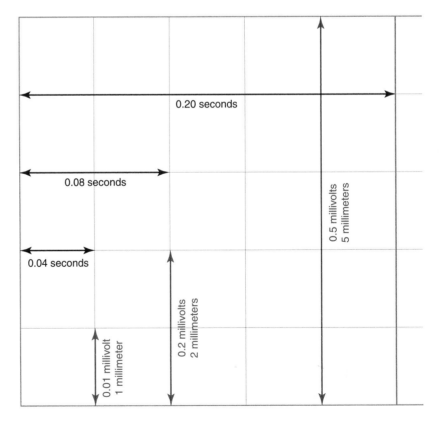

If something interferes with heart energy, causing the heart to contract less forcefully as in *cardiac tamponade*, voltage will be decreased. This will be indicated by decreased height of the waveforms.

Voltage is more closely assessed with the analysis of a 12-lead ECG. For a patient's heartbeat to be counted by a monitor, the voltage of the main tall waveform needs to be at least 5 mm.

In the clinical setting, voltage is measured in millimeters, not millivolts. For example, when describing the height of an R wave, it is more correct to say that the R wave is 4 mm tall, not 0.04 mV.

TAKE HOME POINTS

Energy (voltage) of the heartbeat is measured up and down on the ECG paper. Each small box (up or down) is 0.1 mV, or 1.0 mm. Each large box (up or down) is 0.5 mV, or 5 mm.

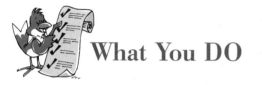

What You DO

Measuring different waveforms and intervals across time in the cardiac cycle requires you to measure distances across the horizontal line.

- To measure time accurately, use ECG calipers.

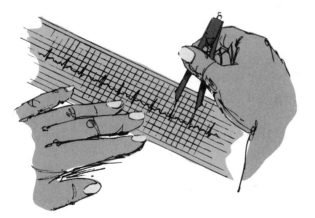

- Hold the calipers in your dominant hand, with your thumb over the upper-middle-front section and your index finger just behind the back of the calipers.
- Use your middle finger to prevent the two tips from slipping. This technique is not unlike holding a pencil when writing.

To measure from point A to point B on the rhythm strip provided on the following page.

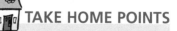

TAKE HOME POINTS

Do not use an engineer's caliper with a wheel in the center. It will make it more difficult to adjust the caliper to the interval being measured.

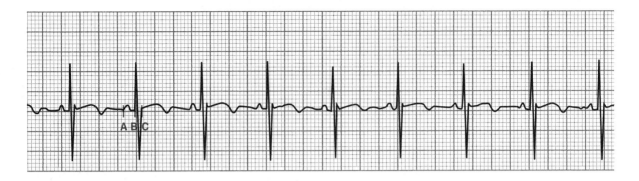

- Place the left tip of your caliper on point A and the right tip of your caliper on point B. Remember, measurements are always done on the baseline.
- Do not try to count the number of boxes between the calipers from these two points. Instead, hold your calipers to prevent movement.
- Without changing the width of the caliper tips, raise them from the ECG tracing to an area of the graph paper where there is a clear view of the horizontal lines.

There should be three small boxes from A to B. This indicates that 0.12 seconds ($3 \times 0.04 = 0.12$) passed during this area of electrical stimulation. On the same strip, look at the parts labeled B and C.

- Place the left tip of your caliper on point B and the right tip on point C.
- Carefully lift the caliper to the top of the graphics without changing the distance between caliper tips.
- Count the number of boxes between the two tips.

There should be two small boxes between B and C. This indicates it took 0.08 seconds for this wave of stimulation to travel down the heart's conduction system.

To measure an ECG rhythm strip without calipers:

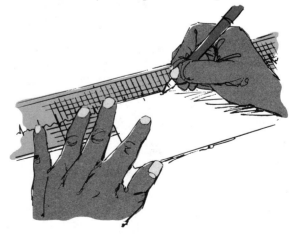

- Take a clean piece of paper and line it up under the baseline of the heartbeat you are measuring.
- Place a small vertical mark on the beginning of the waveform that you want to measure (on the left) and another at the end of the waveform (on the right).
- Bring the paper to the top of the graphic area, and count the number of boxes between the two marks you have made.

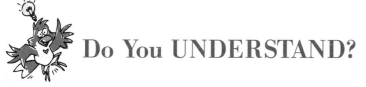

Do You UNDERSTAND?

DIRECTIONS: Fill-in the blanks with the correct number of seconds.

1. Each small box on the horizontal line equals _____ seconds.
2. Three small boxes on the horizontal line equals _____ seconds.
3. One large box on the horizontal line equals _____ seconds.
4. How long does it take for the QRS complex shown in the following figure to occur?

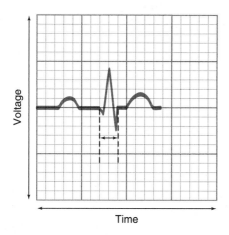

DIRECTIONS: Fill-in the correct word or number.

5. Fifteen large boxes equal _____ seconds in time.
6. Second markers are located on the _____ or _____ margins of ECG paper.
7. Second markers can occur every 1, 3, or _____ seconds on ECG paper.

Answers: 1. 0.04; 2. 0.12; 3. 0.20; 4. 0.04 seconds × 2 = 0.08 seconds; 5. 3; 6. top, bottom; 7. 6.

DIRECTIONS: **Fill-in the correct word or number.**

8. Five small boxes vertically from the baseline on the ECG paper equal _____ mm.

9. Decreased strength of heart contraction will result in decreased _____ of the ECG waveforms.

DIRECTIONS: **Look at the rhythm strip below and measure the points from A to E as indicated. Write your findings.**

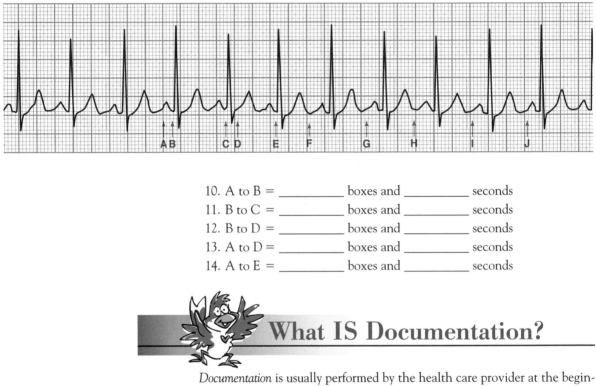

10. A to B = _____ boxes and _____ seconds
11. B to C = _____ boxes and _____ seconds
12. B to D = _____ boxes and _____ seconds
13. A to D = _____ boxes and _____ seconds
14. A to E = _____ boxes and _____ seconds

What IS Documentation?

Documentation is usually performed by the health care provider at the beginning of each shift. In addition to documenting the various waveforms and intervals, you may be responsible for documenting the consistent, sustained rhythm of the patient's heart. You will gather this information by examining the patient's rhythm strip.

What You NEED TO KNOW

Most monitoring systems are computerized and include the patient's name, room number, date, time, heart rate, and lead in which the patient is being monitored. If this information is not recorded on the patient's rhythm strip, you need to write it in an area of the strip that is free of electrical tracing. You also need to verify that you ran and analyzed the strip by signing your name on the strip or in the patient's chart.

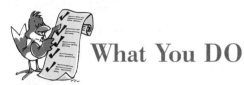

What You DO

When there is a change in ectopy or in the heart rhythm (dysrhythmia), you are responsible for printing a 6-second strip that includes the abnormality. You may also need to notify a physician (depending on the severity of the change). You should then include an entry in the patient's chart that includes:

- Date and time
- Rhythm change and analysis
- Patient assessment changes
- Treatment initiated
- Patient response to treatment
- Name of the health care provider who verified the rhythm

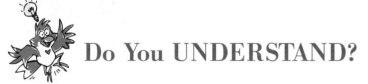

Do You UNDERSTAND?

Case Study

A 65-year-old man is admitted to your telemetry unit for acute exacerbation of asthma. His baseline vital signs are: 99, 110, 22, blood pressure (BP) 130/80. He has been in a sinus rhythm, but the alarms have just rung. When you enter the room, he is out of bed, sitting in a chair, and receiving his hand-held nebulizer treatment of albuterol (Proventil). The monitor indicates that he has gone into a sinus tachycardia, with frequent, premature ventricular contractions. He is complaining of palpitations and a flushed feeling. Vital signs are 100.4°, 140, 36, BP 160/90. He is sweating and has an ashen color.

DIRECTIONS: Give a sample of what you would document on the chart.

_____

_____

_____

_____

_____

_____

Answer: Date: 02/00; **time:** 1000. Calls patient's room. Finishes nebulizer of Proventil. Patient reports palpitation and flushed feeling, "I can't catch my breath." Patient is flushed, looks ashen, and is diaphoretic and warm to the touch. Vital signs: 100.4°, 140, 36. Pulse is weak and thready. BP is elevated from normal by 30 mm/Hg at 160/90. Pulse and respirations are elevated. Rhythm strip has changed from sinus rhythm to sinus tachycardia with premature ventricular contractions. Nebulizers d/c and patient back to bed. Physician and nurse practitioner notified for further direction.

4 Measuring Atrial and Ventricular Rates

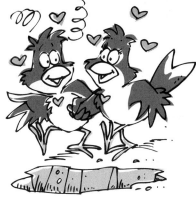

Now that you understand waveforms and how to measure time on ECG paper, it is time to learn how to count atrial and ventricular rates on an ECG printout. This chapter describes three simple and rapid methods of estimating heart rate: (1) the 6-second method, (2) the rule of 1500s, and (3) the rule of 300s.

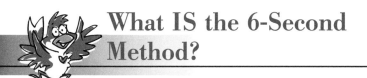

What IS the 6-Second Method?

The easiest method of counting atrial and ventricular rates is with the 6-second method. This is also called the *rule of 10s*. The 6-second method is used for quick assessments when an approximate rate is needed, whether the heart rate is regular or irregular.

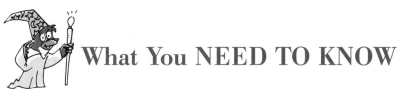

What You NEED TO KNOW

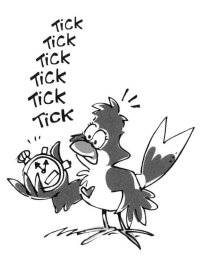

To determine heart rates using the 6-second method:
- Print out ECG paper covering a 6-second block of time (6-second strip).
- Remember to check the second markers on the top or bottom of the strip to identify a period of exactly 6 seconds. After every fifth large box is a 1-second marker, after every fifteenth large box there is a 3-second marker, and 6-second markers are after every thirtieth large box.

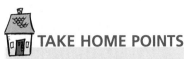

TAKE HOME POINTS

- Markers at the top or bottom of the strip will tell you over how many seconds an event has taken place.
- To identify a 6-second strip, it is important to check your ECG paper to see if markers occur every 1, 3, or 6 seconds. (See Chapter 3 for a review of second markers.)

The 6-second method will provide an estimate of your patient's heart rate. In a patient with a normal heart, the atrial and ventricular rates should be the same. This method can also be used for patients with regular or irregular rhythms.

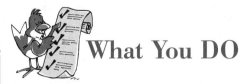

What You DO

To determine the atrial rate using the 6-second method:
- Count the number of P waves on a 6-second strip.
- Multiply that number by 10 to determine the full-minute rate. There are 10 6-second intervals in a minute.
  To determine the ventricular rate using the 6-second method:
- Count the number of R waves in a 6-second strip and multiply that number by 10. The entire QRS complex must fit within the 6-second marks to count the R wave as a beat.

Example 1

In the following strip, the atrial rate is 60 beats per minute (bpm), because there are six P waves in the 6-second strip (6 × 10 = 60). The ventricular rate is 60 bpm, because there are six QRS complexes in the 6-second strip (6 × 10 = 60).

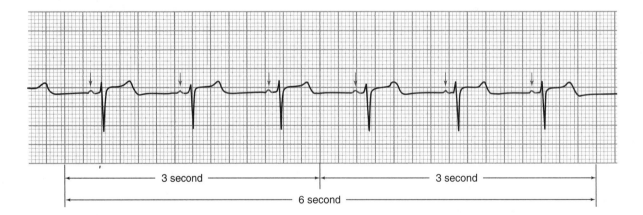

3 second ——————— 3 second
6 second

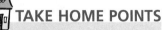

TAKE HOME POINTS

- A heart rate of above 100 is considered a tachycardia, and a heart rate below 60 is considered a bradycardia.
- When determining heart rate, the ventricular rate is preferred.
- The 6-second method is also referred to as the rule of 10s.

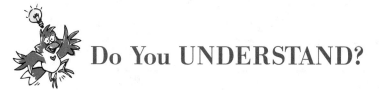

Do You UNDERSTAND?

DIRECTIONS: Use the 6-second rule to calculate the atrial and ventricular rates in strip 1 and strip 2.

> If the rhythm is a tachycardia or bradycardia, the patient needs to be assessed right away. Rates that are too slow or too fast can cause heart failure.

1.

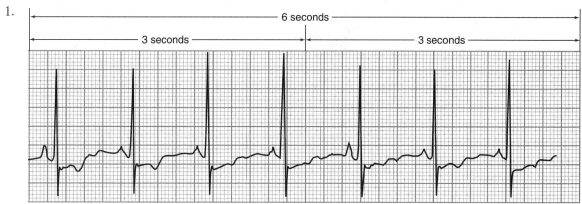

2.

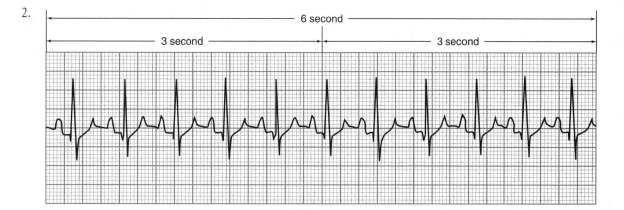

Answers: 1. Atrial rate is 70, because there are seven P waves in the 6-second strip; the ventricular rate is 70, because there are 7 complete QRS complexes in a 6-second strip; this is a normal rate. 2. There are 11 P waves in this 6-second strip; therefore the atrial rate is 110 (11 × 10 = 110); the ventricular rate is 110, because there are 11 QRS complexes in a 6-second strip; this is a tachycardia.

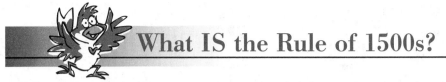

What IS the Rule of 1500s?

The *rule of 1500s* is a more accurate but slightly more complicated method of counting heart rates.

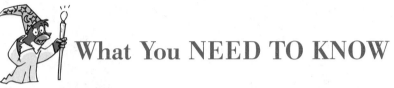

What You NEED TO KNOW

- The rule of 1500s may only be used for counting regular rates.
- Atrial and ventricular rates should be equal in the normal heart.

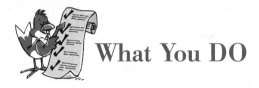

What You DO

Atrial Rate

To determine the atrial rate using the rule of 1500s:
- Count the number of small blocks between the tallest point of two consecutive P waves.
- Divide that number (denominator) into 1500 (numerator).

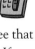

Ventricular rate

To determine the ventricular rate using the rule of 1500s:
- Count the number of small blocks between the peaks of two consecutive R waves.
- Divide this number into 1500.

Examine the ECG strip at the top of the following page. You will see that there are 23 small boxes between the last two P waves on the strip. If you want to determine the atrial rate using the rule of 1500s, you would divide 1500 by 23 (1500 ÷ 23 = 65). Therefore this strip indicates that the patient's atrial rate is 65 bpm.

 The rule of 1500s is used for regular rates only. Atrial and ventricular rates should be equal in the normal heart.

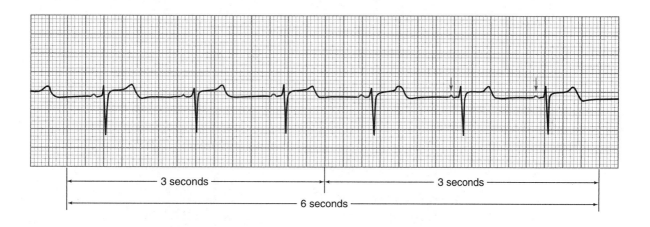

|← 3 seconds →|← 3 seconds →|
|← 6 seconds →|

If you want to determine the ventricular rate using the rule of 1500s, you would count the small boxes between each R wave. In this case, there are 23 small boxes between each R wave on the strip. Once again, you would divide 1500 by 23. This means the ventricular rate indicated on the strip is also 65 bpm.

TAKE HOME POINTS

Regardless of the method you use to determine a patient's heart rate, you should always use the ventricular rate to analyze whether the rate is normal, fast, or slow.

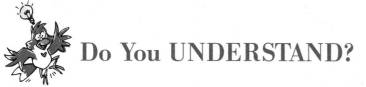

Do You UNDERSTAND?

DIRECTIONS: **Examine the next two rhythm strip examples and calculate the ventricular rates using the rule of 1500s.**

1.

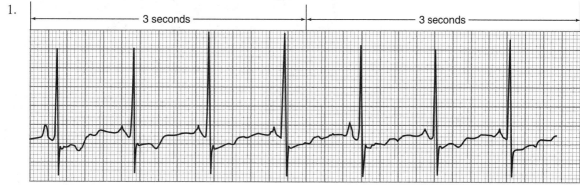

|← 3 seconds →|← 3 seconds →|

Answer: 1. There are 20.5 small boxes between the R waves in this strip; therefore 1500 ÷ 20.5 = 73.1, or 73 bpm; this is a normal rate.

2.

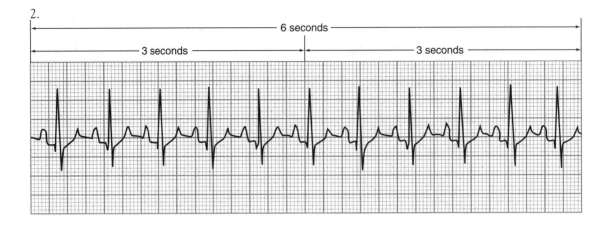

What IS the Rule of 300s?

The *rule of 300s* is a common method used to calculate regular heart rhythms. This method depends on observation and memorization. It is quick, simple, and does not require a calculator.

What You NEED TO KNOW

To use the rule of 300s, two sets of numbers must be memorized.

First set is 300, 150, and 100
Second set is 75, 60, and 50

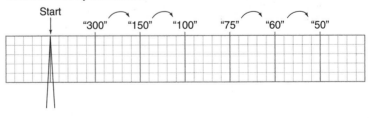

Determine rate by observation

The heart rate can be determined by attaching these numbers to the heavy horizontal lines between the peaks of two R waves. The theory behind the rule of 300s is that the distance between two heavy horizontal lines is $^1\!/_{300}$ of a minute. Therefore the number of large boxes between two R waves into 300 are divided to discover the rate per minute.

If the space between two R waves is three large boxes, 300 is divided by 3 ($300 \div 3 = 100$). This means that your patient's heart rate is 100 bpm. If the space between two R waves is eight large boxes, 300 is divided by 8 ($300 \div 8 = 37$). This means that your patient's heart rate is 37 bpm. You are not expected to memorize the numbers on the fine, horizontal lines of the ECG, just to understand how to read them and use them to calculate your patient's heart rates. The 6-second method is easier to use when estimating slow heart rates (rates below 50 bpm).

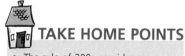

300	150	100	75	60	50	43	37	33
250	136	94	71	58	48	42	37	
214	125	88	68	56	47	41	36	
187	115	83	65	54	45	39	35	
167	107	79	62	52	44	38	34	

What You DO

- Find an R wave that peaks on a heavy horizontal line.
- Name that line "Start."
- Name each consecutive heavy horizontal line according to the numbers that you have memorized until you have reached the second R wave. See the following examples:

1.

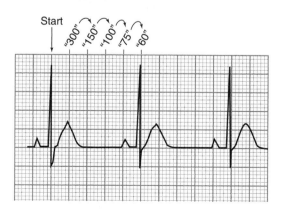

Start "300" "150" "100" "75" "60"

TAKE HOME POINTS

- The rule of 300s provides an estimation of heart rate, not the exact heart rate.
- If the second R wave does not fall exactly on the heavy line, use the number on the heavy line closest to it.

The rule of 300s should only be used to calculate the heart rates of those with regular heart rhythms.

2.

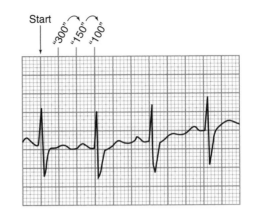

3.

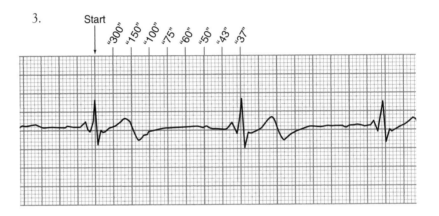

4.

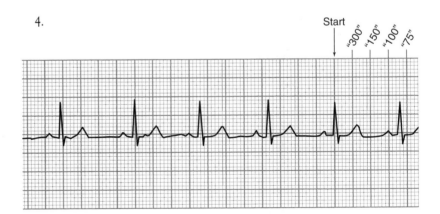

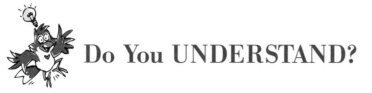

Do You UNDERSTAND?

DIRECTIONS: Calculate the heart rate on the following rhythm strip using the rule of 300s.

1.

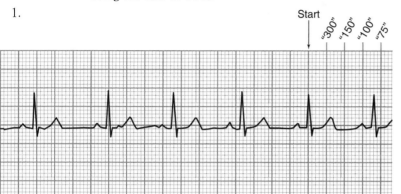

Start

"300" "150" "100" "75"

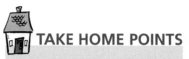

TAKE HOME POINTS

- Remember, "Start"; then 300, 150, 100; then 75, 60, 50.
- If your patient's heart rate is below 50, use the 6-second method.
- It is not necessary to memorize the numbers on the fine horizontal lines of the ECG strip.

www.americanheart.org
www.atlcard.com
www.wices.com/icescardiac

5 Analyzing the Rhythm Strip

The previous chapters have discussed waveforms, electrocardiographic (ECG) paper, and measuring atrial and ventricular rates. Now you are ready to apply this information to analyzing a rhythm strip. This chapter covers a step-by-step approach to rhythm strip interpretation known as the 8-step method.

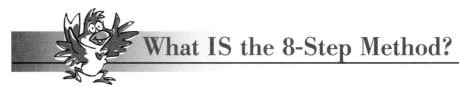

What IS the 8-Step Method?

The *8-step method* of interpreting rhythms is a good way to identify the origin of an impulse on a rhythm strip, describe the conduction sequence of the rhythm, and define the salient features of the rhythm. To interpret information on a rhythm strip using this method, you would take the following eight steps:

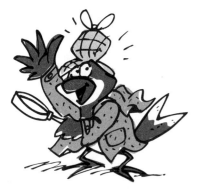

1. Identify the waveforms and assess the morphology and location of the P waves, QRS complexes, and T waves.
2. Count the atrial rate.
3. Count the ventricular rate.
4. Determine whether the atrial rhythm is regular or irregular.
5. Determine whether the ventricular rhythm is regular or irregular.
6. Measure the PR interval to determine whether it is within normal limits, and ensure that all of the PR intervals are consistent.
7. Measure the width of the QRS complex to determine whether it is within normal limits. Ensure that all the QRS complexes are consistent.
8. Assess the clinical significance of the rhythm.

What You NEED TO KNOW

To complete the first step of rhythm strip analysis (identification of the waveforms), you should ask the following questions:

- Is there one P wave before every QRS complex?
- Is the P wave upright in lead II?
- Do all the P waves look alike or have the same shape?
- Can the waveforms representing ventricular depolarization be identified (the QRS complex)?
- Is there a Q, R, or an S wave present?
- Do all the QRS complexes look alike?
- Can the T waves be identified? Do all the T waves look alike?

Once you have identified the waveforms, you should count the atrial and ventricular rates (see Chapter 4). Next, you should determine whether the atrial rhythm is regular. To do this, you should measure P-to-P intervals. A regular atrial rhythm is one in which each P-to-P interval plots out the same distance.

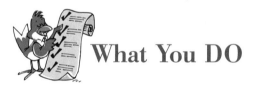

What You DO

Atrial regularity is determined by plotting P-to-P intervals using calipers.

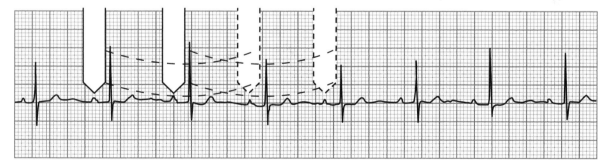

- Place the left caliper tip at the beginning of the P wave, and place the right caliper tip at the beginning of the very next P wave. This is the P-to-P interval.
- Without changing the width of the caliper tips, lift the calipers and place them on the next P wave.

TAKE HOME POINTS

- The 8-step method looks at rate, rhythm, conduction times, and the clinical significance of the rhythm.
- It is essential to compare all intervals in the rhythm to each other to make sure they are consistent.

TAKE HOME POINTS

- P waves should occur before the QRS complex.
- T waves should follow the QRS complex.
- In most cases, the QRS complex is the largest waveform in the rhythm strip. (Therefore you should look for P waves where they are supposed to be: in front of the QRS complex.)
- Remember, if the rhythm is fast, P waves may be sitting on top of the T waves.
- Because the sinoatrial (SA) node should initiate the impulse and conduct to the ventricles, there should be one P wave before every QRS complex. Therefore the atrial and ventricular rates should be the same.

- If the caliper tips fall on the next P wave, the atrial rhythm is considered regular.
- If the caliper tips do not fall on the next P wave (off more than one small block), the atrial rhythm is considered irregular.

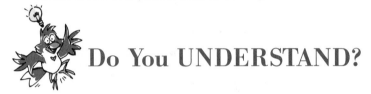

Do You UNDERSTAND?

DIRECTIONS: **Measure the P-to-P intervals in the examples that follow. Is the ventricular rhythm regular or irregular?**

1.

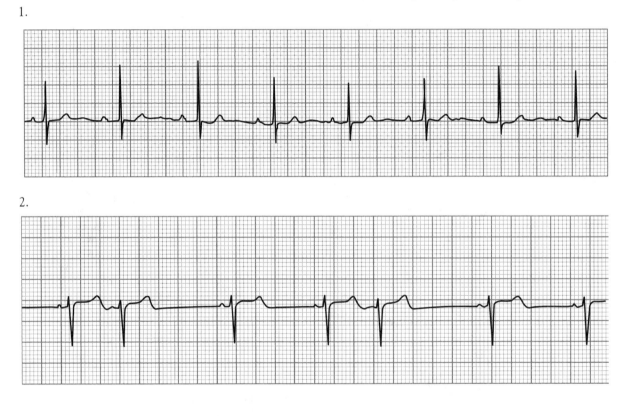

2.

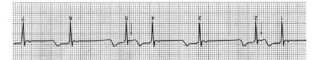

Answers: 1. Regular; therefore the atrial rhythm is regular; 2. Irregular; the P-to-P interval is off at the second and fifth beats; therefore the atrial rhythm is irregular.

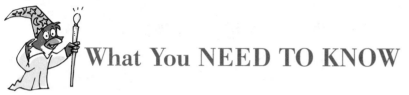

What IS Determining the Ventricular Rhythm?

The next step is to determine whether the ventricular rhythm is regular or irregular. A regular ventricular rhythm reveals whether the ventricles are firing in a normal, even manner.

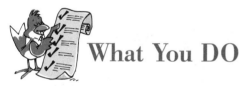

What You NEED TO KNOW

Determining the regularity of the ventricular rhythm is similar to determining atrial rhythm. However, instead of measuring P-to-P intervals, the R-to-R intervals are measured (QRS complex to QRS complex).

What You DO

Measuring ventricular regularity (rhythm) is similar to measuring atrial rhythm. However, the R-to-R intervals are measured, instead of the P-to-P intervals.

- Use calipers.
- Place the right caliper tip on top of an R wave and the left tip on top of the next R wave.
- Without changing the width of the calipers tips, lift the calipers and place them on the next R wave.
- If the caliper tips fall on the next R wave, the ventricular rhythm is considered regular.
- If the caliper tips do not fall on the next R wave (off more than one small block), the ventricular rhythm is considered irregular.

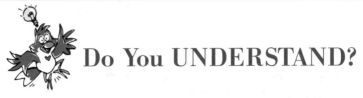

Do You UNDERSTAND?

DIRECTIONS: Measure the R-to-R intervals in the following examples.
Is the ventricular rhythm regular or irregular?

1.

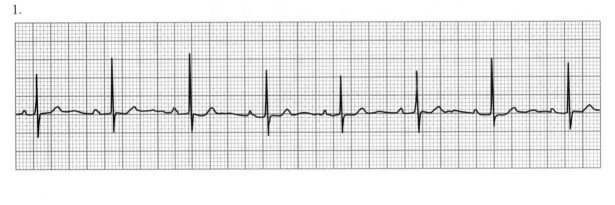

2.

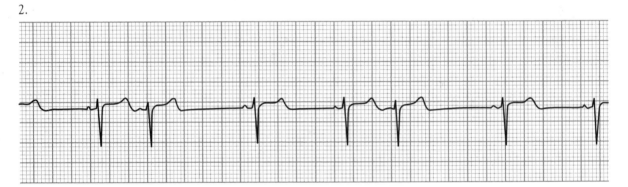

Answers: 1. Regular; 2. Irregular (at the second and fifth beats).

What IS PR Interval Measurement

Once you have determined the ventricular rhythm, it is time to determine whether the PR interval measurement is within normal limits. The PR interval includes the time it takes for atrial depolarization and AV holding to occur.

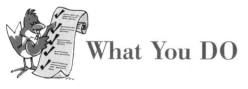

What You NEED TO KNOW

A normal PR interval is between 0.12 and 0.20 seconds (between three and five small boxes on the ECG paper).

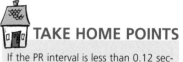

TAKE HOME POINTS

If the PR interval is less than 0.12 seconds or greater than 0.20 seconds, it is abnormal.

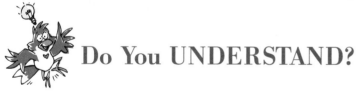

What You DO

You should measure the PR interval from the beginning of the P wave to the end of the PR segment, which is the beginning of the QRS complex.

Do You UNDERSTAND?

DIRECTIONS: Identify the PR intervals in the following examples, and identify the abnormal PR intervals.

1.

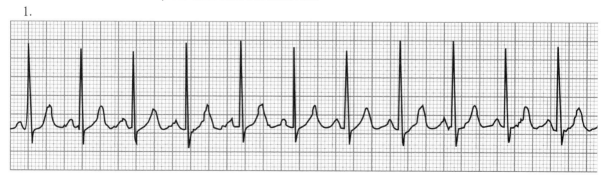

Answer: 1. 0.16 seconds.

2.

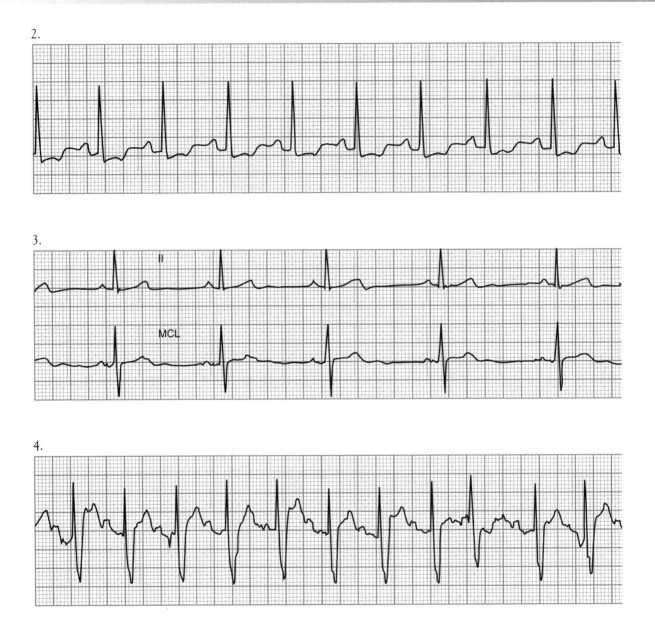

3.

4.

Answers: 2. 0.22 seconds (abnormal); 3. 0.14 seconds; 4. 0.24 seconds (abnormal).

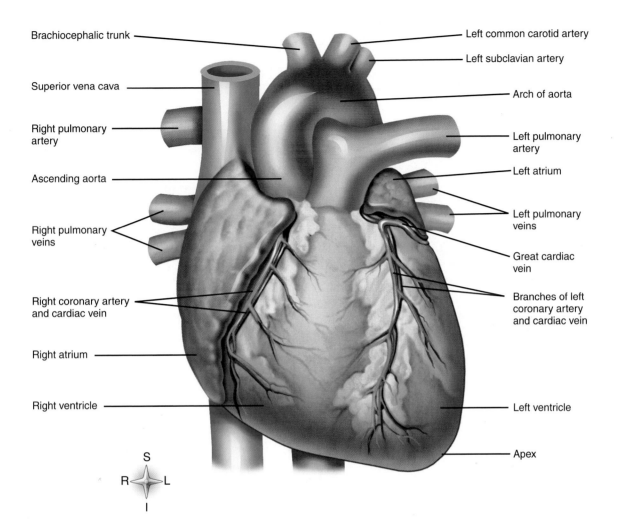

Brachiocephalic trunk

Superior vena cava

Right pulmonary
artery

Ascending aorta

Right pulmonary
veins

Right coronary artery
and cardiac vein

Right atrium

Right ventricle

Left common carotid artery

Left subclavian artery

Arch of aorta

Left pulmonary
artery

Left atrium

Left pulmonary
veins

Great cardiac
vein

Branches of left
coronary artery
and cardiac vein

Left ventricle

Apex

S

R   L

I

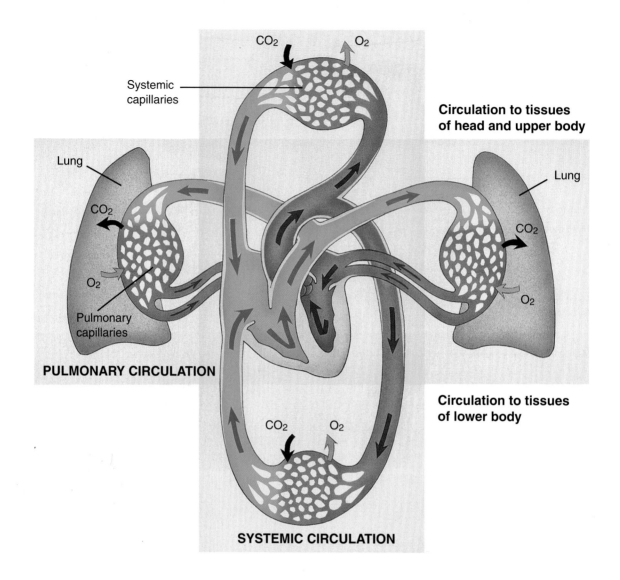

Systemic capillaries

Circulation to tissues of head and upper body

Lung

CO_2

O_2

Pulmonary capillaries

PULMONARY CIRCULATION

Lung

CO_2

O_2

Circulation to tissues of lower body

CO_2

O_2

SYSTEMIC CIRCULATION

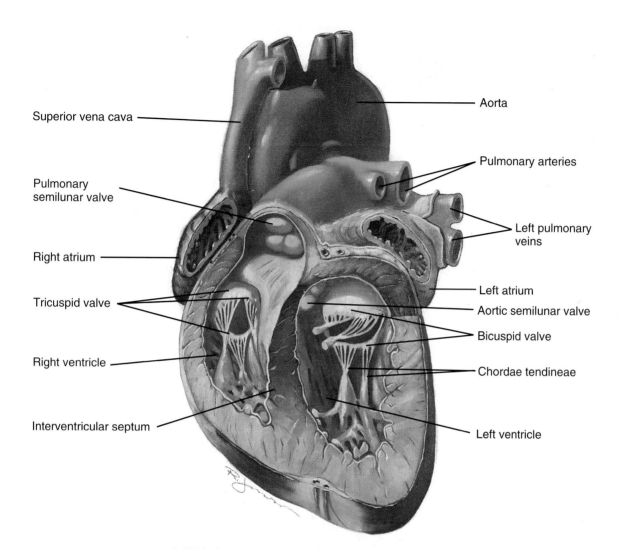

Superior vena cava

Pulmonary
semilunar valve

Right atrium

Tricuspid valve

Right ventricle

Interventricular septum

Aorta

Pulmonary arteries

Left pulmonary
veins

Left atrium

Aortic semilunar valve

Bicuspid valve

Chordae tendineae

Left ventricle

Atrial Fibrillation and Atrial Flutter Algorithm

Perform Primary ABCD Survey (Basic Life Support)
- Correct critical problems IMMEDIATELY as they are identified)
- Assess responsiveness, **A**irway, **B**reathing, **C**irculation; ensure availability of monitor and **D**efibrillator

Perform Secondary ABCD Survey (Advanced Life Support)
- Administer oxygen, establish IV access, attach cardiac monitor, administer fluids as needed (O_2, IV, monitor, fluids)
- Assess vital signs, attach pulse oximeter, and monitor blood pressure
- Obtain and review 12-lead ECG and portable chest x-ray; perform a focused history and physical examination

Is the patient stable or unstable? Is the patient experiencing serious signs and symptoms caused by tachycardia? Is the patient's cardiac function normal or impaired? Attempt to identify patient's cardiac rhythm using 12-lead ECG and clinical information. Is Wolff-Parkinson-White syndrome (WPW) present? If yes, see WPW syndrome, Chapter 20, page 231. Has atrial fibrillation or atrial flutter been present for more or less than 48 hours?

Stable Patient

Normal Cardiac Function		Impaired Cardiac Function	
Onset < 48 hours	Onset > 48 hours	Onset < 48 hours	Onset > 48 hours
Control Rate	**Control Rate**	**Control Rate**	**Control Rate**
Calcium channel blocker (Class I) OR Beta-blocker (Class I) OR Digoxin (IIb)	Calcium channel blocker (Class I) OR Beta-blocker (Class I) OR Digoxin (IIb)	Diltiazem (IIb) OR Amiodarone (IIb) OR Digoxin (IIb)	Diltiazem (IIb) OR Amiodarone (IIb) OR Digoxin (IIb)
Convert Rhythm	**Convert Rhythm**	**Convert Rhythm**	**Convert Rhythm**
Cardioversion OR Amiodarone (IIa) OR Procainamide (IIa) OR Ibutilide (IIa) OR Flecainide (IIa) OR Propafenone (IIa)	Delayed cardioversion OR Early cardioversion	Cardioversion OR amiodarone (IIb)	Delayed cardioversion OR Early cardioversion

Delayed cardioversion: Anticoagulation therapy for 3 weeks before cardioversion for at least 48 hours in conjunction with cardioversion and for at least 4 weeks after successful cardioversion.

Early cardioversion: IV heparin immediately, transesophageal echocardiography (TEE) to rule out atrial thrombus; cardioversion within 24 hours; anticoagulation for 4 weeks

Unstable Patient

If hemodynamically unstable, perform synchronized cardioversion:
> **Atrial fibrillation:** 100, 200, 300, or 360 J, or equivalent biphasic energy
> **Atrial flutter:** 50, 100, 200, 300, or 360 J, or equivalent biphasic energy

Medication dosing: Amiodarone—150 mg IV bolus over 10 minutes, followed by an infusion of 1 mg/min for 6 hours and then a maintenance infusion of 0.5 mg/min. Repeat supplementary infusions of 150 mg as necessary for recurrent or resistant dysrhythmias. Maximum total daily dose 2.2 g. **Beta blockers**—*Esmolol:* 0.5 mg/kg over 1 minute followed by a maintenance infusion at 50 µg/kg/min for 4 minutes. If inadequate response, administer a second bolus of 0.5 mg/kg over 1 minute and increase maintenance infusion to 100 µg/kg/min. The bolus dose (0.5 mg/kg) and titration of the maintenance infusion (addition of 50 µg/kg/min) can be repeated every 4 minutes to a maximum infusion of 300 µg/kg/min. *Metoprolol:* 5 mg slow IV push over 5 minutes three times as needed to a total dose of 15 mg over 15 minutes. *Propranolol:* 0.1 mg/kg slow IV push divided in three equal doses at 2 to 3 minute intervals. Do not exceed 1 mg/min. Repeat after 2 minutes if necessary. *Atenolol:* 5 mg slow IV (over 5 minutes). Wait 10 minutes; then give second dose of 5 mg slow IV (over 5 minutes). **Calcium channel blockers**—*Diltiazem:* 0.25 mg/kg over 2 minutes (e.g., 15 to 20 mg). If ineffective, 0.35 mg/kg over 2 minutes (e.g., 20 to 25 mg) in 15 minutes. Maintenance infusion 5 to 15 mg/hr, titrated to heart rate if chemical conversion is successful. Calcium chloride (2 to 4 mg/kg) may be given slow IV push if borderline hypotension exists before diltiazem administration. *Verapamil:* 2.5 to 5.0 mg slow IV push over 2 minutes. May repeat with 5 to 10 mg in 15 to 30 minutes. Maximum dose 20 mg. **Ibutilide**—Adults ≥ 60 kg: 1 mg (10 mL) over 10 minutes. May repeat once in 10 minutes. Adults < 60 kg: 0.01 mg/kg IV over 10 minutes. **Procainamide**—100 mg over 5 minutes (20 mg/min). Maximum total dose 17 mg/kg. Maintenance infusion 1 to 4 mg/min. **Flecainide, propafenone**—IV form not currently approved for use in the United States. **Sotalol**—1.0 to 1.5 mg/kg IV slowly at a rate of 10 mg/min.

See credits, page 270.

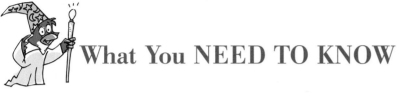

What IS Assessing the QRS Complex?

The QRS complex represents ventricular depolarization. After determining whether the PR interval is normal, the QRS complex is assessed to see whether it is within normal limits.

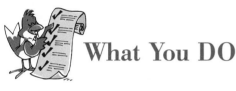

What You NEED TO KNOW

The QRS complex may have a Q , R, or an S wave (or any combination of these waves).

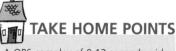

TAKE HOME POINTS

A QRS complex of 0.12 seconds wide or wider indicates that the rhythm originates in the ventricles or that some interventricular conduction delay has occurred.

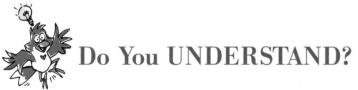

What You DO

- You should measure a QRS complex from the end of the PR interval, which is the waveform that begins the QRS complex and includes all of the waveforms that represent ventricular depolarization.
- A normal QRS complex should be less than 0.12 seconds or less than 3 small boxes on the ECG paper.

Do You UNDERSTAND?

DIRECTIONS: Measure the duration of the QRS complex in the following examples, and identify the abnormal QRS complexes.

1.

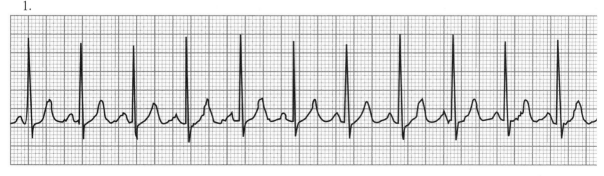

Answer: 1. 0.08 seconds.

2.

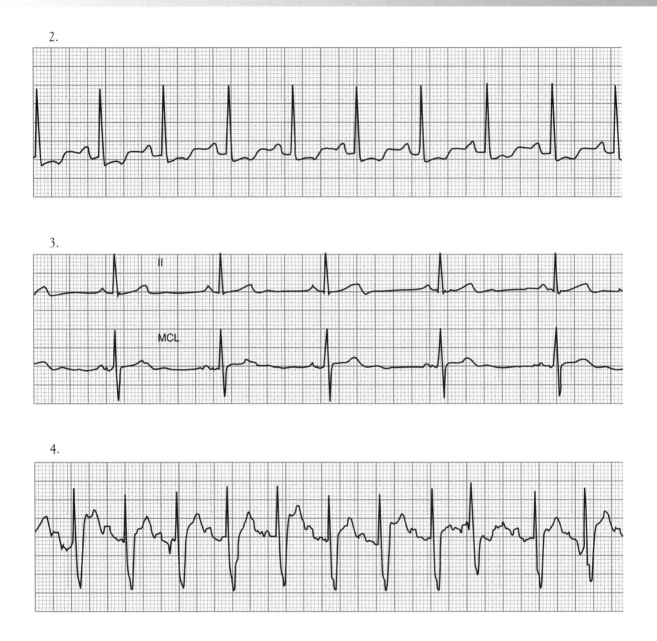

3.

II

MCL

4.

Answers: 2. 0.08 seconds; 3. 0.08 seconds; 4. 0.12 seconds (abnormal).

What IS Measurement of the QT Interval?

The QT interval represents the amount of time that it takes for ventricular depolarization and repolarization to occur. Although measurement of the QT interval is not always included in the 8-step method of rhythm interpretation, it is important to note a baseline QT interval.

What You NEED TO KNOW

Normal QT intervals are rate dependent, and most measure between 0.36 and 0.44 seconds. (See the following examples of QT interval measurement.)

   1. QT interval = 0.34 seconds (abnormal)

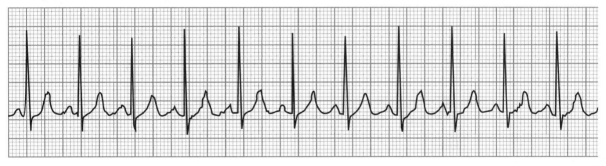

   2. QT interval = 0.34 seconds (abnormal)

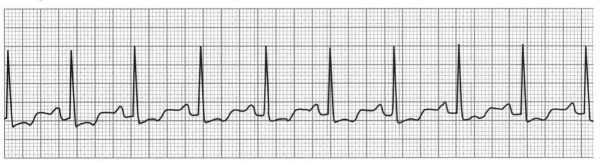

3. QT interval = 0.44 seconds

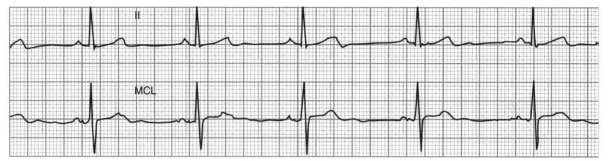

4. QT interval = 0.36 seconds

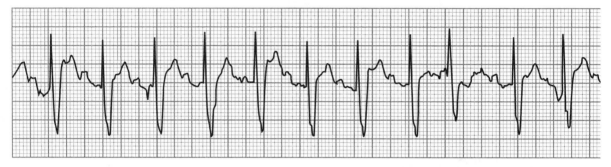

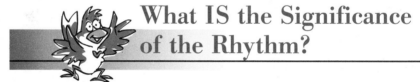

What IS the Significance of the Rhythm?

The final step in rhythm strip analysis is to determine the clinical significance of the rhythm. This is an essential step in evaluating the patient's condition.

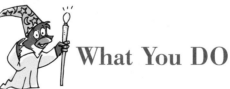

What You DO

Notify the health care professional if your patient experiences any signs or symptoms of instability. You should be prepared to treat the rhythm, based on your institution's protocols.

If a patient experiences any signs or symptoms of instability, such as hypotension, light headedness, shortness of breath, chest pain, or changes in levels of consciousness, you should notify the health care professional and be prepared to treat the rhythm, based on your institution's protocols.

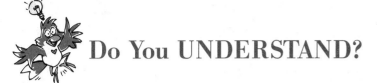

Do You UNDERSTAND?

DIRECTIONS: Examine the following rhythm strips. Using the 8-step
method, note the following characteristics: location
and shape of waveforms, atrial rate, ventricular rate,
atrial and ventricular rhythms, PR interval, and QRS
complex width. You should also practice measuring
QT intervals.

1.

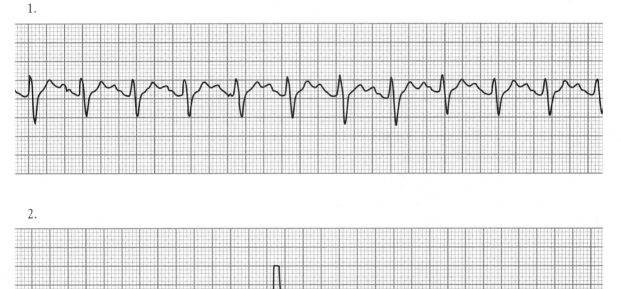

2.

has no P wave in front of it—otherwise bradycardia.
after fourth beat, PR—0.16, QRS—0.08, QT—0.40, appearance of waves, third beat is premature and
QRS, normal; 2. Atrial rate—50, ventricular rate—60, atrial and ventricular rhythm—regular, except
regular, PR—0.12 seconds, QRS—0.12 seconds, QT—0.32 seconds, appearance of waves—1 P to 1
Answers: 1. Atrial rate—100, ventricular rate—100, atrial rhythm—regular, ventricular rhythm—

3.

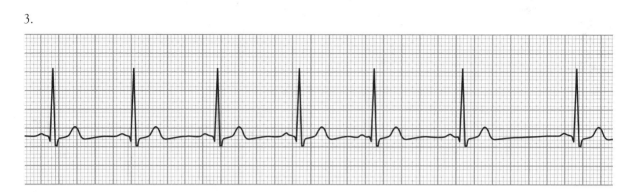

4.

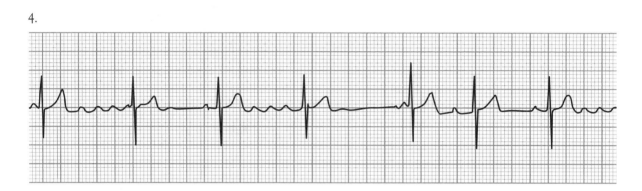

5.

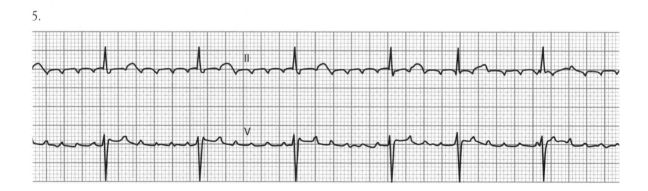

Answers: 3. Atrial rate—60, ventricular rate—60, atrial and ventricular rhythm—regular until last three beats, PR—0.16, QRS—0.08, QT—0.40, appearance of waves—normal; 4. Ventricular rate—50, atrial rhythm—irregular, ventricular rhythm—irregular, PR—varies with each beat, QRS—0.08, QT—0.36, appearance of waves—very irregular; 5. Artial Ps but regular after first, third, and last beat; 5. Atrial rate—260, ventricular rate—50, atrial rhythm—irregular, ventricular rhythm—irregular, QRS—106, QT—0.44, appearance of waves, multiple P waves—bradycardia.

CHAPTER 6
Troubleshooting Problems in Waveforms

To analyze an electrocardiographic (ECG) recording accurately, it is necessary to have a clear, well-produced tracing with a stationary isoelectric baseline (baseline without drift). Common technical problems that require troubleshooting are artifact, 60-cycle interference, weak signal, and wandering baselines. This chapter discusses the recognition of artifact and provides you with tips for troubleshooting waveform problems.

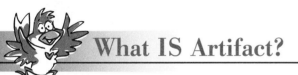

What IS Artifact?

Artifact is an artificial disturbance of the ECG signal that interferes with high-quality capture of the ECG tracing. Often it is caused by electrical interference (60-cycle interference), muscular activity, movement, or mechanical problems. Artifact can be compared with the noise you hear when making tuning adjustments to a radio. These signal distortions may be continual or intermittent.

What You NEED TO KNOW

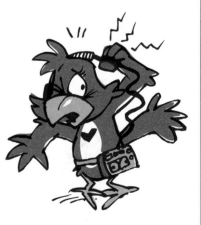

One of the most common causes of artifact is patient movement. Hiccups, shivering, convulsions, and chest movements that occur during respirations can interfere with waveforms and cause the baseline of the ECG tracing to wander.

The ECG strip on the following page demonstrates artifact resulting from patient movement. This type of interference may trigger the monitor's heart rate alarm.

> ⚠ **Patient movements cause interference that may trigger the monitor's heart rate alarm.**

53

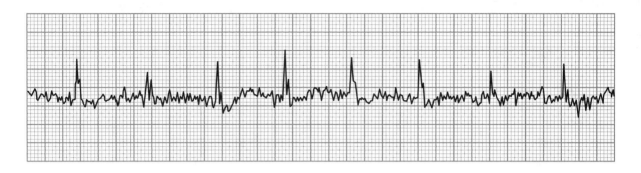

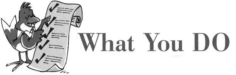

What You DO

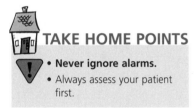

TAKE HOME POINTS

- **Never ignore alarms.**
- Always assess your patient first.

When an ECG artifact is discovered, you need to do the following:

- Assess the patient and ensure his or her safety.
- Differentiate between a patient problem and a mechanical problem by working in an organized fashion, from the patient back to the monitoring system.
- If the patient is in any distress, initiate further assessment and treatment if necessary.
- Ensure that the electrode pads and lead wires are attached to the patient. Patient movement can cause electrodes and lead wires to detach. Keep in mind that they should be changed and repositioned every 3 days (sooner if problematic).
- Inspect the lead wires for corrosion or worn areas. Normally, lead wires are cleaned and reused between patients. However, if they are corroded or frayed, they should be discarded and replaced.
- Work with one piece of equipment at a time, checking for a clean tracing between each intervention. For persistent problems, a portable monitor may be needed to monitor the rhythm at the bedside while troubleshooting.

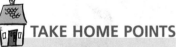

TAKE HOME POINTS

If unable to find the source of the ECG artifact, call the appropriate biomedical or maintenance personnel and have them check the equipment for potential hazards or defects.

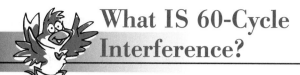

What IS 60-Cycle Interference?

Interference that is attributed to improper grounding of electrical equipment placed near the patient is known as *60-cycle* or *alternating current* (AC) *interference*. The result of this type of interference is a wide, fuzzy baseline.

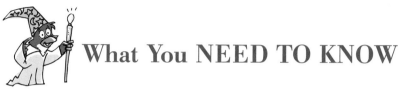

What You NEED TO KNOW

The hallmarks of this type of artifact are 60 small, regular spikes in a 1-second interval tracing.

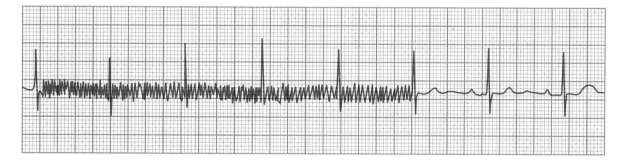

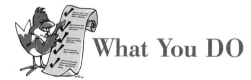

What You DO

When you discover an ECG with 60-cycle interference:

- Assess the patient, and ensure his or her safety.
- Unplug one piece of electrical equipment at a time, and note whether the tracing clears while the equipment is unplugged.
- Once you have determined which piece of equipment is responsible for the interference, you should plug it into a different outlet.
- Check to see whether any new equipment has been added to the bedside, such as electric shavers or radios brought from home. This type of equipment should be evaluated by the biomedical department to determine whether it is responsible for the interference.

> ⚠ **If the patient is on mechanical ventilation that has no battery back-up, ensure that oxygen delivery and ventilation is provided by ambu bag before you assess the plug. Ensure that there is battery back-up when troubleshooting intravenous (IV) pump plugs. The delivery of IV vasoactive and antiarrhythmic drugs should not be interrupted during troubleshooting.**

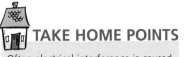

TAKE HOME POINTS

Often electrical interference is caused by a damaged plug on the patient's bed.

- If the equipment continues to cause interference when placed in the new location, replace it.
- Send any defective equipment to the biomedical department for inspection and repair.

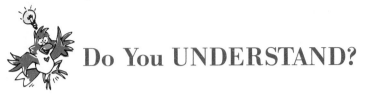

Do You UNDERSTAND?

DIRECTIONS: On the lines provided, list four possible causes for artifacts.

1. _____

_____

_____

_____

DIRECTIONS: On the lines provided, list the steps you would take to troubleshoot an artifact problem.

2. _____

_____

_____

_____

_____

_____

_____

Answers: 1. Hiccups, shivering, convulsions, strong respiratory movements; 2. Assess the patient and ensure safety, initiate further assessment and treatment (if necessary), check to see that electrode pads and lead wires are attached to patient, inspect lead wires and clean or replace (if necessary), send any faulty equipment to the biomedical department.

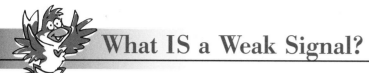

What IS a Weak Signal?

Occasionally, the monitor will not pick up the patient's actual heart rate because of a *weak signal*. This may be caused by an improperly placed, loose, or dry electrode. Weak signals may also be caused by obesity, because electrical impulse from the patient's heart must travel through a greater amount of subcutaneous tissue to reach the electrode.

What You NEED TO KNOW

The QRS (the largest waveform) must be a certain height for the monitor to count it as a heartbeat. In some conditions, like cardiac tamponade, the mechanical compression of the heart may prevent a strong heartbeat. However, keep in mind that the QRS complex may appear too small if the health care provider has forgotten to turn up the gain or the size-adjustment knob, which makes the complex height taller.

You should always assess the patient first, because a change in clinical status could signal serious problems. For example, a patient who becomes unstable and has distant, muffled heart sounds and a weak ECG signal may be experiencing cardiac tamponade.

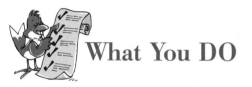

What You DO

When you discover a weak signal:

- Assess the patient to determine whether there is any change in his or her condition.
- Systematically check the electrodes, connections, and lead wires for any damage.
- Count the patient's apical heart rate for 1 minute, and compare it with the rate on the monitor.
- Turn the gain or size-adjustment knob up until the monitor picks up each heartbeat.
- Change the lead select button on the monitoring system to a lead that allows for better visualization of the heart rhythm.

TAKE HOME POINTS

To ensure proper functioning of the monitoring system, the patient's apical heart rate should be checked and compared against the rate reported on the monitor.

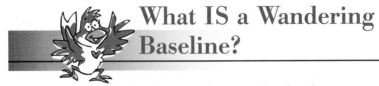

What IS a Wandering Baseline?

A *wandering baseline* is another type of artifact that can cause problems in the analysis of ECG recording. The baseline of the patient's rhythm is determined by drawing a flat line through the ECG complex.

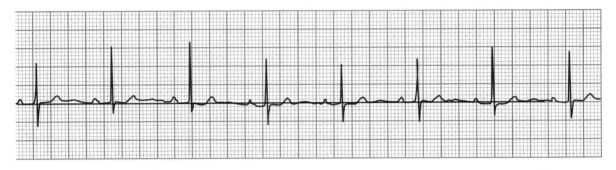

When the patient is restless or breathing heavily, the baseline will not be straight. Rather, it will appear to ride up and down in a wavy manner.

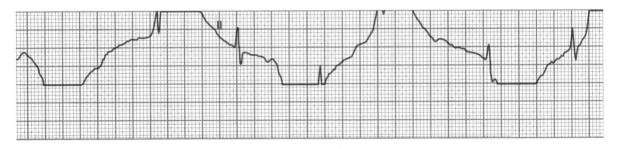

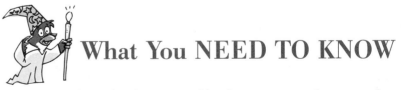

What You NEED TO KNOW

Often a wandering baseline is caused by chest movement that occurs during respiration. Anxiety or pain may contribute to a wandering baseline.

⚠️ The up and down movement of the baseline can make it difficult to obtain accurate measurements when assessing the rhythm strip, which can lead to misinterpretation.

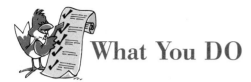

What You DO

- Remember to always assess the patient first.
- If your patient is experiencing pain, you should evaluate the pain and institute appropriate pain-relieving measures, including medication and positioning.
- Document your assessment, interventions, and patient response.
- Reposition any electrodes that have been placed over bony areas or areas of skin that move during respiration. If electrodes are placed on your patient's arms and legs, it may help to bring them closer to the heart.
- Continue to maintain the placement area required for the lead wire.

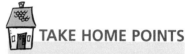

TAKE HOME POINTS

The lead wires and cables should not be so tight that they pull on the electrodes.

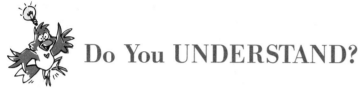

Do You UNDERSTAND?

DIRECTIONS: Define the following types of artifact.

1. Weak signal: _____

_____

2. AC (60-cycle) interference: _____

_____

3. Wandering baseline: _____

_____

4. Artifact: _____

_____

DIRECTIONS: Unscramble the words in parentheses to fill in the blanks.

5. To ensure proper functioning of the cardiac-monitoring system, you should always compare the heart rate on the ECG with the patient's _____ pulse. *(ipaacl)*

6. If a patient's ECG has a wandering baseline, the electrodes may have been placed over _____ areas. *(yonb)*

Answers: 1. A weak signal is an ECG complex that is not picked up when the monitor counts the patient's heart rate; 2. AC or 60-cycle interference is leakage of electricity from improperly grounded devices; 3. A wandering baseline rides up and down, within and between the ECG complexes; 4. Artifact is an artificial disturbance that interferes with high-quality capture of the ECG tracing; 5. apical; 6. bony.

Electrocardiogram: Monitoring and Electrode Placement

This chapter discusses the differences between continuous and 12-lead monitoring. You'll also learn how to place electrodes on a patient.

The *electrocardiogram* (ECG) is a graphic display of the electrical activity of the heart. Electrical activity, depolarization, and repolarization can be picked up by electrodes placed on the skin. This electrical activity is transmitted via leads (wires) to a monitoring device. The monitoring device converts the electrical activity to a graphic waveform (oscilloscope) display. An oscilloscope is the part of the monitor that magnifies (over 1000 times) the electrical activity of the heart and displays it as a continuous waveform recording on the monitor screen.

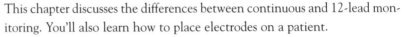

What ARE the Components of the ECG Equipment?

Leads

www.americanheart.org
www.atlcard.com/introekg.
html
www.wices.com/icescardiac

The word *lead* can have two different meanings. It can refer to the small, flexible, color-coded wires leading from the electrodes to the monitoring device. Leads are coded with letters on the head of the lead, and the colors indicate where they are to be placed on the body:

LETTERS	MEANING	COLOR
RA	Right arm	White
LA	Left arm	Black
RL	Right leg	Green
LL	Left leg	Red

There may also be a C lead (that indicates chest) on some systems. A C lead is always brown.

Lead can also refer to the standardized patterns of electrode placement. Electrodes are placed on different parts of the body (chest, arms, legs) to allow the electrical activity of the heart to be viewed from different angles. Leads are discussed in detail later in this chapter.

Electrodes

Electrodes are small, sticky discs or tabs that are strategically placed on the patient's chest and extremities. They pick up and transmit the *millivolts* (mV) of electrical energy produced by the heart during depolarization and repolarization via the lead wire to a monitoring device. Disc-shaped electrodes have an inner, moist, conductive gel, surrounded by an outside ring of sticky adhesive. A common use for this type of electrode is for continuous bedside monitoring.

Tab-shaped electrodes are used with 12-lead ECG monitoring and are $1^1/_2$ inches long with adhesive on the long side to allow for attachment to the skin. The opposite side permits attachment of an alligator-type clip to the patient cable.

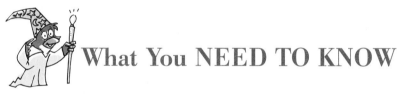

What You NEED TO KNOW

Electrodes must be attached to the patient correctly to obtain a clear and accurate picture of heart function.

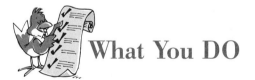

What You DO

To attach electrodes to a patient, you should do the following:
- Explain what you are doing. Reassure the patient that he or she will not receive an electrical shock and that alarms do not always mean that there is a problem with his or her heartbeat.
- Provide privacy for electrode application.
- Wash your hands.
- Identify the patient by checking his or her ident-a-band and asking his or her name.

Older adults may not tolerate alcohol on the skin. Sensitivity to the conductive gel on the electrode may also occur. If skin irritation is present, the electrode site should be checked and rotated more frequently than every 3 days.

Do not place electrodes in the right second ICS or under the left breast. This site is used to defibrillate (electrically shock) the patient during a cardiac arrest. Shocking over an electrode will cause the force of electricity to follow the lead wires, causing damage to the patient and the equipment. It may also prevent proper voltage from being delivered to the patient. Artifact or abnormal electrical patterns on the recorded rhythm may occur if these instructions are not followed.

- Electrodes transmit best when they are in direct contact with skin. Avoid placing electrodes on hairy areas. Hair will interfere with contact between the skin and the electrode. Shaving is no longer an acceptable practice; it may irritate the patient's skin. Clipping the hair is preferred.
- If the skin is moist or soiled, cleanse the area with an alcohol wipe or soap and water; allow it to dry. This will remove any excess skin oils and promote good skin contact.
- Allow the area to dry thoroughly before applying the electrodes. If the patient is continuously sweating or moist (diaphoretic), you can apply a thin coat of benzoin. However, be sure that the benzoin is dry before attaching the disc.
- Keep in mind that electrodes will dry out in about 3 days and that they should be changed every 2 to 3 days.
- Avoid bony prominences. Intercostal spaces (ICSs) are good electrical conductors and are easy to find by palpating between the ribs.
- Avoid the ribs and sternum. Also avoid skin folds, breast tissue, and bony areas. These body areas interfere with electrical conduction and have a tendency to produce more artifact.
- Remove the electrodes from their packages.
- Snap the lead wire to the metal snap on the outside of the disc before applying. This avoids having to compress the lead wire to the electrode on the patient, which could possibly cause pain.
- Remove the paper backing from the electrode without touching the sticky adhesive. Examine the center of the disc to check if the gel is moist. If it is dry, discard and use a new disc.

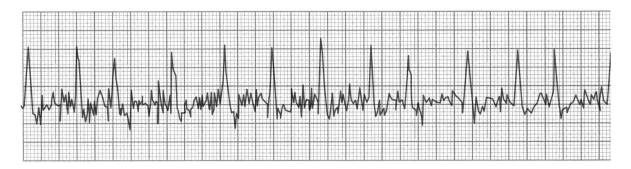

- Place each electrode on the prepared site by tracing and pressing firmly around the adhesive. If your system comes with an alligator clip (a clip with a type of jaw attachment on the lead wire), place the tab electrode on the skin first. Squeeze the jaws of the clip open and attach it to the electrode.
- Connect the color-coded lead wires to the corresponding color on the monitor cable. For example, white lead wire goes to white monitor cable.

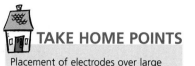

TAKE HOME POINTS

Placement of electrodes over large muscles may interfere with an accurate ECG analysis.

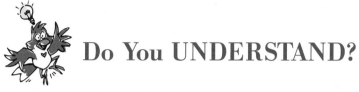

Do You UNDERSTAND?

DIRECTIONS: Fill in the blanks.

1. Electrical energy generated from the heart is measured in

   _____.

2. Thin, flexible wires that connect electrodes to the patient cable are

   called _____.

3. An _____ is a sticky

   pad that helps conduct electrical energy to the monitor.

4. An _____ displays

   waveforms of the heart's electrical activity.

DIRECTIONS: Indicate in the spaces provided whether the following statements are *true* or *false*.

5. _____   Bony areas increase transmission of heart impulses.
6. _____   Chest hair does not have to be removed for electrode placement.
7. _____   Large muscle groups and skin folds increase artifact.
8. _____   Electrodes should be changed every 4 to 5 days.

Answers: 1. millivolts; 2. leads; 3. electrode; 4. oscilloscope; 5. false; 6. false; 7. true; 8. false.

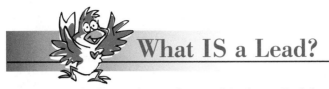

What IS a Lead?

A *lead* is an electrical view of the heart. Each lead represents a view from a different position. Leads consist of two *poles*: a negative pole and a positive pole. Electrical activity that flows within the heart can be recorded between the negative and positive poles (electricity flows from negative to positive).

The two poles are identified by either two electrodes, one at each pole (*bipolar*), or they are identified as one electrode and a mathematically determined reference point (*unipolar*). A pair of electrodes, one positive and one negative, or a single electrode and a reference point form a lead.

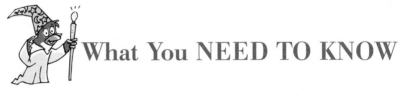

What You NEED TO KNOW

Normally, the electrical impulse produced in the heart starts in the sinoatrial (SA) node, which is located in the right upper chest. The impulse then moves toward the ventricles in the left lower chest. Therefore electrical flow is downward and to the left. This flow pattern is known as normal *axis*. Axis refers to the general direction of the flow of electrical activity (depolarization) as it spreads through the heart.

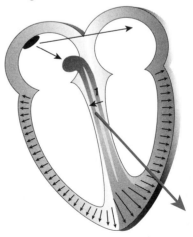

As the flow of electrical activity moves *from* the *negative* electrode *toward* the *positive* electrode, an upward (positive) wave is produced. If the flow of electrical activity moves away from the positive electrode, a downward (negative) wave is produced.

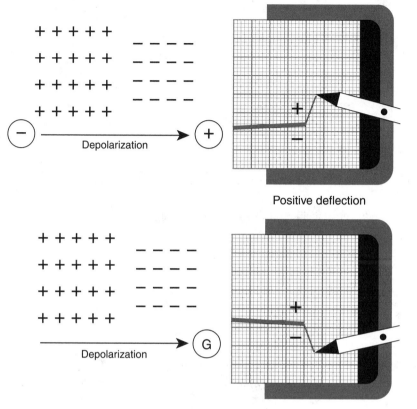

Positive deflection

Negtive deflection

The camera analogy is frequently used to describe a lead (view). Consider the positive electrode the camera lens or the recording electrode. The negative electrode would then be the director, telling the camera in which direction to shoot the picture.

In addition to positive and negative electrodes, a *ground* electrode is also used. Because leakage of electricity from faulty wires can generate a shock, a *ground electrode* is needed to absorb any excess electricity. For this reason, all monitoring systems have a ground electrode and a three-pronged plug to protect the patient.

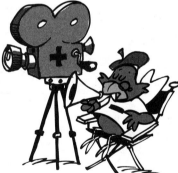

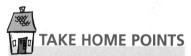

TAKE HOME POINTS

- To avoid confusion and misinterpretation of data, electrodes must be placed on the patient correctly.
- The flow of electrical activity in the heart does not change (the view changes with each lead).

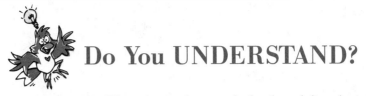

Do You UNDERSTAND?

DIRECTIONS: **Write the word or words that best define the information in each sentence.**

1. An electrode is placed at the positive pole, and a corresponding electrode is placed at the negative pole.

   _____

2. Prevents accidental shock to the patient.

   _____

3. General direction of electrical flow in the heart.

   _____

4. The direction of the deflection that will occur if the flow of electrical activity (depolarization) moves away from the positive electrode.

   _____

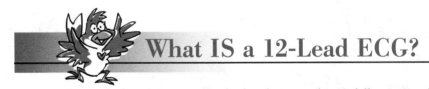

What IS a 12-Lead ECG?

A *12-lead* ECG is a graphic display that provides 12 different, simultaneous views of the heart's electrical activity. The 12-lead ECG is used to diagnose the cause of dysrhythmia, determine conduction defects, diagnose and monitor myocardial infarction (MI), diagnose myocardial ischemia and injury, and determine cardiac position and size. It is also used to diagnose particular diseases, such as pericarditis and Wolff-Parkinson-White syndrome, and evaluate electrolyte abnormalities and the effects of drug therapy.

Answers: 1. bipolar; 2. ground electrode; 3. axis; 4. downward (negative).

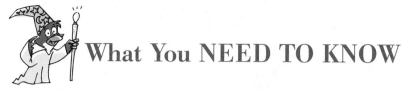

What You NEED TO KNOW

The heart can be viewed from four major or general surfaces. The front of the heart is considered the *anterior surface*; the back of the heart is considered the *posterior surface*; the bottom of the heart is considered the *inferior surface*; and the side of the heart is considered the *lateral surface*.

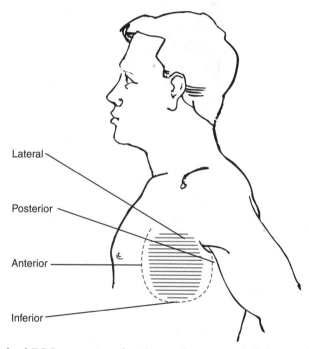

The 12-lead ECG can assess the electrical activity of all four surfaces of the heart. For example, if the health care provider wants to examine the anterior surface of the heart, the lead or leads that best assess this particular heart surface is selected.

The 12 leads of the ECG test are divided into two subgroups: the *limb leads*, which include standard limb leads and augmented limb leads; and the *chest leads*, known as *precordial leads* or *V leads*. Electrode placement knowledge is essential in performing a 12-lead ECG.

Four electrodes are attached to the patient's upper and lower extremities, and six electrodes are positioned in specific locations across the upper chest. Although only 10 electrode pads are attached, the ECG machine (via computer), obtains 12 views of the heart by changing poles.

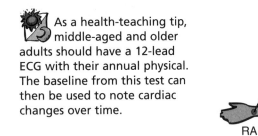
As a health-teaching tip, middle-aged and older adults should have a 12-lead ECG with their annual physical. The baseline from this test can then be used to note cardiac changes over time.

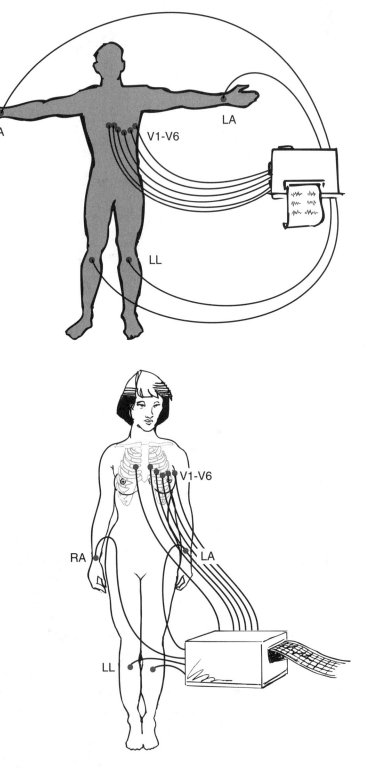

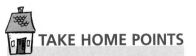
TAKE HOME POINTS

The 12-lead ECG provides multiple views of the heart's electrical activity from each of the four major heart surfaces.

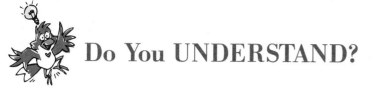

Do You UNDERSTAND?

DIRECTIONS: Fill in the blanks.

1. The bottom of the heart is considered the _____ surface.
2. The front of the heart is considered the _____ surface.
3. The side of the heart is considered the _____ surface.
4. The back of the heart is considered the _____ surface.

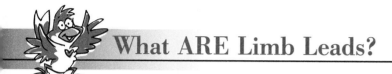

What ARE Limb Leads?

Limb leads are the first six views of a 12-lead ECG. They are divided into *standard limb leads* and *augmented limb leads.* Limb leads record electrical activity from top to bottom and from right to left on a frontal plane of the chest. To record electrical activity from the limb leads, electrodes are placed on the right and left arms and on the left leg or foot. The placement of these electrodes forms a triangle, known as *Einthoven's triangle.* If this triangle is shortened and centered, it forms a plane over the chest.

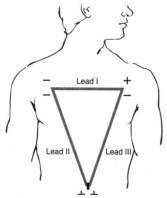

Standard Limb Leads

Standard limb leads are *bipolar;* therefore they have two electrodes: one at the positive pole and one at the negative pole. One lead wire is attached to a positive electrode on one limb, and the other is attached to a negative electrode on the other limb. Standard limb leads are designated as leads I, II and III.

Lead I. Lead I views electrical activity from the right upper chest to the left upper chest. Electrodes are placed on the right arm (negative) and the left arm (positive).

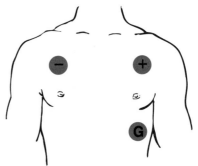

Lead II. Lead II views electrical activity from the right upper chest to the left leg. Electrodes are placed on the right arm (negative) and the left leg (positive).

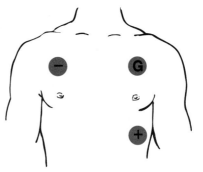

Lead III. Lead III views electrical activity from the left upper chest to the left leg. Electrodes are placed on the left arm (negative) and the left leg (positive).

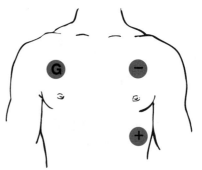

Augmented Limb Leads

Augmented limb leads are designated as *augmented voltage right arm (aVR)*, *augmented voltage left arm (aVL)*, and *augmented voltage foot (aVF)*. They are called *augmented* because the voltage must be amplified 1.5 fold by the ECG machine to produce waves of the same magnitude as those of leads I, II, III. Augmented limb leads are unipolar, because they have one positive pole and a reference point in the center of the heart. However, they use the same electrode placement as the standard limb leads (right and left arm, left foot).

aVR. Lead aVR views electrical activity from a reference point in the center of the heart to the right arm (the right-arm electrode is positive). The electrical wave of depolarization moves away from the positive electrode. The waveforms produced on the ECG paper are downward (negative).

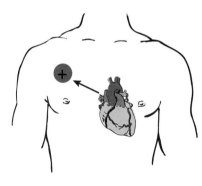

aVL. Lead aVL views electrical activity from a reference point in the center of the heart to the left arm (the left arm electrode is positive). The QRS waveform produced in aVL will be eqiphasic (half above the isoelectric line and half below the isoelectric line), because the flow of electricity moves toward the positive electrode and then away from it.

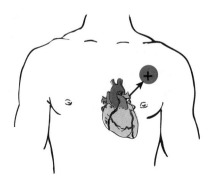

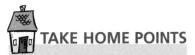

TAKE HOME POINTS

- The small *a* represents the word augmented.
- The *V* represents the word *voltage*.
- The *capitalized third* letter tells the health care provider where to place the positive electrode pad or tab.
- Normally, aVR produces only negative waveforms.
- Augmented leads also form intersecting lines on a plane. They view the heart from different angles than the standard leads.

aVF. Lead aVF views electrical activity from a reference point in the center of the heart to the left foot (the left-foot electrode is positive). The waveforms produced in aVF will always be upward (positive), because the general flow of electricity moves toward the positive electrode.

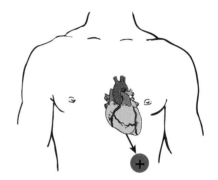

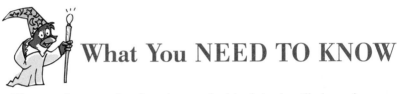

What You NEED TO KNOW

The waveforms produced in the standard limb leads will always be upward (positive), because the general flow of electricity moves toward the positive electrode.

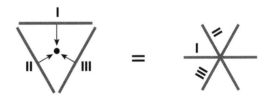

By pushing leads I, II, and III to the center of the Einthoven's triangle, three intersecting lines are formed. Each line provides a different view of the patient's chest (see the following figure).

Limb leads provide views of the heart from six different angles in the *frontal plane*. This is accomplished by superimposing the intersecting lines of the standard limb leads over the intersecting lines of the augmented limb leads.

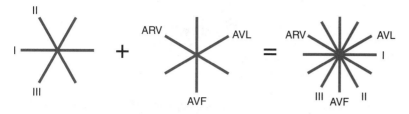

The frontal plane represents a vertical view of the heart, from superior to inferior (up to down) and from right to left.

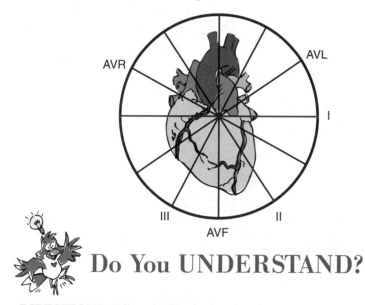

Do You UNDERSTAND?

DIRECTIONS: **Fill in the blanks for the placement of the positive electrodes in standard and augmented leads.**

1. Lead I   _____

2. Lead II   _____

3. Lead III   _____

4. Lead aVR _____

5. Lead aVL _____

6. Lead aVF _____

Answers: 1. left arm; 2. left foot; 3. left foot; 4. right arm; 5. left arm; 6. foot.

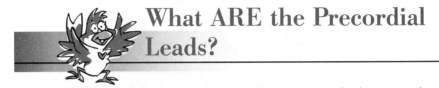

What ARE the Precordial Leads?

The last six leads of the ECG look at events in the heart on a horizontal plane. These are called the precordial, chest, or V leads. They are positioned directly over the heart, viewing the anterior and lateral surfaces. The positive poles are areas on the anterior and lateral chest. The negative pole is considered the opposite side of the positive pole or to the posterior and lateral of the chest. Similar to the augmented leads, these leads are unipolar. Therefore one electrode is placed on the anterior chest (the positive electrode). To obtain the six leads, six electrodes are placed in six different positions across the anterior and lateral chest wall.

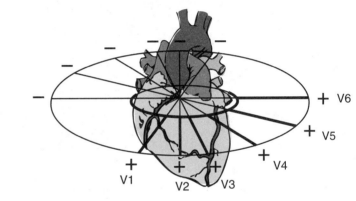

What You NEED TO KNOW

The precordial leads are placed from the right to the left of the heart. They are called *V1, V2, V3, V4, V5,* and *V6.*

- **V1.** The positive electrode is placed directly over the right atrium. Mainly the QRS complex is negative, and the R wave is small in V1, because the flow of electricity moves away from the positive electrode.
- **V2.** The positive electrode is placed just anterior to the atrioventricular (AV) node. Mainly the QRS complex is negative, and the R wave is slightly taller than in V1.

- **V3.** The positive electrode is placed over the ventricular septum. The QRS complex is isoelectric, which means half is above the baseline and half is below the baseline.
- **V4.** The positive electrode is also placed over the ventricular septum but to the left of V3. The QRS complex is more positive than in V3.
- **V5 and V6.** The positive electrodes are placed over the lateral surface of the left ventricle. The QRS complexes are more positive than in V4.

Placement of electrodes for the precordial leads is guided by the ICSs as follows:

- **V1.** Fourth ICS, right sternal boarder
- **V2.** Fourth ICS, left sternal boarder
- **V3.** Halfway between V2 and V4
- **V4.** Fifth ICS, left midclavicular line
- **V5.** Fifth ICS, left anterior axillary line
- **V6.** Fifth ICS, left midaxillary line

The intersecting lines of the precordial leads form a horizontal plane providing six views, from anterior to posterior and from right to left. The R wave gets progressively larger from V1 to V6 as more of the ventricles are viewed. This is called R *wave progression*.

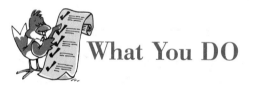

What You DO

Correct electrode placement is crucial in obtaining the correct waveforms. To place precordial leads correctly:

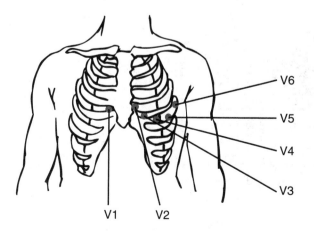

- Place the V1 electrode over the fourth ICS, to the right of the sternum.
- Place the V2 electrode just lateral to V1, at the left of the sternum at the fourth ICS.
- Skip to V4, and place the V4 electrode over the fifth ICS and midclavicular line or the point of maximal impulse (PMI).
- Find V3 (halfway between V2 and V4).
- Place the V6 electrode at the left midaxillary line (level with V4).
- Place the V5 electrode halfway between V4 and V6, at the anterior axillary line.

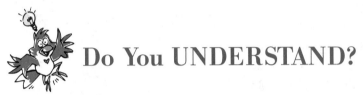

Do You UNDERSTAND?

DIRECTIONS: **Describe the location of the precordial leads.**

1. V1 _____

2. V2 _____

3. V3 _____

4. V4 _____

5. V5 _____

6. V6 _____

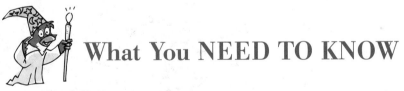

What You NEED TO KNOW

The 12-lead ECG takes several seconds to conduct, once you have placed the electrodes on the patient. It records the electrical activity of the heart from 12 points (6 limb leads and 6 chest leads), and documentation is provided on standard-sized paper.

Answers: 1. **Fourth ICS, to the right of the sternum;** 2. **Fourth ICS, to the left of the sternum;** 3. **Find V4 first, halfway between V2 and V4;** 4. **Fifth ICS, midclavicular line;** 5. **Find V6 first, halfway between V4 and V6;** 6. **Fifth ICS, lateral to V4, midaxillary line.**

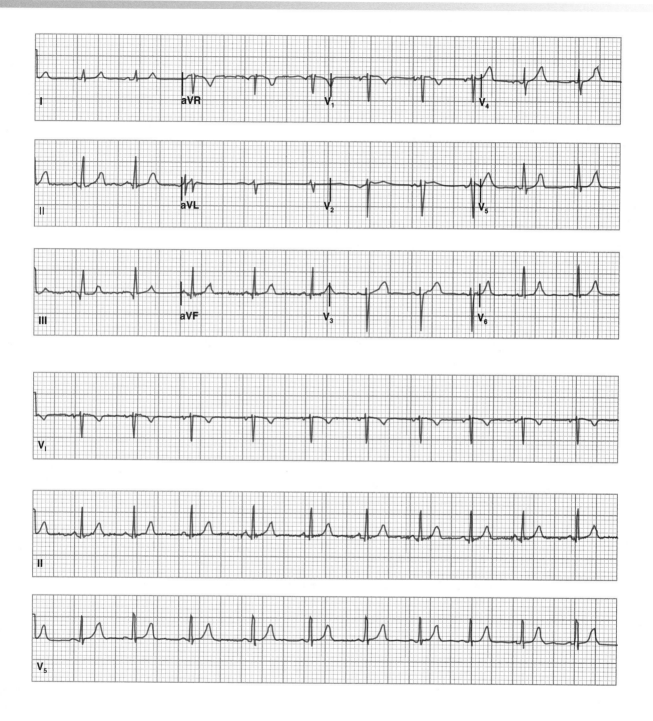

This test is performed during routine physical examinations, admission to the hospital, and when cardiac, electrical, or mechanical problems are suggested. An ECG may be prescribed by the physician or by an advanced practical nurse, or the unit may have standing orders for the provider to perform this test when the patient's condition warrants it.

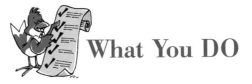

What You DO

- If serial 12 leads will be obtained, it may be helpful to mark the electrode positions with permanent ink.
- Connect all cables to the designated electrodes. The patient cable is already attached to the ECG machine.
- Confirm that the 10 electrodes and cables are in the correct position.
- Enter the name, date, and patient number on the ECG.
- To avoid artifact and obtain the best quality, ask the patient to remain still during the procedure.
- Run the test according to the manufacturer's directions.

Information about the patient (name, date, time, medical record number, physician) need to be confirmed on the ECG printout. It is also important to include any symptoms that the patient may be experiencing.

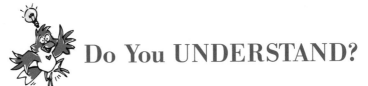

Do You UNDERSTAND?

DIRECTIONS: **Indicate in the spaces provided whether the following statements are *true* or *false*.**

1. _____ The 12-lead ECG may take several hours to perform.
2. _____ To perform the 12-lead ECG, 12 electrodes are placed on various parts of the body to obtain multiple views.
3. _____ The patient should remain still while the actual ECG is being performed.

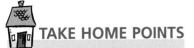

TAKE HOME POINTS

Consistent placement of all electrodes is essential to detect changes in the anterior, posterior, inferior, and lateral surfaces of the heart.

Answers: 1. false; 2. false; 3. true.

What IS Continuous ECG Monitoring?

Continuous ECG monitoring, also referred to as continuous cardiac monitoring, is the continuous recording of the heart's electrical activity. Continuous ECG monitoring is mainly used to assess the heart rate, rhythm, and ST segment. Its primary function is to check for ectopy (abnormal heart beat) or dysrhythmia. Continuous cardiac monitoring is accomplished using either a 3- or 5-lead system.

The 3-lead system is limited to single-channel recording, which means only one lead can be viewed on the monitor at a time. A 5-lead system allows for dual-channel recording, which means that two leads can be viewed on the monitor at the same time. Continuous ECG monitoring can be accomplished either by a hardwire system (bedside monitoring) or by telemetry. Continuous ECG monitoring by telemetry uses radio waves rather than electricity to deliver information about the heart's electrical activity to a monitor.

What You NEED TO KNOW

With continuous monitoring, the limb leads are placed on the chest, not on the limbs as in standard 12-lead ECG monitoring. Arm leads should be placed on the shoulders, close to where the limbs join the body. The *RA* is placed in the right shoulder area, and the *LA* is placed in the left shoulder area. The *RL* is moved up to the right abdominal area, and the *LL* is moved up to the left abdominal area.

Hardwire or Bedside Monitoring

Continuous ECG monitoring or *bedside cardiac monitoring* by hardwire requires the patient to be directly connected to a large monitoring device at the bedside. This system is used when patients are limited to bedrest, and it operates on electricity. Information is transmitted to the bedside monitor via lead wires and cables and to the central station by hardwire (electrically). There are many settings in which this type of monitoring is used, including intensive care units (ICUs), emergency departments (EDs), operating rooms (ORs), day surgery centers, and cardiac catheterization laboratories.

Cellular phones can disrupt the transmission of radio waves. Therefore the use of cellular phones is not permitted on or near telemetry units.

Telemetry

Telemetry is accomplished by using short cables, which are connected to a small, portable radio transmitter. The heart's electrical activity is transmitted by radio waves from the transmitter to ceiling antennas. This information is then transmitted to a central monitoring station. The transmitter is battery powered and can be carried by the patient in a pocket or pouch, allowing the patient to freely move around. Telemetry monitoring is used on units where patients no longer require intensive care but still require close cardiac surveillance.

 ## What IS a 3-Lead System?

A *3-lead* or *3-electrode system* is a continuous monitoring system with three patient wires. These electrode systems are the easiest to learn and are used wherever quick monitoring is needed (in EDs, telemetry units, first responder units). The advantage of the 3-lead system is that it is less expensive and requires less memory than other systems, since only three electrodes and three patient leads are required. This system is limited to single-channel (one lead) viewing.

What You NEED TO KNOW

The standard placement for electrodes in a 3-lead system are on the right shoulder area under the clavicle and on the left shoulder area under the clavicle on the lower left chest area, below the fifth ICS or apex of the heart. The three leads are color coded white, black, and red.

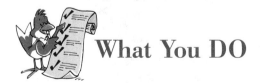 ## What You DO

The color-coded leads are connected as follows:
- The white lead wire, designated RA, is attached to the right arm electrode.
- The black lead wire, designated LA, is attached to the left arm electrode.
- The red lead wire, designated LL, is attached to the electrode on the left lower chest.

With this pattern of electrode placement, the 3-lead system can be used to monitor the standard limb leads I, II, or III by turning the selector dial. No electrodes need to be moved. The selector on the monitoring device automatically adjusts which electrode will be positive, which will be negative, and which will be the ground.

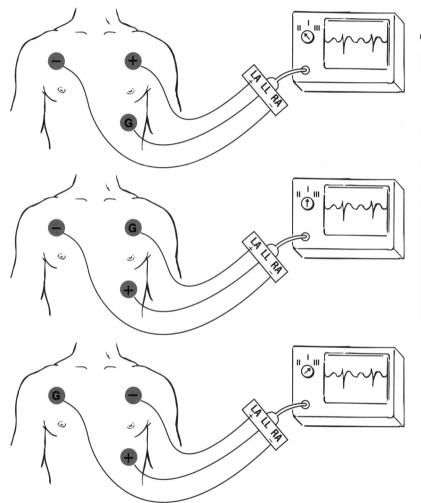

TAKE HOME POINTS

- The left lower electrode must be placed below the level of the heart.
- To recall lead placement for the 3-lead system, remember "white is right" and "smoke over fire." The white lead goes on the right arm, and the black lead goes over the red lead on the left.
- Lead I is useful for patients with respiratory distress, because chest wall motion is least affected in this lead.
- Lead II is preferred for observing the patient's underlying rhythm, because lead II produces the most upright waveforms. Lead II is a primary monitoring lead for dysrhythmia detection.

A patient may need to receive defibrillation. If defibrillator pads are placed over electrodes, the electricity produced from defibrillation will travel through the lead wires and electrodes and could cause harm to the patient and equipment. When placing electrodes on a patient, avoid the apex of the heart to ensure that the defibrillator pads fit in these areas.

Standard Lead Placement in a 3-Lead System

LEAD	POSITIVE	NEGATIVE	GROUND
Lead I	Left arm	Right arm	Left lower chest
Lead II	Right arm	Right arm	Left arm
Lead III	Left arm	Left arm	Right arm

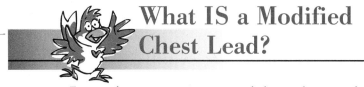

What IS a Modified Chest Lead?

Frequently, it is necessary to record electrical activity from the heart's anterior or lateral surface to assess ventricular rhythm disturbances. Modified chest lead 1 (MCL1) and modified chest lead 6 (MCL6) are useful for identifying bundle branch blocks and for differentiating supraventricular tachycardia from ventricular tachycardia.

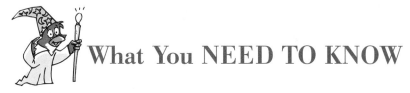

What You NEED TO KNOW

Lead MCL1 is the modified version of the precordial lead V1. Lead MCL6 is the modified version of the precordial lead V6. To obtain these views with a 3-lead system, you must move the electrodes.

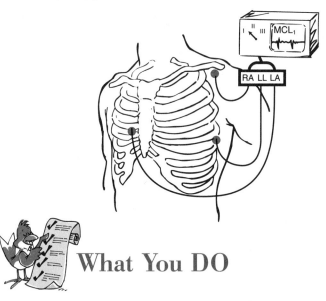

What You DO

To use MCL1 and MCL6 to record electrical activity from the heart's anterior or lateral surface:

- Connect one electrode to the *LA* lead wire, and place it in the V1 position. This becomes the positive electrode.
- Connect one electrode to the *RA* lead wire, and place it in the right arm position. This becomes the negative electrode.

- Connect one electrode to the *LL* lead wire, and place it in the V6 position. This becomes the ground electrode.
- Turn the monitor's selector dial to lead 1.

Once these electrodes are in place, you may also monitor lead MCL6. To obtain a lateral surface view, turn the selector dial to lead II.

> ⚠️ **Obtain a 12-lead ECG to confirm any significant rhythm disturbances. Remember, it is the correct attachment to the correct color and the proper placement of electrodes that determine the accuracy of the ECG waveform.**

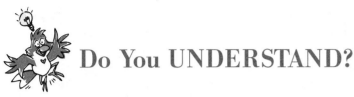

Do You UNDERSTAND?

DIRECTIONS: **On the diagrams that follow, label the negative, positive, and ground electrode placement for leads II and MCL1.**

1. Lead II

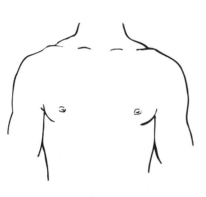

2. Lead MCL

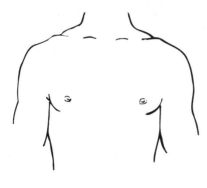

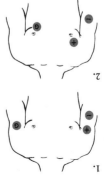

Answers:

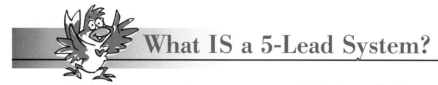

What IS a 5-Lead System?

A *5-lead system* is used in recovery rooms, ICUs, EDs, and telemetry units. This system includes five electrodes and five leads that attach to a patient cable, and it allows for continuous monitoring of the patient's electrical heart rhythm in two leads at the same time (*dual lead* monitoring).

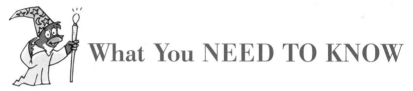

What You NEED TO KNOW

The 5-lead system adds a right leg (*RL*) and a chest electrode (*V1 position*) to the previous 3-lead standard electrode placement. By adding the *RL* electrode, any of the six limb leads can be viewed. The *chest* electrode can be moved to any of the precordial V positions to obtain all six precordial views. Review the sections on limb leads and precordial leads.

TAKE HOME POINTS

The 5-lead system can provide all 12 views of the 12-lead ECG. However, it requires that the chest electrode be moved to obtain all of the V leads.

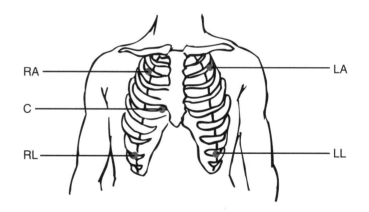

In the 5-lead system, leads II and V1 are used the most.

To confirm and document a dysrhythmia before starting treatment, the use of more than one lead may be necessary.

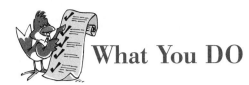

What You DO

- In a 5-lead system, electrodes are placed in the right and left second ICS spaces, and they are placed at the right and left seventh ICS spaces.
- These four electrodes are placed vertically at the midaxillary line.
- The chest electrode is placed at the fourth ICS space to the right of the sternum.

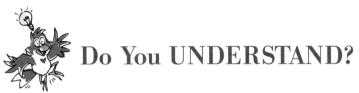

Do You UNDERSTAND?

DIRECTIONS: **List the advantages of a 3-lead system and a 5-lead system.**

Advantages of a 3-lead system

1. _____

2. _____

3. _____

Advantages of a 5-lead system

4. _____

5. _____

6. _____

TAKE HOME POINTS

Color-coded lead wire system

Right upper arm = white

Left upper arm = black

Right fourth ICS = brown

Right lower chest = green

Left lower chest = red

TAKE HOME POINTS

The monitor internally changes the designation of positive and negative electrodes when you turn the selector dial to a specific lead.

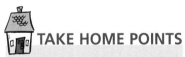

Examine lead wires, patient cables, and monitors for loose connections and physical damage to avoid potential electrical shock to the patient.

DIRECTIONS: Write the placement and color of the electrodes in a
5-lead monitoring system on the following illustration
of the patient's torso.

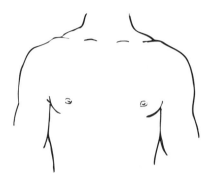

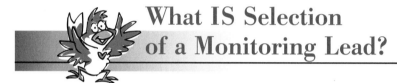

What IS Selection
of a Monitoring Lead?

Systems monitor and record the patient's heart rhythm in more than one
view at the same time. You will need to select a monitoring lead based on
your patient's that will be different from patient to patient depending on the
abnormality.

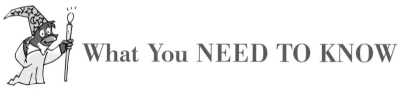

What You NEED TO KNOW

Lead II remains the preferred lead for monitoring a patient's underlying
rhythm. MCL1 and MCL6 are preferred for identifying bundle branch
blocks and ventricular ectopy. See the following table for suggested monitoring lead selection.

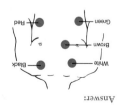

Answer:

Suggested Monitoring Lead Selection

LEAD	RATIONALE FOR USE
II	Produces large, upright visible P waves and QRS complexes for determining underlying rhythm
V1 or MCL1	Helpful for detecting right bundle branch block and for differentiating ventricular ectopy from supraventricular rhythm aberrantly conducted in the ventricles
V6 or MCL6	Helpful lead for detecting left bundle branch block for differentiating ventricular ectopy from supraventricular rhythm aberrantly conducted in the ventricles
III, aVF, V1	Produce visible P waves; useful in detecting atrial dysrhythmias; useful in patients with respiratory distress; involved left and right arm electrodes placements are less affected by chest motion compared with other leads
II, III, aVF	Helpful in detecting ischemia, injury, and infarction in the inferior wall
I, aVL, V5, V6	Helpful in detecting ischemia, injury, and infarction in the lateral wall
V1 through V4	Helpful in detecting ischemia, injury, and infarction in the anterior wall

Vectorcardiography

Newer 5-lead systems have the capability of monitoring 12-leads simultaneously. Conventional ECGs provide flat, frontal, and horizontal views. However, Dr. E. Frank developed *vectorcardiography* to obtain three-dimensional (3-D) views.

The 3-D views are obtained in the following way:
- Frontal plane—right to left (X) and head to foot (Y)
- Horizontal plane—right to left (X) and anterior to posterior (Z)
- Sagittal plane—head to foot (Y) and anterior to posterior (Z)

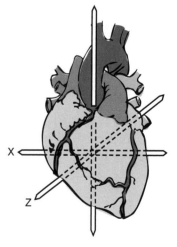

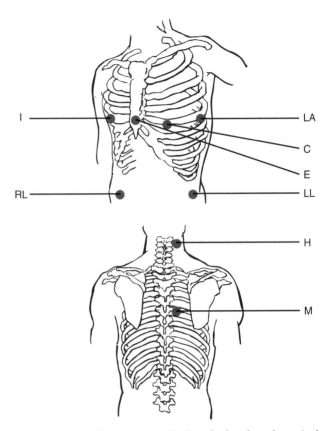

To obtain multiple 3-D views, Dr. E. Frank developed an 8-electrode placement system.

This system that has been modified to perform 12-lead ECG monitoring with a 5-lead continuous monitoring system. A 5-lead continuous monitoring system can derive a 12-lead ECG by using three of Frank's electrode sites: *E, A,* and *I.* An *S* site is added to the upper sternum, and a ground is added to the right lower area. This is called the *EASI method.*

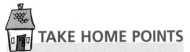

TAKE HOME POINTS

Because this new technology has not been accepted by the entire medical community, the 12-lead ECG remains the *gold standard* for ECG monitoring.

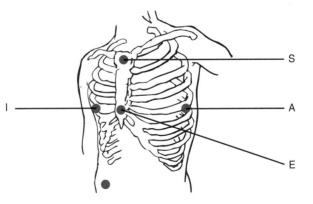

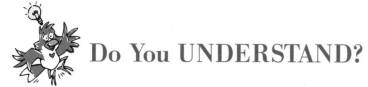

Do You UNDERSTAND?

DIRECTIONS: **Indicate in the spaces provided whether the following statements are *true* or *false*.**

1. _____ Newer 5-lead continuous-monitoring systems have the capability to perform a 12-lead ECG.

2. _____ With the EASI method of electrode placement, the S electrode is placed in the V1 position.

3. _____ Vectorcardiography views the heart in three dimensions, rather than on planes as in standard 12-lead monitoring.

8

Sinus Dysrhythmias: Rhythms of the Sinoatrial Node

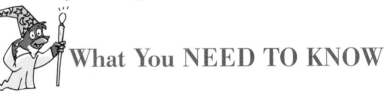

What IS the Sinoatrial Node?

The *sinoatrial* (SA) *node* is the normal pacemaker of the heart. It consists of a small group of cardiac cells that generate an electrical impulse. This impulse is conducted down the normal conduction pathway causing depolarization of the heart, which is normally followed by contraction (see Chapter 1). The SA node initiates this pacing impulse at a regular rate of 60 to 100 beats per minute (bpm).

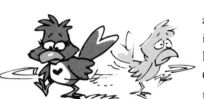

What You NEED TO KNOW

SA node stimulation results in the following:
- Electrocardiogram (ECG) that shows uniform (consistent in shape) P waves
- Constant PR of 0.12 to 0.20 seconds
- Constant QT intervals
- Uniform QRS complexes of 0.04 to 0.11 seconds
- Regular rate of 60 to 100 bpm, producing a normal rhythm

This physiologic pattern of heart rhythm produced by the SA node is considered normal and therefore called *normal sinus rhythm* (NSR).

Basically, the heart conduction system begins at the SA node and travels through atrial tissue to the atrioventricular (AV) node. Then it travels to the bundle of His, through the Purkinje fibers, and to the ventricular tissue.

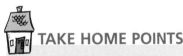

TAKE HOME POINTS

Although all cardiac cells have the ability to initiate a heartbeat, the SA node provides the best physiologic rate and rhythm to sustain adequate cardiac output. The SA node is therefore considered the *"Master Pacemaker."*

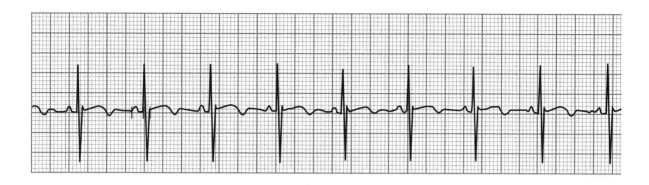

Any change or disturbance in the heart's conduction system (or from NSR) is called either an abnormal heart rhythm (cardiac dysrhythmia) or abnormal heart beat (cardiac ectopy).

Dysrhythmia

A *dysrhythmia* of the SA node primarily results from overactivity of either the sympathetic nervous system (SNS) or the parasympathetic nervous system (PNS). Damage to the SA node after a heart attack or administration of certain drugs (epinephrine) may also influence sinus node functioning.

Now let us examine various dysrhythmias of the SA node in detail to learn about their characteristics, causes, treatments, expected outcomes, and complications.

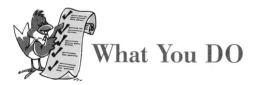

What You DO

- Assess the previous ECG strip for uniformity in the P wave, PR interval, and QRS complexes.
- Determine atrial and ventricular rates.
- Check the ECG strip for NSR.
- Assess patient health factors that may cause changes in the heart's conduction (e.g., heart disease, thyroid disease, noncompliance with medications, use of illicit drugs).

TAKE HOME POINTS

NSR is the rhythm with which all the dysrhythmias are compared.

Criteria for identifying normal sinus rhythm

- **P waves:** Rounded and consistent in shape; one in front of every QRS complex
- **Rate:** Between 60 and 100 bpm
- **Rhythm:** Regular
- **PR intervals:** 0.12 to 0.20 seconds
- **QRS complex:** 0.04 to 0.11 seconds

Sinus dysrhythmia occurs more commonly in children and adolescents. Bradycardia can occur postoperatively in children because of inflammation or permanent injury of the SA node. They are, however, often asymptomatic because they can increase their stroke volumes and maintain their cardiac outputs. Bradycardia, sinus arrest, or sinus block may occur in older adults, because long-term hypertension or atherosclerosis affects the blood supply to the SA node.

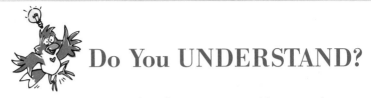

Do You UNDERSTAND?

DIRECTIONS: **Number the components of heart conduction in the correct sequence.**

1. _____ a. AV node
   _____ b. Atrial tissue
   _____ c. Purkinje fibers
   _____ d. SA node
   _____ e. Bundle of His
   _____ f. Ventricular tissue

DIRECTIONS: **Use different colored pens or pencils to trace the components of conduction.**

2. a. SA node to AV node
   b. AV node to Purkinje fibers
   c. Purkinje fibers to ventricular tissue

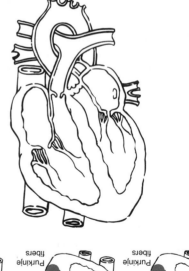

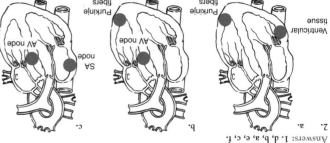

Answers: 1. d, b, a, e, c, f.
2. a.   b.   c.

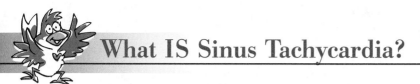

What IS Sinus Tachycardia?

A *sinus tachycardia* occurs when the SA node discharges impulses at a rate of 101 to 150 impulses per minute and when each impulse is conducted through the normal conduction pathway, followed by contraction. Sinus tachycardia therefore follows all the same criteria of the NSR, *except for the rate* of 101 to 150 bpm.

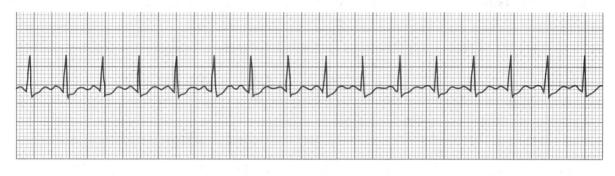

What You NEED TO KNOW

The patient may report a sensation of rapid heartbeat (palpitations), complain of dizziness, or become short of breath. These symptoms occur because the rapid rate decreases ventricular filling time, causing a decreased stroke volume and lower blood pressure, which results in a reduction of cardiac output and inadequate tissue perfusion. Thus less blood will be available to the body for its use.

Sinus tachycardia is most commonly caused by SNS stimulation (the fight-or-flight response). It may be triggered by fear, anxiety, exercise, excitement, pain, some drugs, fever, hypovolemic shock (from bleeding or dehydration), or heart failure.

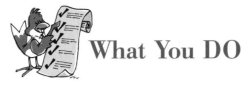

What You DO

In a person with cardiac disease, this rapid heart rate could trigger congestive heart failure or a heart attack if the cardiac muscle is unable to sustain the rapid rate.

If you suspect that a patient has sinus tachycardia, you should:

- Treat the underlying cause. For example, identify and control the source of fear, anxiety, or pain to reduce or eliminate the source of the fight-or-flight response; give antipyretics as prescribed to reduce fever; identify the drug source for which sympathetic stimulation is a known side effect (aminophylline). Sinus tachycardia is usually not treated with heart medication.
- Once the underlying cause is identified and removed, the heart rate will return to normal and, if experienced, palpitations, shortness of breath (dyspnea), and dizziness should subside. In the person with an otherwise normal heart, no complications should arise.
- Identify the rapid rate as sinus tachycardia and document it.
- Consider possible causes most applicable to the patient's unique situation; investigate further through collection of subjective and objective data, and share results with the primary care provider.
- Be alert for signs and symptoms heralding other problems, such as lack of perfusion caused by inadequate blood volume (hypovolemic shock) that results in restlessness; decreased blood pressure; pallor; thirst; weak pulse; or early heart failure, resulting in restlessness and the need to sit up to breathe easier (orthopnea) or to cough.

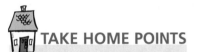

TAKE HOME POINTS

To determine whether a rhythm is sinus tachycardia, observe for the following:

- **Rate:** A rapid heart rate is between 101 and 150 bpm.
- **Rhythm:** Regular; P-to-P intervals and R-to-R intervals are equal.
- **P wave:** P wave should be uniform in shape and present before each QRS complex.
- **QRS:** QRS complexes should look alike and be 0.04 to 0.11 seconds apart.
- **PR interval:** The interval is between 0.12 and 0.20 seconds.

Sinus tachycardia results in decreased ventricular filling time.

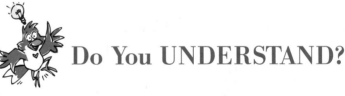

Do You UNDERSTAND?

DIRECTIONS: **Place a check by the characteristics, causes, or treatments that apply to sinus tachycardia.**

1. _____ a. Rate less than 60 bpm
   _____ b. Rate greater than 100 bpm
   _____ c. Results from SNS stimulation
   _____ d. Results from PNS stimulation
   _____ e. Results in irregularities in waveforms and rhythms
   _____ f. Waveforms and rhythms remain regular
   _____ g. Caused by fear, anxiety, pain
   _____ h. Caused by medications, such as sympathetic blockers
   _____ i. First, give medications to reduce the rate
   _____ j. Identify underlying cause and attempt to treat it

Answers: 1. b, c, f, g, j.

DIRECTIONS: Indicate in the spaces provided whether the following
statements related to sinus tachycardia are *true* or
false.

2. _____ Sinus tachycardia decreases the workload of the heart.

3. _____ The first intervention for sinus tachycardia is an appropriate
drug.

4. _____ Sinus tachycardia can be initiated by physical or emotional
causes.

5. _____ Sinus tachycardia can be a sign of more serious health problems, such as hemorrhage or heart failure.

DIRECTIONS: **The following strip is an example of sinus tachycardia.
Prove this by comparing it with the information in the
previous "Take Home Points" section. Place your findings on the spaces provided.**

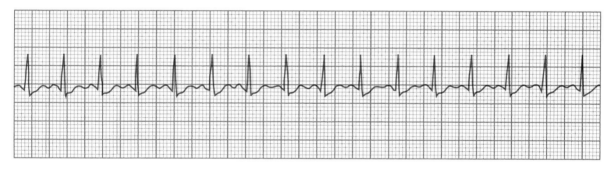

6. Rate: between 101 and 150 bpm _____

7. Rhythm regular _____

8. PR: P wave is uniform before each QRS with constant PR intervals

_____

9. QRS: uniform (0.04 to 0.11 seconds) _____

10. PR: measurable within normal limits _____

Answers: 2. false (tachycardia increases workload); 3. false (first attempt to identify the cause);
4. true; 5. true; 6. 120; 7. regular; 8. 0.16 seconds and constant; 9. 0.08 seconds; 10. 0.14 seconds.

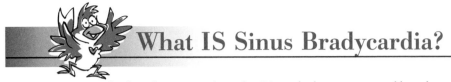

What IS Sinus Bradycardia?

A *sinus bradycardia* occurs when the SA node fires at a rate of less than 60 times per minute and each impulse is conducted through the normal conduction pathway, followed by contraction. Sinus bradycardia therefore follows all the same criteria of the NSR, except for the rate, which is less than 60 bpm.

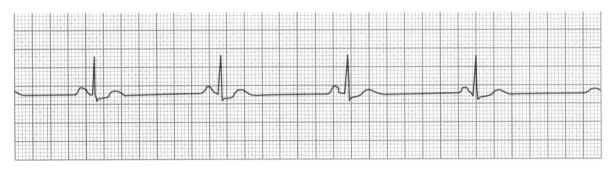

What You NEED TO KNOW

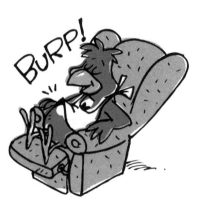

Parasympathetic stimulation or vagal dominance over the SA node most commonly causes sinus bradycardia. The PNS is responsible for the "rest and digest" response. During rest, the PNS through the vagus nerve causes the heart rate to slow down. Vagus nerve stimulation can occur when bearing down (Valsalva's maneuver), such as in defecation or as a result of coughing, vomiting, suctioning, gagging, or carotid sinus massage. An injured SA node, caused by infarction or ischemia (in or surrounding the node) may also cause sinus bradycardia. A sinus bradycardia is often found as a side effect in patient's receiving cardiac medications.

Sinus bradycardia can be "normal" in athletes who exercise regularly. The heart chambers increase their capacities as the heart muscle thickens (hypertrophies) to maintain an adequate cardiac output despite the lower heart rate.

However, a significant sinus bradycardia will cause cardiac output to be insufficient, and therefore cerebral and coronary blood flow will be compromised. This can result in decreased cerebral perfusion leading to fainting (Stokes-Adams syndrome). It can also lead to decreased coronary perfusion, leading to chest pain (angina).

Sinus bradycardia is treated only if the patient develops signs of decreased perfusion (e.g., hypotension, decreased level of consciousness, chest pain, shortness of breath). If the patient is stable, as in the case of the patient with an athletic heart, no treatment is necessary.

An antidysrhythmic medication (atropine) is the first-line drug for the treatment of a symptomatic bradycardia. Atropine is classified as a vagolytic, which blocks the influence of the vagus (tenth cranial) nerve (vagal effects) on the SA node, thereby allowing the heart rate to increase. If drug therapy fails, a temporary or permanent pacemaker may be necessary. (Pacemakers are also used in conjunction with drug therapy.) Drugs that stimulate the SNS (e.g., dopamine, epinephrine, isoproterenol) may also be used.

If sinus bradycardia occurs because of frequent constipation, stool softeners (docusate sodium) are prescribed to reduce straining during bowel movements. In addition, the health care provider may need to offer nutritional information about fiber and fluid intake.

If treatment is effective, the heart rate will increase to between 60 and 100 bpm, while retaining its NSR pattern.

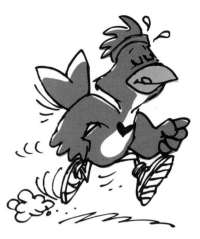

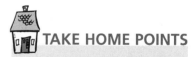 **Sinus bradycardia may indicate the onset of a sinus arrest; therefore its presence should always be investigated and a cause determined.**

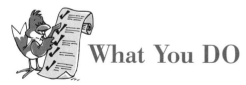 # What You DO

To evaluate patients with sinus dysrhythmia, you should do the following:
- Carefully evaluate an ECG strip to determine that the heart rhythm is otherwise normal (except for the slow rate); document it. Severe sinus bradycardia can cause decreased perfusion to vital tissues, leading to fainting (Stokes-Adams syndrome) or organ damage or both.
- If known bradycardic medications (digoxin) are given, record the rate frequently for comparative purposes.

TAKE HOME POINTS

To determine whether a rhythm is sinus bradycardia, you should observe for the following:
- **Rate:** Slow pulse rate with fewer than 60 bpm
- **Rhythm:** Regular (P-to-P intervals and R-to-R intervals are equal)
- **P wave:** Uniform in shape and present before each QRS complex
- **QRS:** Complexes look alike; 0.04 to 0.11 seconds apart
- **PR interval:** 0.12 to 0.20 seconds

- Observe the rhythm frequently for the presence of ectopic or abnormal beats that suggest that another pacemaker is firing. If ectopic or abnormal beats are present or if the patient is symptomatic (dizziness, fainting), contact the health care provider immediately.
- Counsel the patient about dietary interventions that will reduce constipation (e.g., drink eight 8-ounce glasses of water per day unless contraindicated, increase dietary fiber). These interventions may reduce straining for bowel movements that may stimulate the vagus nerve, reduce heart rate, and cause fainting, particularly in older adults.

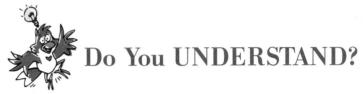

Do You UNDERSTAND?

DIRECTIONS: **Examine the following ECG strip. Specify the heart rate and, using the terms** *normal,* *abnormal,* *regular,* **and** *irregular,* **specify the ECG features of sinus bradycardia.**

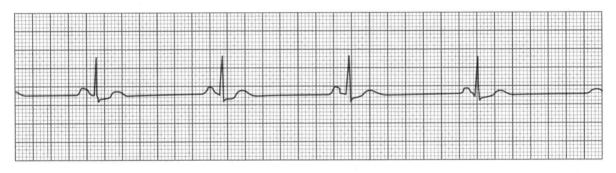

1. Rate: _____
2. P waves: _____
3. QRS: _____
4. Rhythm: _____
5. PR interval: _____

Answers: 1. 60; 2. normal; 3. normal; 4. regular; 5. 0.18.

DIRECTIONS: **List the four cases in which sinus bradycardia may**
occur.

6. _____

  _____

  _____

  _____

What IS Sinus Dysrhythmia?

A *sinus dysrhythmia* is a slight irregularity in rhythm associated with respiration. The SA node fires but not in a regular fashion. Heart rate speeds up with inspiration and slows down with expiration.

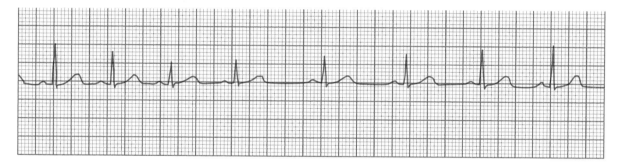

During inspiration the thoracic cavity enlarges, allowing more blood to enter the heart. The heart rate increases in an attempt to pump out this increased volume. During expiration, the thoracic cavity returns to normal and blood flow and heart rate slow.

Answers: 6. in the well-developed athlete; after certain medications (e.g., morphine, propranolol); in the patient with constipation; in a patient known to have SA node disease (the firing is unpredictable).

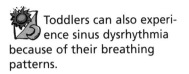 Toddlers can also experience sinus dysrhythmia because of their breathing patterns.

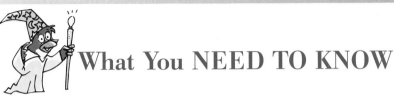

What You NEED TO KNOW

Sinus dysrhythmia is a normal variant and not considered a cardiac risk, because the rate and rhythm are sufficient to sustain the regular cardiac output and retain the SA node as the pacemaker. It is more typically seen in adolescents and women during periods of extreme stress or exercise.

By documenting the occurrence of sinus dysrhythmia, the baseline pattern for a patient is known and other dysrhythmias can be judged accordingly.

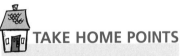
TAKE HOME POINTS

To determine whether a rhythm is a sinus dysrhythmia, you should observe for the following:

- **Rate:** Between 60 and 100 bpm
- **Rhythm:** Slightly irregular or phasic with respiration; the P-to-P intervals and R-to-R intervals may vary by 0.12 seconds or more (between the longest and shortest intervals)
- **P wave:** Uniform in shape and present before each QRS complex
- **QRS:** Complexes look alike; 0.04 to 0.11 seconds apart
- **PR interval:** 0.12 to 0.20 seconds

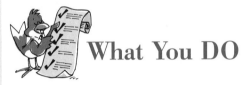

What You DO

If you suspect sinus dysrhythmia, you should do the following:

- Ask the patient to hold his or her breath, and document a rhythm strip showing this slight variation in rate. (The heart rate should increase during inspiration and decrease during expiration.)
- Document the ECG-obtained rhythm for future comparisons.
- If dysrhythmia occurs occasionally, no treatment is indicated.

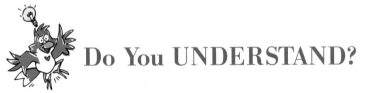

Do You UNDERSTAND?

DIRECTIONS: **Answer the following exercise.**

1. What do NSR, sinus tachycardia, and sinus bradycardia have in common that is not true of sinus dysrhythmia?

_____

_____

_____

Answer: 1. They have equal P-to-P and R-to-R intervals, whereas in sinus arrhythmia these intervals may vary 0.12 seconds or more.

DIRECTIONS: Review the following rhythm strips and place a check
mark on the lines below, indicating the characteristics
they reveal:

2.

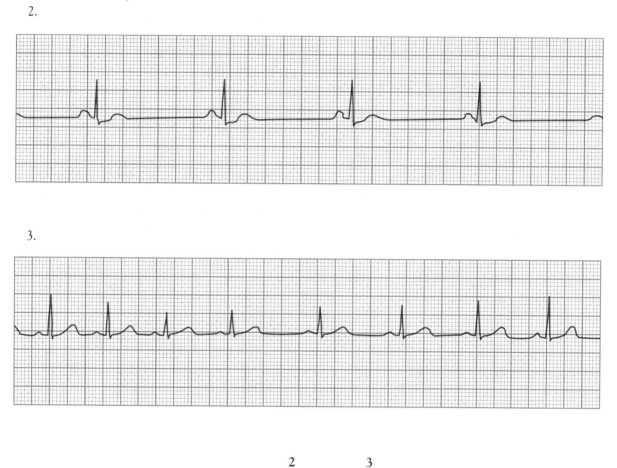

3.

	2		3	
	Yes	No	Yes	No
a. Rate: 60 to 100 bpm	___	___	___	___
b. Rhythm: Regular	___	___	___	___
c. P wave: Uniform	___	___	___	___
d. P wave: Before QRS	___	___	___	___
e. PR intervals: Within 0.12 to 0.20 sec	___	___	___	___

Answers: 2. a. no, b. yes, c. yes, d. yes, e. yes; 3. a. yes, b. no, c. yes, d. yes, e. yes.

4.

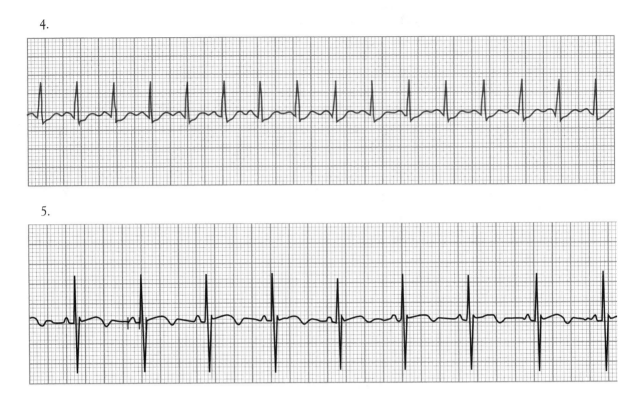

5.

	4		5	
	Yes	No	Yes	No
a. Rate: 60 to 100 bpm	__	__	__	__
b. Rhythm: Regular	__	__	__	__
c. P wave: Uniform	__	__	__	__
d. P wave: Before QRS	__	__	__	__
e. PR intervals: Within 0.12 to 0.20 sec	__	__	__	__

6. What two characteristics did the four strips have in common?

_____

_____

7. Assuming that the duration of the PR interval, QRS complex, and QT interval are within normal limits, name these four rhythms:

a. _____

b. _____

c. _____

d. _____

Answers: 4. a. no, b. yes, c. yes, d. yes, e. yes; 5. a. yes, b. yes, c. yes, d. yes, e. yes; 6. P waves are uniform and precede each QRS (this means that the SA node initiated each beat); 7. a. sinus bradycardia, b. sinus dysrhythmia, c. sinus tachycardia, d. NSR.

What IS Sinoatrial Arrest or Block?

An SA arrest or block occurs when one or more heart beats are dropped within an NSR sequence.

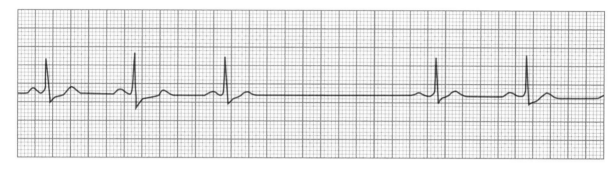

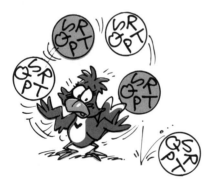

If the SA node fails to fire, it is called a *sinus arrest*. No impulse is generated; therefore there are no P, QRS, or T waves produced. This creates a pause, or flat line, in the ECG for an unpredictable length of time (until the failed SA node recovers and starts to work again). If the pause is too long, a backup pacemaker may generate an escape beat (i.e., a beat or impulse from another site, such as the AV node, atrium, or ventricle, that is generated to prevent compromise to the body from the slowed heart rate).

TAKE HOME POINTS

- Both sinus block and sinus arrest result in depolarization failure of atria and ventricles.
- The loss of the P, QRS, and T waveforms creates a pause or flat line on the ECG.
- Sinus blocks and arrests are treated in the same manner.

If the sinus node fires but the impulse is blocked from exiting the SA nodal tissue, it is termed a *sinus block*. The impulse is generated but not conducted. This may occur for one or more beats; however, the pause is of a predictable length. Because the SA node continue to fire at its regular rate, the pause lasts exactly the same time interval as the previously conducted beats. P waves can be plotted through the pause. It is this characteristic that differentiates the sinus block from the sinus arrest.

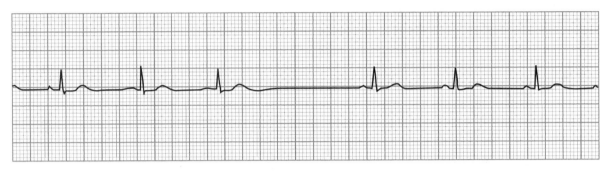

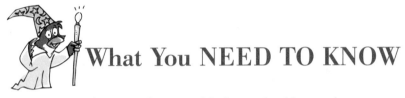

What You NEED TO KNOW

In patients with sinoatrial arrest or block, you should remember:

- Treatment is aimed at removing the underlying cause.
- Using calipers or some other reliable form of measurement, you should note whether the next regular beat after the pause maintains the usual P-to-P and R-to-R intervals (cycle length) in the NSR pattern.
- The usual cause of sinus dysrhythmia is excessive vagal stimulation of the SA node; this may be evident with overdoses of digitalis glycosides (digoxin), with an antidysrhythmic group IA medication (quinidine), or with SA node ischemia. (Review the section on *What IS Sinus Bradycardia* for discussion on vagal stimulation.)
- High serum potassium levels (i.e., greater than 5.0 mEq/L), stress, and severe vasoconstriction may also be responsible for sinus dysrhythmia.
- Tight neckwear, heavy lifting, and even hyperextension and rotation of the neck have been known to cause sinus arrest or block.

Heart rhythms need to be carefully monitored whenever new drug therapies are initiated, such as digitalis after a heart attack.

- If a drug effect is suggested, the drug should be discontinued promptly.
- Heart rhythms need to be carefully monitored whenever new drug therapies are initiated, such as digitalis after a heart attack. In this case, large loading doses of the medication are given and an overdose is possible as reflected in sinus arrest or block.
- The expected outcome of treatment is that the dropped beat or beats will cease or not result in any noticeable change in cardiac output or patient comfort.
- If sinoatrial arrest or block only occurs occasionally, no treatment is indicated.

If prolonged (lasting longer than 3 seconds) or frequent (generally more than 6 per minute, but check hospital policy), an antidysrhythmic (atropine) may be given to inhibit the vagal effect on the SA node. Pacemaker therapy may be needed if other therapy fails.

Heart monitor rate limitations are typically set at 60 for the lower limit and at 100 at the upper limit so that sudden rate changes will trigger the monitor's alarm to sound.

Missed beats may occur frequently or sequentially enough to cause the patient to experience the signs and symptoms of a significant bradycardia and its sequela. If this occurs, Atropine or a permanent pacemaker may be necessary.

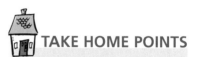

Never turn off heart monitor alarms, and be sure to check individual hospital policies for the acceptable monitor limits.

TAKE HOME POINTS

To determine whether a rhythm is SA arrest or block, you should observe the following:

- **Rate:** Usually normal but may be in bradycardic range
- **Rhythm:** Regular except for missing beats
- **P wave:** Present and uniform except during the missing beats
- **QRS:** No complex when beat is missed

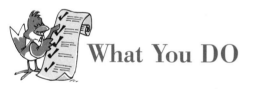

What You DO

When SA arrest or block is noted, you should:

- Document the rhythm.
- Modify such things as tight neckwear or head hyperextension or rotation to avoid sinus arrest instances (if these are the causes).
- Notify the health care provider if it occurs with any regularity or two consecutive beats are missed.
- Notify the health care provider if SA block occurs in relation to giving cardiac medications.

Do You UNDERSTAND?

DIRECTIONS: Indicate in the spaces provided whether the following statements related to sinus block or arrest are *true* or *false*. Suggest a correction for *false* statements.

1. _____ Rate is usually normal but frequently in a bradycardic range.

_____

_____

2. _____ P wave is present, but there is no QRS complex.

_____

_____

3. _____ There is no QRS complex for the missed beat.

_____

_____

DIRECTIONS: Fill in the blanks.

4. Sinus arrest or block can be caused by _____,

_____, or _____ of the SA node.

Answers: 1. true; 2. false (P wave is absent); 3. true; 4. excessive vagal stimulation, overdoses of drugs (digitalis, quinidine), or ischemia.

9 Atrial Dysrhythmias

The dominant pacemaker of the heart is the sinoatrial (SA) node, because it normally discharges impulses at a rate and rhythm most compatible with human needs. In the heart there are many groups of cells (sites) other than the SA node that have the ability to perform as a pacemaker. These sites, called automaticity foci, act as backup or escape pacemakers if the SA node were to fail. (See "Automaticity" in Chapter 1.)

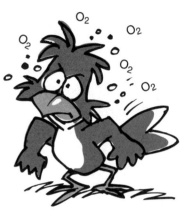

In atrial dysrhythmias, however, a pacemaker site (automaticity focus) in the atria takes over as pacemaker because of irritability, overriding the SA node, either intermittently or continuously. Because this focus (pacemaker) is abnormally firing, it is called an ectopic focus or an ectopic pacemaker. Ectopy or etopic means outside the normal place and is used to describe any beat originating outside the SA node because of irritability. It is also used to describe a focus that is not functioning as a backup pacemaker.

When a pacemaker other than the SA node fires, the waveforms produced will be different in shape (morphology) than the normal waves of SA node. If the ectopic focus is at the top of the atria, the P wave will be upright but shaped differently. If the ectopic focus is near or below the AV node, the P wave may be negative or absent.

Ectopic foci primarily result from irritability of atrial tissue that is most often caused by increased stimulation of the sympathetic nervous system (SNS) stimulation (adrenergic stimulation).

Conditions such as stress and hyperthyroidism increase SNS stimulation by initiating the fight-or-flight response, causing the release of natural adrenergic substances (e.g., epinephrine, norepinephrine). Caffeine, amphetamines, cocaine, alcohol, or other SNS stimulants are also frequently implicated. Lack of oxygen (hypoxia) to atrial tissue, electrolyte imbalances (especially hypokalemia), hypothermia, and digitalis toxicity have also been found to cause atrial irritability.

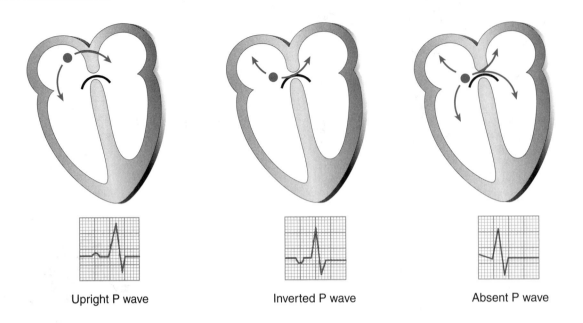

Upright P wave   Inverted P wave   Absent P wave

Once identified, atrial dysrhythmias are usually treated promptly to pre-serve cardiac function and control rate. Now let us discuss atrial dysrhythmias in detail to learn about their characteristics, causes, treatments, expected outcomes, and complications.

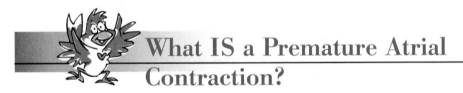

What IS a Premature Atrial Contraction?

A *premature atrial contraction* (PAC) occurs when an ectopic focus in the atria fires before the next SA node impulse is due. This premature impulse causes atrial depolarization, producing an abnormally shaped P wave on the electrocardiogram (ECG), followed by atrial contraction.

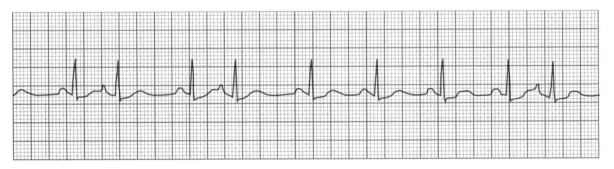

The impulse is then conducted to the atrioventricular (AV) node and then to the ventricles, followed by ventricular contraction. The contraction is called *premature* because it happens *before* the next expected heart beat initiated by the SA node. A slight *noncompensatory pause* occurs after the PAC. It may also occur before the next normal beat. This pause permits baroreceptors to adjust and the SA node to "reset," reestablishing its rhythm.

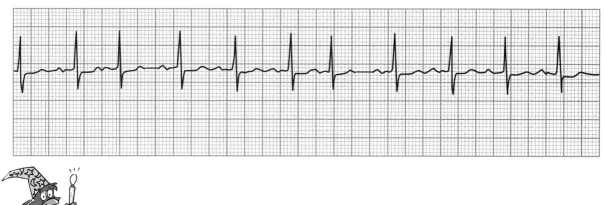

What You NEED TO KNOW

PACs are quite common. Most patients are generally unaware of the PAC and do not experience symptoms. Occasionally, the patient may complain of palpitations or skipped beats. The cause is irritability of the atrial tissue. This irritability may be caused by SNS stimulation, as in anxiety, hypoxia, or ischemia.

Although conducted PACs are most common, some can be nonconducted or aberrantly conducted, producing different waveforms. *Nonconducted PACs* are premature beats that result in only atrial depolarization. This occurs when the AV node from the previous beat does not have time to repolarize before the next impulse arrives. This means that the impulse arrives when the AV node is in the refractory period of repolarization, during which time it cannot be stimulated. Remember, cardiac cells must repolarize for the next depolarization to occur. In this case the premature impulse is not conducted to the ventricles; therefore neither a QRS complex nor the T wave is recorded on the ECG and no ventricular contraction occurs.

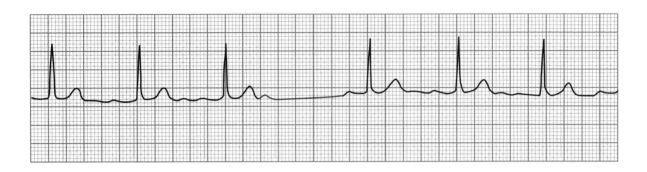

Aberrantly conducted PACs occur when only one of the ventricles from the previous beat has time to repolarize—the other ventricle does not. In this case, one ventricle depolarizes immediately in response to the premature impulse and the other ventricle's response is delayed until its repolarization is complete. Aberrantly conducted PACs produce a widened QRS complex on ECG because the ventricles repolarize separately.

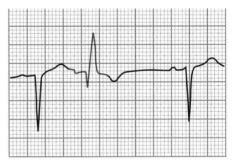

Watch for the development of more serious atrial dysrhythmias like atrial tachycardia, flutter, or fibrillation. These indicate more serious atrial irritability.

When a PAC occurs every other beat (after each normal beat), it is called *atrial bigeminy*. When a PAC occurs every third beat (after every two normal beats) it is called *atrial trigeminy*.

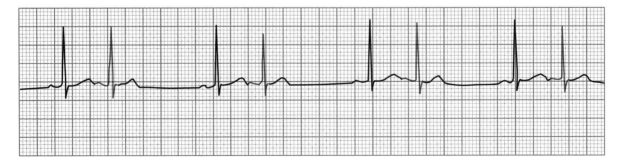

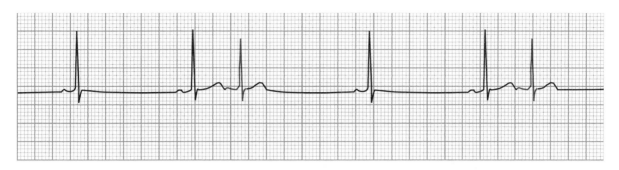

Drugs such as caffeine, nicotine, amphetamines, marijuana, catecholamines, and anesthetic agents or diseases (hyperthyroidism) may enhance PACs.

If PACs occur infrequently and do not increase to more than six per minute, treatment is usually unnecessary. However, if PACs occur with increased frequency, antidysrhythmic Group IA drugs (e.g., quinidine) may be given.

The expected outcome of treatment is that the PACs will cause no changes in cardiac output or patient comfort and will not increase to more than six per minute. Increased frequency of PACs may lead to more serious dysrhythmias, such as atrial fibrillation.

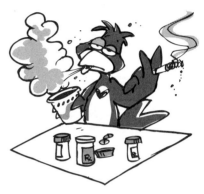

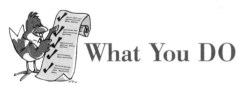

What You DO

- Identify and document the rhythm.
- Distinguish PACs from other forms of irregular rhythms; that is, look for P waves, check their shapes, and determine whether they are followed by QRS complexes and noncompensatory pauses.
- Document PACs via ECG strips.
- Count the number of PACs occurring per minute, and notify the health care provider if there are more than six per minute or a progressive increase from the occasional PAC. Treatment is usually not required unless the patient is symptomatic.
- Once identified, teach the patient about lifestyle changes that can and should be used, such as stress reduction, limiting caffeine and alcohol intake, adequate rest with exercise.

TAKE HOME POINTS

To determine whether a rhythm includes a PAC, you should observe for the following:

- **Rate:** Usually unaffected
- **Rhythm:** Normal except for the premature beat and noncompensatory pause
- **P wave:** Either abnormally shaped or inverted; will be different in shape (i.e., morphology) from sinus node P waves; may also be buried in T wave of the preceding beat
- **PR interval:** Can be shortened or prolonged but will be different from the PR intervals of SA node
- **QRS:** Usually unaffected (i.e., 0.04 to 0.11) and follows the P wave; may be aberrantly conducted (>.0.11) or nonconducted

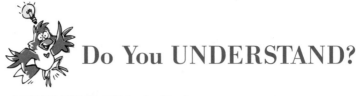

Do You UNDERSTAND?

DIRECTIONS: **Fill in the blanks.**

1. A beat is called _____ when some ectopic pacemaker fires ahead of the SA node.

2. A contraction called a PAC occurs when the _____ tissue is irritable.

3. In most instances, a _____ complex follows a P wave in the PAC.

DIRECTIONS: **Complete the following exercises.**

4. Which of the numbered complexes are PACs?

   _____

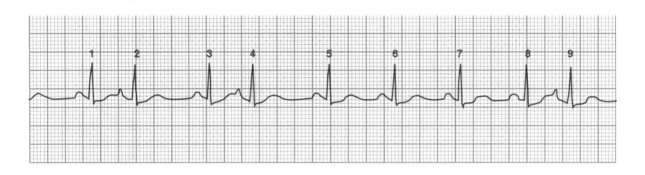

5. Compare the T waves preceding QRS complexes three and four. Why are they different?

   _____

   _____

DIRECTIONS: **Fill in the blanks.**

6. The larger space between complex four and five is called the

   _____

   and occurs because _____

   _____.

Answers: 1. premature; 2. atrial; 3. QRS; 4. 2, 4, 9; 5. The T wave for QRS complex four contains the P wave of the PAC and therefore looks larger or is shaped differently from the other T waves; 6. noncompensatory pause, the SA node is reset to reestablish the ventricular rate.

What IS a Wandering Atrial Pacemaker?

A wandering atrial pacemaker (WAP) occurs when the pacemaker site shifts or *wanders* from the SA node to different pacemaker sites in the atria and back again. The morphology of the P wave changes according to the pacemaker site where the impulse has originated. It is caused by increased parasympathetic (vagal) stimulation that causes the SA node to slow down, allowing another pacemaker to take over. There are usually at least three different foci firing in the atria, so there will be at least three different shapes of P waves on the ECG. The firing rate will vary slightly, but it usually remains between 60 and 100 beats per minute (bpm). If the rate increases to greater than 100 bpm, the dysrhythmia is called *multifocal atrial tachycardia* (MAT). MAT is seen in patients with chronic obstructive pulmonary disease (COPD) or serious heart disease. It is essentially the same as WAP; however, the rate is greater than 100 bpm.

WAP is not considered serious; it is found in the very young, frequently in athletes.

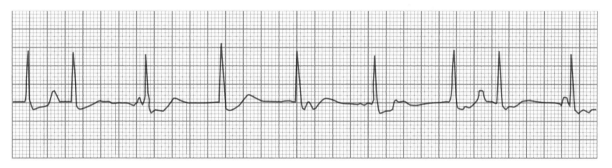

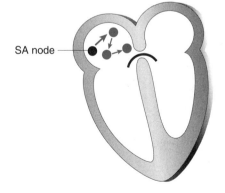

SA node

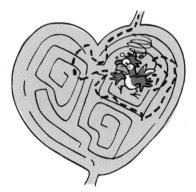

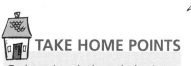

TAKE HOME POINTS

To determine whether a rhythm is a WAP, observe the following:

- **Rate:** Usually normal (between 60 and 100 bpm); however, it may slow if there is vagal dominance. If greater than 100 bpm, it is a MAT.
- **Rhythm:** Irregular; intervals increase and decrease as the pacemaker shifts between the SA node and other atrial pacemakers.
- **P wave:** Primary characteristic is the differences in the shape of the P waves that reflect different sites of origin.
- **PR interval:** Variable and may be difficult to measure at times.
- **QRS complexes:** Follows all P waves.
- **QT:** Measurable and within normal limits.
- **MAT:** May be called a supraventricular (i.e., above the ventricles) tachycardia, because the rhythm originates from pacemakers in the atria that are above the ventricles.

What You NEED TO KNOW

There is generally a dominance of vagal stimulation or a drug, such as a digitalis glycoside (e.g., digoxin), has been given to cause WAP. In most cases the patient experiences no symptoms and no treatment is necessary. However, an antidysrhythmic (e.g., atropine) may be prescribed if the rate slows too much (i.e., less than 60).

It is expected that the wandering pacemaker will not result in a permanent shift in the dominant pacemaker and the cardiac output will be sufficiently sustained. If MAT occurs, treatment is directed toward eliminating the irritability and slowing the ventricular rate.

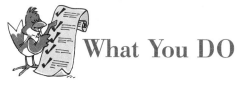

What You DO

- Document rhythm.
- If a drug (e.g., digitalis) is the suggested cause, you should withhold it and monitor the rhythm.

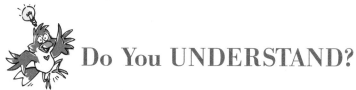

Do You UNDERSTAND?

DIRECTIONS: **Fill in the blanks.**

1. If the health care provider suspects a WAP, what component of waveform should be evaluated?

_____

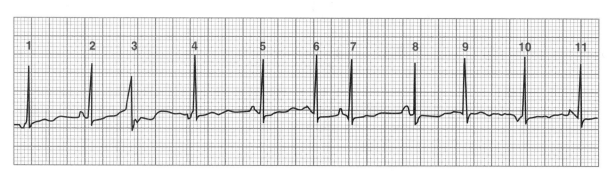

2. The QRS complexes are numbered 1 through 11.

   a. Which complexes are most likely to have been initiated by the atria above the AV node?

   _____

   b. Which complexes are most likely to have been initiated by the atria at or below the AV node?

   _____

   c. Which complexes are most likely to have been initiated by the ventricle?

   _____

What Is Paroxysmal Atrial Tachycardia?

Paroxysmal atrial tachycardia (PAT) is the *sudden* onset of a rapid, ectopic, atrial rhythm. A very irritable ectopic focus in the atria takes over as pacemaker, firing at rates of 150 to 250 bpm. Because the impulse is generated from a different pacemaker than the SA node, the P waves produced are different in shape from the SA node–generated P waves. The impulse travels down the normal conduction pathway, producing normal QRS and T waves followed by contraction. In contrast to sinus tachycardia, in which the SA node gradually increases rate in response to exercise or excitement, PAT begins and ends abruptly. One or more PACs usually precede PAT.

   In patients with no history of cardiac disease, PAT is caused by SNS stimulation as seen with emotional stress and anxiety, excessive caffeine, and alcohol and tobacco use. PAT may also be seen with myocardial infarction and states of hypoxia.

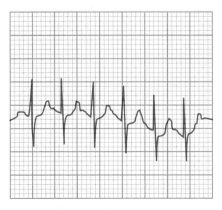

What You NEED TO KNOW

In patients with rapid rates (greater than 200 bpm), hypokalemia, or high blood levels of digitalis, conduction may be blocked, which is called *PAT with block*. PAT with block occurs when the AV node is not able to respond to the rapid number of impulses being sent from the ectopic atrial focus. When this happens, the AV node will selectively conduct only a certain number of impulses down to the ventricles; all others will be blocked. PAT with block is identified when there is a P wave with no QRS or T wave after it, because conduction to the ventricles was blocked at the AV node. Blocks may occur with every other P wave (i.e., a 2:1 ratio of P wave to QRS) or variably.

The young may tolerate PAT because of their normal fast heart rate and their ability to compensate; however, it may make older patients feel light headed and fatigued.

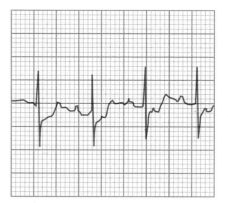

The rapid rate decreases ventricular filling time resulting in decreased cardiac output and increased myocardial oxygen consumption. Treatment goals for PAT are aimed at reducing the ventricular rate and decreasing the cause of irritability.

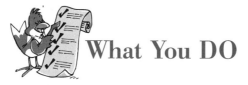

What You DO

- Identify and document the rhythm. Note whether PAT is occurring with block.
- Monitor for signs of hypoperfusion and myocardial ischemia, such as syncope, hypotension, and chest pain.

- For stable patients, maneuvers to stimulate the vagus nerve (vagal maneuvers) of the parasympathetic nervous system (PNS), such as bearing down or tightening abdominal muscles (Valsalva's maneuver) or carotid massage, are used. Vagal maneuvers suppress automaticity and decrease conduction through the AV node, resulting in a slower heart rate.
- If vagal maneuvers fail, drug therapy with an antidysrhythmic (adenosine) can be initiated. Adenosine is the drug of choice for PAT; however, digoxin may be used to slow the ventricular rate and convert the rhythm-to-sinus rhythm, but it must be used with caution because it may cause PAT with block. Beta blockers or calcium channel blockers may also be used to slow the ventricular rate and convert the rhythm. Quinidine may be added to prevent the recurrence of PAT.
- For the unstable patient (i.e., the patient exhibiting syncope, hypotension, or chest pain), cardioversion will be necessary.

Cardioversion is similar to defibrillation, but less wattage is used (i.e., 50 to 360 J), and it is not considered an emergency procedure. The patient is premedicated with a sedative (usually diazepam) but is conscious (the shock may be momentarily painful). The shock is synchronized with the R wave of the ECG pattern to avoid precipitating ventricular fibrillation.

> ⚠️ **Carotid massage is another form of vagal maneuver, but it should not be performed by nurses.**

> ⚠️ **A life-threatening dysrhythmia may occur if the shock is delivered at the peak or downward slope of the T wave. Cardioversion is used if the patient is unstable or if drug therapy failed.**

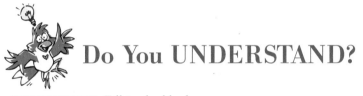

Do You UNDERSTAND?

DIRECTIONS: Fill in the blanks.

1. Paroxysmal means _____.
2. In PAT the atrial rate ranges from 150 to _____ bpm.
3. PAT with block occurs in patients with high blood levels of
   _____.
4. Aberrant conduction through the ventricles will produce a QRS complex that is _____.
5. PAT can be seen in patients with _____ cardiac history.

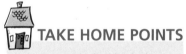

TAKE HOME POINTS

To determine whether the rhythm is PAT, you should observe for the following:

- **Rate:** *Atrial:* 150 to 250 bpm
  Ventricular: Varies, depending on whether there is any degree of AV block
- **Rhythm:** Regular, unless there is a variable block
- **P wave:** Different in morphology to the SA node–generated P wave (May be hidden in the T wave of the preceding beat.)
- **PR interval:** Difficult to measure
- **QRS:** Normal 0.04 to 0.11 (Conduction beyond the AV node is normal; QRS may be absent if the conduction is blocked, and it may be wide if aberrantly conducted.)

Answers: 1. sudden; 2. 250; 3. digitalis; 4. wide; 5. no.

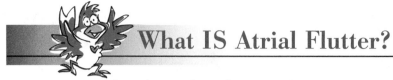

What IS Atrial Flutter?

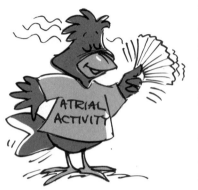

In *atrial flutter* the atria fire and contract 250 to 400 times per minute with a variable ventricular response of 60 to 150 bpm. This is the result of a single, extremely irritable atrial focus. Between ventricular contractions, the atrial activity is seen as *saw tooth* or flutter waves at a rate of 250 to 400 per minute. The AV node is not able to respond to the large number of impulses from the ectopic atrial focus; therefore it selectively conducts only a certain number of impulses down to the ventricles; all others will be blocked.

Depending on the number of saw tooth waves between ventricular contractions, the rhythm is referred to as atrial flutter with 2:1, 3:1, or 4:1 block. If the ventricular block rate or *conduction ratio* remains the same (fixed), the rhythm will then be regular. If the ventricular block rate or conduction ratio varies, the heart rate will be irregular.

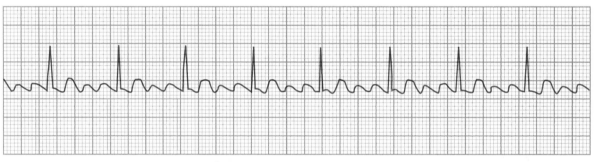

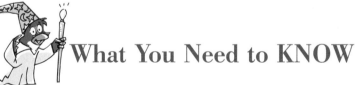

What You Need to KNOW

⚠ Rapid ventricular rates result in decreased ventricular filling time, which diminishes cardiac output and increases myocardial oxygen consumption. This decrease in cardiac output with increased workload can result in chest pain or left ventricular heart failure if the condition remains untreated.

The presence of atrial flutter can only be documented via ECG and not by listening to or counting the pulse (even an apical pulse). The rhythm of the pulse can be regular or irregular. If there is a high degree of block (e.g., an atrial rate of 300 with a 4:1 block that yields a ventricular rate of 75), the effect on the ventricle may be minimal.

Atrial flutter can occur alone, but it tends to occur in association with COPD, high blood pressure, heart muscle abnormalities, heart failure, coronary artery disease, and hyperthyroidism. Atrial flutter can be treated pharmacologically or by cardioversion (see the discussion of cardioversion earlier in the chapter).

Pharmacologic therapy involves the use of digitalis glycosides (e.g., digoxin), beta-adrenergic blockers (e.g., labetalol), or calcium channel blockers (e.g., diltiazem) to slow the ventricular response.

If the ventricular response is rapid, the patient may complain of palpitations, angina, or dizziness. With rapid ventricular rates, cardiac output is diminished and myocardial oxygen consumption is increased. A flutter with a ventricular rate greater than 100 bpm may be called a *supraventricular tachycardia*, because the rhythm originates from a pacemaker in the atrium that is above the ventricles.

Once the ventricular rate is under control, an antidysrhythmic (e.g., quinidine) is added to slow the atrial rate. If treatment is effective, it is expected that the patient will return to normal sinus rhythm (NSR) with sufficient cardiac output.

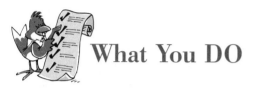

What You DO

- Identify the dysrhythmia, document via ECG strip, and notify the health care provider.
- Determine whether the patient is symptomatic (i.e., the patient has chest pain or dizziness) and assess vital signs.
- If drugs are used, monitor rhythm for effectiveness in converting or sustaining NSR.
- Assist with cardioversion as necessary.

Observe the cardiac monitor carefully. Depending on the degree of block, the high rate alarm may or may not sound.

Do You UNDERSTAND?

DIRECTIONS: **Complete the following exercises.**

1. Specify the ventricular rate for each of the following situations.
   a. Atrial rate of 300 with 3:1 block = _____
   b. Atrial rate of 240 with 4:1 block = _____
   c. Atrial rate of 250 with 2:1 block = _____
   d. Atrial rate of 150 with 1:1 block = _____

DIRECTIONS: **Atrial flutter can occur with varying degrees of ventricular block. Examine the following ECG strip and fill in the blanks.**

2. a. Identify the occurrences of 2:1 block

_____

b. Identify the occurrences of 3:1 block

_____

c. What is the ventricular rate for 1 minute?

_____

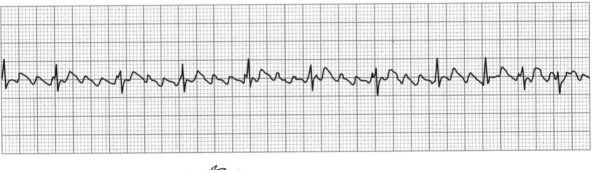

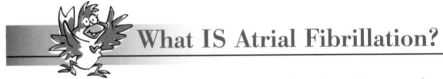

What IS Atrial Fibrillation?

In *atrial fibrillation*, multiple foci or pacemakers fire in the atria at the same time, resulting in chaotic impulse formation and producing impulses at a rate of 400 or more per minute. The atria are not able to recover before additional ectopic pacemakers fire again; thus both atria never fully depolarize. The result is quivering or fibrillation of the atria instead of contraction. Because the atria never fully depolarize, no discernable P waves are produced. Only a series of tiny erratic spikes are produced. Sometimes the spikes are so tiny that they appear to be a wavy baseline.

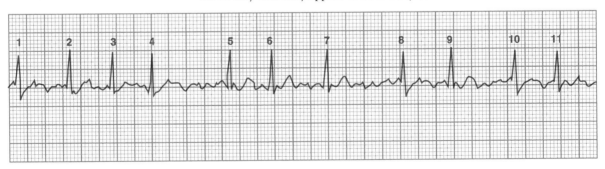

Answers: 2a. 2:1 after complexes 1 and 8; 2b. 3:1 after complexes 2, 3, 4, 5, 6, 7; 2c. rate = 90.

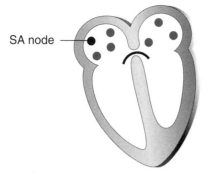

SA node

The AV node is not able to respond to the large number of impulses from the multiple ectopic foci; it conducts impulses in a totally unpredictable or erratic manner, resulting in an irregular ventricular response. The heart rhythm in atrial fibrillation is called *irregularly irregular*, which means that not only is the rhythm irregular, but it also has no predictable pattern. Occasionally the ventricles may respond aberrantly. (See the discussion of aberrantly conducted PAC on page 109.)

Treatment goals for atrial fibrillation are to eliminate or decrease the cause of the atrial irritability and to decrease the ventricular rate.

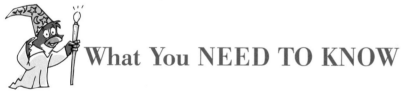

What You NEED TO KNOW

The patient is generally aware of atrial fibrillation when the heart rate is uncontrolled and palpitations may be experienced. In atrial fibrillation, the patient's pulse remains irregular whenever it is palpated, auscultated, or measured. Ventricular rates should be assessed using the *6-second method* (see Chapter 4). If the rate is less than 100 bpm, the rhythm is called atrial fibrillation with a controlled ventricular response or *controlled atrial fibrillation*.

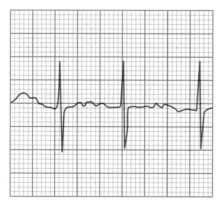

Atrial fibrillation with a rapid ventricular response is considered very serious.

If the rate is greater than 100 bpm, the rhythm is called atrial fibrillation with a rapid ventricular response or *uncontrolled atrial fibrillation.*

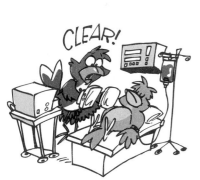

Normal atrial contraction provides 25% to 30% of cardiac output. Atrial contraction is clinically termed *atrial kick.* In atrial fibrillation, atrial contraction or atrial kick is lost. As such, the atria do not completely fill the ventricles with blood. This results in blood pooling in the atria and decreased cardiac output. The treatment for atrial fibrillation is dependent on the rate of ventricular response and the degree of circulatory insufficiency the patient experiences.

If the patient is unstable (i.e. experiencing chest pain or heart failure) or if drug therapy fails, cardioversion to restore the SA node as pacemaker may be attempted.

Drug therapy includes the following:

- Digitalis glycoside (digoxin). It increases the refractory or resting time of the AV node, resulting in a controlled ventricular response that the patient can then tolerate.
- Beta-adrenergic blockers (labetalol).
- Calcium channel blockers (diltiazem) slow the ventricular response. An antidysrhythmic (quinidine) may decrease atrial irritability.

Treatment for controlled atrial fibrillation of long-standing origin may be solely directed toward eliminating the cause of the atrial irritability. As a result of treatment, it is expected that the patient will sustain a controlled ventricular response with adequate evidence of sufficient overall circulation.

The major threat, particularly in the instance of a heart attack, is inadequacy of cardiac output. This output is decreased about 25% when atrial contraction is not contributing to ventricular filling.

The major threat, particularly in the instance of a heart attack, is inadequacy of cardiac output. This output is decreased about 25% when atrial contraction is not contributing to ventricular filling. Therefore heart failure and further ischemia are of grave concern.

Another major threat is the formation of small blood clots (mural thrombi) that accumulate on the walls of the atria as a result of pooling. In addition to the problem with pooling, the blood is also agitated by the fibrillation, which accelerates normal clotting. Thrombi can become emboli, resulting in pulmonary emboli, heart attack, or stroke depending on their final resting place. Anticoagulants (e.g., heparin sulfate, warfarin sodium) may be prescribed to reduce the threat of clot formation, particularly around heart valves in long-standing atrial fibrillation.

Atrial fibrillation with a rapid ventricular response may be called a supraventricular tachycardia, because the rhythm originates from pacemakers in the atria that are above the ventricles.

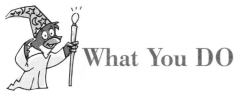

What You DO

- If atrial fibrillation develops suddenly, document it, notify the physician and prepare for the possibility of cardioversion, administration of intravenous digitalis glycoside (e.g., digoxin), or both.
- Whether acute or chronic, you should monitor the vital signs for evidence of sufficiency of cardiac output.
- Be alert for any signs that emboli have been released from atria walls, such as sudden onset of chest pain or shortness of breath (heart attack or pulmonary emboli), cool extremities (clots to lower arterial system), or change in level of consciousness or muscle movement (stroke).
- Monitor coagulation studies (Heparin = partial thromboplastin time [PTT]; warfarin sodium = prothrombin time [PT]) and the international normalized ratio (INR) if anticoagulants are prescribed. Patients with chronic atrial fibrillation who then become bedridden or sedentary for other health problems add the risk of emboli to their health concerns.
- If digitalis glycoside (e.g., digoxin) or antidysrhythmia group IA medication (e.g., quinidine) is given, monitor the patient for toxicity if the heart rate suddenly increases or decreases. This monitoring is done through blood level determinations.
- Monitor the radial or apical pulse. The palpated radial pulse may feel not only irregular in rhythm but also irregular in volume because irregular amounts of blood are being circulated.

! The formation of small blood clots that accumulate on the walls of the atria as a result of pooling is a major threat. In addition to this problem, the blood is also agitated by the fibrillation, which accelerates normal clotting. Thrombi can become emboli, resulting in pulmonary emboli, heart attack, or stroke depending on their final resting place. Anticoagulants may be prescribed.

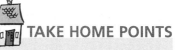

TAKE HOME POINTS

To determine whether a rhythm is atrial fibrillation, you should observe for the following:

- **Rate:** Varies according to ventricular response (<100 = controlled atrial fibrillation; >100 = uncontrolled atrial fibrillation; <100 increases stroke volume for each ventricular contraction, thus improves overall circulation with each heart beat)
- **Rhythm:** Irregularly irregular
- **P wave:** No true P waves (Varying F waves (from course to fine) may be seen
- **PR interval:** Not measurable
- **QRS:** Usually normal but may be aberrant

TAKE HOME POINTS

Generally, patients will know if their heart rate is irregular. Immediate concerns of the health care provider can be dispelled by asking this simple question, "Has anyone ever told you that your heart beat is irregular?"

Do You UNDERSTAND?

DIRECTIONS: **Complete the following exercises.**

1. Name three ways that atrial fibrillation differs from atrial flutter.

_____

_____

_____

Atrial flutter and fibrillation may occur more often in the older patient who has a history of hypertension, coronary artery disease, and myocardial infarctions. These health problems may damage the conduction system over time, and the arrhythmia may be treated as a chronic problem. Older patients should also be cautioned about sudden postural changes (e.g., quickly moving from a lying to a sitting or standing position). These sudden movements may result in fainting if atrial dysrhythmias have altered cerebral blood supply and perfusion.

2. In a patient in NSR, if there is electrical interference on the monitor or the patient is moving, the tracing between QRS complexes can be erratic or nondistinct. What could the health care provider do to test the difference between that interference situation and atrial fibrillation?

_____

_____

_____

_____

_____

Answers: 1. Atrial rate (400 bpm versus 250 to 400 bpm), degree of AV block (no set pattern versus 1:1, 2:1, 3:1, or 4:1), can be chronic and not treated versus an acute situation that requires cardioversion or drugs; **2.** The QRS complexes in atrial fibrillation will be irregularly irregular, although those in NSR will be equidistant. The ventricular rate will be relatively constant in NSR, although the rate in atrial fibrillation may vary.

10 Junctional Dysrhythmias

The atrioventricular (AV) node is an area of tissue located on the posterior floor of the right atrium. This tissue is a connector between the atrial and ventricular conduction pathways. The AV junctional tissue includes the AV node and the tissue immediately surrounding it.

Junctional rhythms, which are sometimes referred to as nodal rhythms, are the result of two primary causes: (1) failure of the sinoatrial (SA) node to generate an impulse and (2) increased automaticity of the junctional tissue. If the SA node fails to generate an impulse either because of a disease or suppression by drugs, it may cease to serve as the primary pacemaker of the heart, and the AV node will work as a compensatory pacemaker to generate an impulse. Normally when the AV junction acts as a compensatory pacemaker, it has the ability to generate impulses at a rate of 40 to 60 beats per minute (bpm). Rhythms also originate from the AV junctional tissue because of increased automaticity of this tissue resulting from electrolyte disturbances, ischemia, or toxic drug levels, particularly digitalis (see Chapter 19).

One of the primary effects of junctional rhythms is a decreased cardiac output resulting from ineffective depolarization of the atria and loss of atrial contraction (atrial kick).

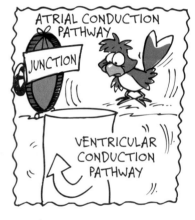

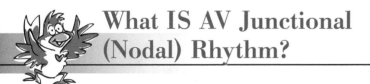

What IS AV Junctional (Nodal) Rhythm?

Because of the anatomic location of the junctional tissue between the atria and the ventricular conduction pathways, impulses that originate in this area may conduct several ways.

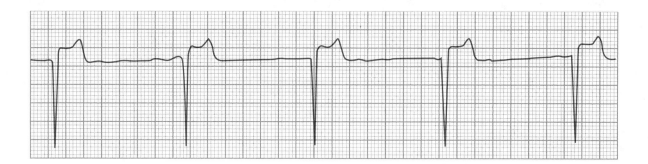

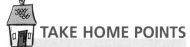

TAKE HOME POINTS

If a rhythm meets the criteria for being defined as junctional (i.e., no P wave, inverted P wave before or after the QRS, or a short PR interval with a normal QRS complex and a rate between 40 and 60 bpm), it is referred to as a junctional rhythm or a junctional escape rhythm.

Impulses may originate in the AV tissue and conduct down the bundle of His, right and left bundle branches, Purkinje fibers, and ventricular cells, resulting in no P wave and a normal width QRS complex (i.e., less than 0.12 seconds).

Impulses may originate in the AV tissue and conduct in a backward (retrograde) fashion through the atria, resulting in an inverted P wave in lead II, which normally has positive P waves. The inverted P wave may occur before the QRS, indicating retrograde atrial depolarization occurred before ventricular depolarization, or the inverted P wave may occur after the QRS, indicating the retrograde atrial depolarization occurred after the ventricular depolarization.

Impulses may originate in AV tissue, which results in an upright P wave occurring before the QRS; however, the PR interval is shorter than normal (less than 0.20 seconds).

The intrinsic rate for the AV node is between 40 and 60 bpm. If the SA node is damaged or diseased to the point where it will not fire or initiate conduction at a rate greater than the inherent rate of the AV node, the AV node simply takes over the conduction system at that point. If the SA node recovers, the AV node will relinquish its pacemaking activities.

Offending drugs, such as a digitalis glycoside (e.g., digoxin) or a Group IA antidysrhythmic (e.g., quinidine), should be withdrawn promptly. The slower heart rate makes the conduction system more vulnerable to other pacemakers in the cardiac muscle, such as irritable foci in the ventricles that can result in ventricular tachycardias.

What You NEED TO KNOW

Generally, there is no treatment for a junctional rhythm if the rate is sufficient for cardiac output. Transvenous pacing may be necessary for this purpose if it is anticipated that the SA node will not recover and perform its duties.

The patient may be given an antidysrhythmic drug (e.g., atropine) if the slower rate (bradycardia) results in chest pain, shortness of breath (dyspnea), or decreased level of consciousness.

Patients with AV junctional tissue disturbances should be observed closely for degeneration to more serious rhythms, such as heart blocks or ventricular escape rhythms. If the AV node fails as a pacemaker, the inherent rate of the ventricular pacemaker is fewer than 40 bpm.

If treatment is effective the patient will sustain sufficient cardiac output and, if possible, experience restoration of the SA node as the primary pacemaker.

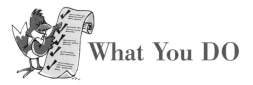

What You DO

When working with a patient with a junctional rhythm, you should:

- Identify the dysrhythmia as junctional (i.e., nodal) in origin as distinguished from sinus bradycardia or advanced heart block. Document it and notify the health care provider if onset is sudden.
- Observe the monitor carefully for any new ectopic activity, such as premature ventricular contractions (PVC).

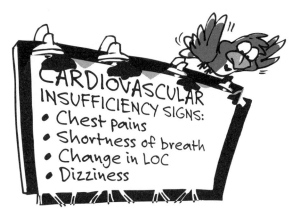

CARDIOVASCULAR INSUFFICIENCY SIGNS:
- Chest pains
- Shortness of breath
- Change in LOC
- Dizziness

- If the patient is taking a drug that is intended to lower heart rate, such as digitalis glycosides (digoxin), consult with the prescribing health care provider before continued drug administration.

 The sudden occurrence of a nodal rhythm when the SA node has previously initiated the cardiac cypate is generally a sign of downward deterioration or displacement of the conduction system. Heart blocks or ventricular dysrhythmias may quickly follow.

TAKE HOME POINTS

Particular attention must be paid to the ECG tracings when the patient has had a heart attack. Inflammation or swelling of heart tissue encasing the conduction system can cause temporary dysfunction, although permanent damage may be evident if oxygen is not restored in time.

TAKE HOME POINTS

To determine whether a rhythm is junctional (nodal), you should observe for the following:

- **Rate:** Between 40 and 60 bpm.
- **Rhythm:** Regular
- **PR interval:** Abnormal P waves; may be inverted or absent (Intervals may occur before, after, or within the QRS complex. PR interval <0.12 seconds if P wave is in the QRS; if not, it is not measurable.)
- **QRS:** Normal
- **QT:** Measurable, within normal limits

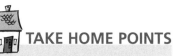 **If the rate is less than 50 per minute, be alert for changes that signal cardiovascular insufficiency (e.g., chest pain, shortness of breath, change in level of consciousness, dizziness).**

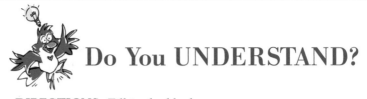

Do You UNDERSTAND?

DIRECTIONS: Fill in the blanks.

1. A rhythm is considered junctional when _____

_____

_____.

2. When the AV node works as a _____ to generate an impulse, it has the ability to generate impulses at a rate of _____ bpm.

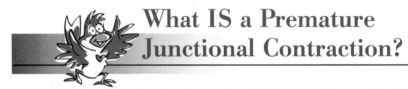

What IS a Premature Junctional Contraction?

A *premature junctional contraction* (PJC) occurs when an irritable area in the junctional tissue generates an impulse before the next SA node-initiated beat, resulting in an early beat. This beat has the features of a junctional beat and occurs sooner than the next normal beat would have occurred.

If the PJCs are infrequent, no treatment is necessary. Frequently occurring PJCs may mean increasing ischemia or irritability. If frequent PJCs result in runs of tachycardias, intravenous (IV) antidysrhythmics may be necessary. If treatment is effective, it is expected that the patient's rhythm will be restored to normal sinus rhythm (NSR) without premature beats or more serious dysrhythmias. Often, the patient is not aware of PJCs unless they occur frequently or cause palpitations.

PJC   PJC

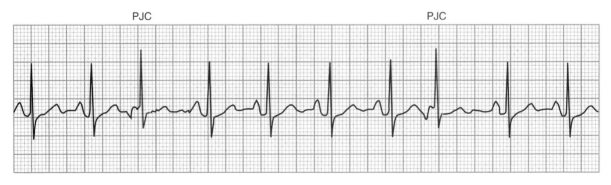

Answers: 1. no P wave, inverted P wave before or after the QRS, or a short PR interval with a normal QRS complex and a rate between 40 and 60 bpm; 2. compensatory pacemaker, 40 to 60 bpm.

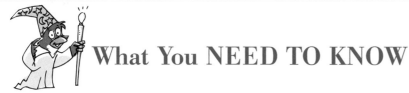

What You NEED TO KNOW

If the PJCs occur infrequently, no treatment is necessary. Frequently occurring PJCs may indicate increasing ischemia or irritability. If frequent PJCs result in runs of tachycardias, intravenous antidysrhythmic medications may be necessary. If treatment is effective, it is expected that the patient's rhythm will be restored to normal sinus rhythm (NSR) without premature beats or more serious dysrhythmias. Often the patient is not aware of a PJC unless they occur frequently or cause palpitations.

When working with a patient with PJC, you should:

- Identify the premature contraction as junctional in nature as distinguished from the more serious PVC. (Remember that PVCs have QRS complexes that are wider than normal [greater than 0.11 seconds].)
- Notify the health care provider if frequency increases or patient becomes symptomatic.
- Give drugs as prescribed and monitor effectiveness.

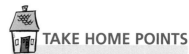

TAKE HOME POINTS

To determine whether a beat is a PJC, you should observe for the following:

- **Rate:** Underlying rhythm
- **Rhythm:** Irregular because of the early beat (PJC)
- **P wave** (associated with PJC): May be absent, inverted before or after the QRS complex; PR interval may be short (< 0.11 seconds)
- **QRS complex:** Within normal limits (< 0.11 seconds)

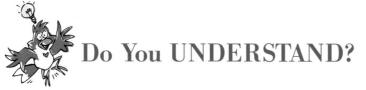

Do You UNDERSTAND?

DIRECTIONS: Cite the characteristics of a PJC.

1. Rate: _____
2. P wave: _____
3. QRS: _____
4. Rhythm: _____

DIRECTIONS: Unscramble the letters in the word jumble to fill in the blanks.

5. If PJCs increase in frequency, there is a possibility that _____ dysrhythmias may arise. (*cetrvniluar*)

6. A PJC causes the rhythm to be _____ because the beat occurs earlier than the next normal beat. (*guirrlear*)

Answers: 1. that of the underlying rhythm; **2.** not identified or occurs after or within QRS complexes; **3.** should be within normal limits (but may be widened if there is an intraventricular conduction delay); **4.** irregular, because of early beat PJC; **5.** ventricular; **6.** irregular.

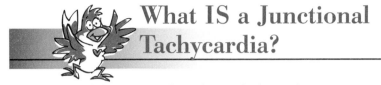

What IS a Junctional Tachycardia?

By definition, a tachycardia is a rhythm with a rate greater than 100 bpm. A *junctional tachycardia* is a rhythm that fits the criteria for being junctional (i.e., no P waves with a normal QRS complex, inverted P waves before or after the QRS complex in a lead where Ps are normally upright, or short PR intervals with a normal QRS complex) and has a rate greater than 100 bpm.

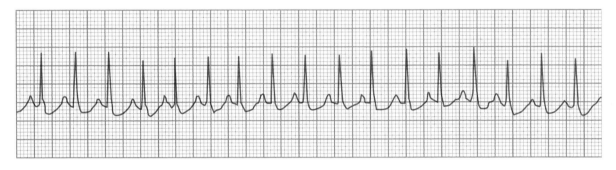

Often in tachycardias, rates get so fast that it becomes difficult to identify P waves and analyze the rhythm strip. Because the QRS is usually the most easily identified waveform in the patient with a cardiac history, the QRS complex width can be measured and determined to be normal or abnormal. If the QRS complex is within normal limits (i.e., less than 0.12 seconds), conduction through the ventricles has occurred normally and the rhythm has had to originate *above* the ventricles.

A rhythm can be classified as supraventricular when the exact origin of the rhythm is uncertain, when it is difficult to identify P waves, and the QRS complex is of normal width. A supraventricular tachycardia (SVT) originates above the ventricles and has a rate greater than 100 bpm. These rhythms often start suddenly and end abruptly; thus the term *paroxysmal*. Paroxysmal supraventricular tachycardia (PSVT) includes atrial tachycardias and junctional tachycardias; however, the term is used when the origin of the tachycardia cannot be specifically identified.

What You NEED TO KNOW

A reentry of the conduction stimulus through the AV node or through a concealed bypass tract is responsible for more than 90% of all PSVTs. Others may be caused by any catecholamine or neurotransmitter release (e.g., epinephrine) or sympathetic response provoked by such events as anxiety, caffeine intake, hypoglycemia, fear, stress, or digitalis toxicity.

If the cause of the catecholamine release can be determined and controlled, the PSVT may end as abruptly as it began without treatment. However, if PSVT is sustained, a health care provider will attempt to induce reflex vagal (tenth cranial nerve) stimulation by massaging the carotid sinuses in the neck, by eyeball pressure, or by inducing Valsalva's maneuver through bearing down as in defecation. If there is no response to these attempts to include reflex vagal stimulation, cardioversion may be used to restore normal sinus rhythm and rate. The antidysrhythmic adenosine may also be given by IV if carotid massage is unsuccessful.

If PSVT occurs repeatedly, drug intervention with digitalis glycosides (e.g., digoxin), Class IA antidysrhythmics (e.g., quinidine), or Group II antidysrhythmic (e.g., propranolol) may be required.

If the PSVT is caused by atrial fibrillation or atrial flutter, the patient should be evaluated for clinical stability, and the duration of the PSVT (either longer or shorter than 48 hours) should be determined. Unstable patients should be treated immediately with cardioversion. Antidysrhythmic agents are used to control the rate and convert the rhythm in stable patients. The American Heart Association's Advanced Cardiac Life Support (ACLS) guidelines promote anticoagulation for these patients.

> **If the duration of the atrial fibrillation is longer than 48 hours, caution should be used when using agents that convert the rhythm in patients not adequately anticoagulated because of the possibility of embolic problems.**

Most patients are immediately aware of PSVT because of the rapid heart action, a fluttering sensation in the chest, and lightheadedness. The dizziness occurs because of the reduced stroke volume (the result of shortened ventricular filling time) with the rapid rate and the small subsequent quantities of blood perfusing the cerebral tissue. Patients are very uncomfortable and will seek immediate relief.

If the tachycardia is sustained, cardiac output may drop. With a decrease in cardiac output and an increase in myocardial oxygen consumption, the patient may experience angina or myocardial ischemia.

PSVT has an abrupt onset and may also subside abruptly without treatment. The expected outcome is that the heart rate will return to NSR without complications.

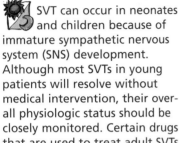 SVT can occur in neonates and children because of immature sympathetic nervous system (SNS) development. Although most SVTs in young patients will resolve without medical intervention, their overall physiologic status should be closely monitored. Certain drugs that are used to treat adult SVTs may be lethal in neonates and very young children.

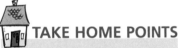

TAKE HOME POINTS

- The term PSVT is used when medical personnel are unable to specifically identify the origin of the tachycardia because of lack of clearly identifiable P waves.
- PSVT can be distinguished from ventricular tachycardia because the QRS complex is not wider than normal. (A normal QRS complex indicates the rhythm originated above the ventricles because ventricular conduction was normal.)

To determine whether a rhythm is PSVT, you should observe for the following:

- **Rate:** Usually greater than 150 bpm
- **P waves:** Difficult to identify; rates are fast and P waves may be hidden or buried in T waves (If the tachycardia is sudden in onset [i.e., paroxysmal], you can find P waves by looking at the very first beat in the run. There may be a visible P wave with the first beat.)
- **Rhythm:** Regular
- **PR interval:** P wave may be hidden in the QRS or sitting on top of T waves
- **QRS:** Usually normal width
- **QT:** Measurable, within normal limits

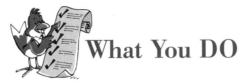

What You DO

When working with a patient with junctional tachycardia, you should:

- Remember that the onset of PSVT will trigger the high-rate alarm, at which time you should assess the patient, verify the rapid pulse rate, and document it.
- Notify the health care provider immediately and observe the patient for signs of chest pain or heart failure.
- Obtain the vital signs.
- If the patient remains stable, keep in mind that vagal maneuvers or IV drugs (e.g., adenosine) may be used to interrupt the rapid rhythm.
- If the patient becomes unstable (e.g., hypotensive) or displays symptoms, such as shortness of breath, chest pain, or changes in level of consciousness, immediate cardioversion is indicated.
- A brief trial of medications may be considered before cardioversion, and sedation should be considered for patients needing cardioversion.

Do You UNDERSTAND?

DIRECTIONS: Check which of the following description pertains to PSVT.

1. _____ a. Normal cardiac rate with early contractions, abnormal P-waves, and regular rhythm.

   _____ b. Cardiac rate of 100 to 140 bpm, regular P waves, compensatory pauses, and regular QRS complexes.

   _____ c. Rates greater than 150 bpm, abnormally shaped and sometimes buried P waves, narrow QRS complexes, and regular rhythm.

   _____ d. Rate greater than 250 bpm, irregular P waves, widened QRS complexes, irregular rhythm.

Answers: 1. c.

Mr. Jones

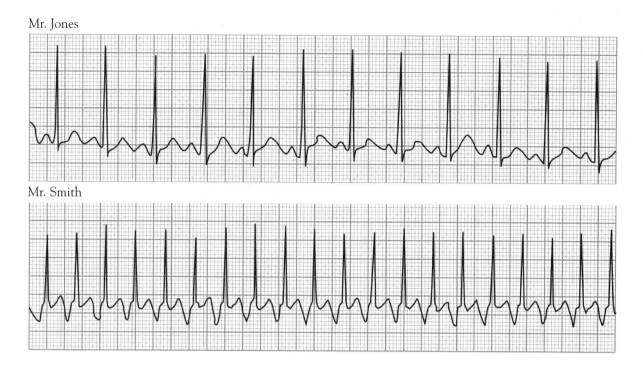

Mr. Smith

DIRECTIONS: Provide the answers to the following questions.

2. When taking vital signs, the nurse notes that Mr. Jones has an apical rate of 120 bpm and Mr. Smith has an apical rate of 200 bpm. Both men are experiencing some type of what?

   _____

3. The nurse then observes the telemetry monitors to view their cardiac rhythms. To determine the probable origin of their rhythms, what observation should the nurse make first?

   _____

   _____

4. Based on these observations, what are the two rhythms?

   Mr. Jones has _____.
   Mr. Smith has _____.

Answers: 2. tachycardia; 3. examine the strips for discernible P waves; 4. Mr. Jones has sinus tachy-cardia, Mr. Smith has PSVT. In both instances, comparison to previous ECGs and consideration of probable causes would be necessary for final identifications.

DIRECTIONS: **Complete the crossword puzzle.**

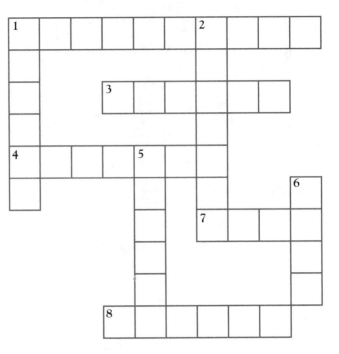

Across

1. In atrial dysrhythmias, stimulus is not from this node.
3. Increased heart rates require greater _____ consumption by the heart muscle.
4. Pressure may be applied to the globe of this organ by a physician to slow the heart rate.
7. 170 to 250 times per minute.
8. Any type can provoke general catecholamine release.

Down

1. Paroxysmal.
2. PSVT rhythm is _____.
5. Can refer to both onset and termination.
6. PSVT may be caused by this.

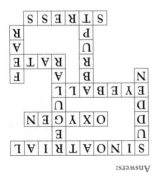

Answers:

What IS an Accelerated Junctional Rhythm?

An accelerated rhythm is one that is faster than the inherent rate for the pacemaker of origin but not fast enough to be a tachycardia. An *accelerated junctional rhythm* is a junctional rhythm with a rate between 60 and 100 bpm. (*Remember, the normal rate for a junctional rhythm is 40 to 60 bpm.*)

What You NEED TO KNOW

- If the SA node is suppressed and the AV junctional tissues act as the compensatory pacemaker, the inherent rate is 40 to 60 bpm.
- Junctional rhythms with rates in excess of 60 bpm are accelerated junctional rhythms and are commonly caused by digitalis toxicity.
- Treatment of accelerated junctional rhythms is aimed at identifying the cause. If the rate is fast enough to be considered an accelerated junctional rhythm, the rhythm may support cardiac output and would not be suppressed unless there is evidence that the SA node will assume the responsibility as primary pacemaker.

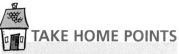 **Be prepared to assist with emergency interventions if patient becomes unstable.**

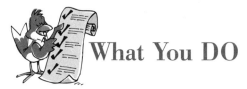

What You DO

When working with a patient with an accelerated junctional rhythm, you should:
- Monitor the heart rate.
- Assess the patient for adequacy of perfusion.
- Assess for the absence of chest pain and an adequate level of consciousness.
- Check the patient for shortness of breath.
- Determine that there is no hypotension.
- Monitor serum digoxin levels and levels of other antidysrhythmic drugs.

TAKE HOME POINTS

- **Rate:** Greater than 60 bpm but less than 100 bpm
- **Rhythm:** Regular
- **P waves:** Absent with a normal width QRS complex, inverted in lead II before or after a normal width QRS complex; PR interval may be shorter than normal (< 0.12 seconds)
- **QRS complex:** Should be normal (< 0.12 seconds); may be wider with an intraventricular-conduction delay

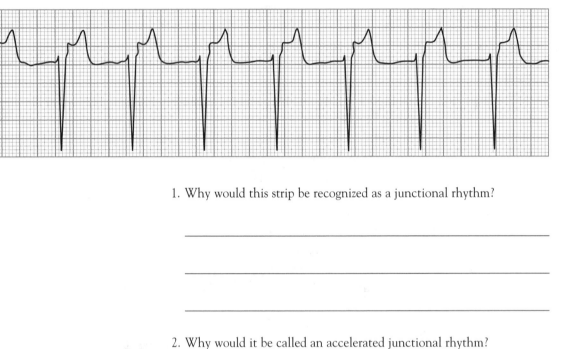

Do You UNDERSTAND?

DIRECTIONS: Examine the sample ECG strip and answer the
following questions.

1. Why would this strip be recognized as a junctional rhythm?

_____

_____

_____

2. Why would it be called an accelerated junctional rhythm?

_____

_____

3. Where are the P waves?

_____

_____

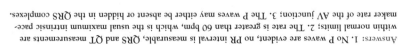

CHAPTER *11*
Premature Ventricular Contractions

What IS a Premature Ventricular Contraction?

A *premature ventricular contraction* (PVC) is an ectopic beat originating in either the left or the right ventricle. It comes early in the cardiac cycle, before the next expected beat (prematurely), and it occurs in the presence of an underlying rhythm, usually a sinus rhythm.

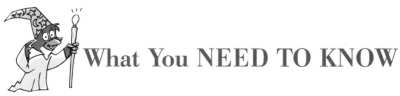

What You NEED TO KNOW

The PVC appears as a premature beat with a wide QRS and a long pause after it. This pause is called a compensatory pause; it occurs because the ventricle is in a refractory phase after the PVC, and it is unable to respond to any stimulus until the next beat.

The QRS is wide because conduction does not travel down the normal pathway. The PVC takes longer to get through the ventricular myocardium when it has to go from one cell to another, instead of staying "on track" in the cells of the conduction system.

PVCs hit prematurely—before the ventricle has had a chance to completely fill with blood. As a result, the ventricle must pump less than the normal amount of blood (stroke volume) with that beat. This is sometimes felt as a *skipped beat*. However, it is really an *extra beat* that is weakly perfused and an apical and radial pulse deficit may be noted. The beat after a PVC is often stronger because the ventricle has a chance to *overfill* after the compensatory pause.

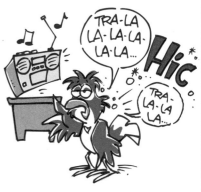

137

In a patient with acute heart disease or lung disease, PVCs can be a warning of increased ventricular irritability that could lead to ventricular tachycardia or ventricular fibrillation.

PVCs are caused by ventricular irritability that may be caused by sympathetic nervous system (SNS) stimulation by caffeine, drugs, or emotional stress. Also, changes in the excitability threshold of the ventricular tissue can be caused by digitalis toxicity, hypoxia, hypokalemia, or myocardial ischemia. Treating the underlying cause is the most important nursing intervention in breaking the rhythm.

Some PVCs are benign, and others are more dangerous. In general, PVCs are only dangerous if they lower the cardiac output or if they lead to more lethal rhythms.

TAKE HOME POINTS

 PVC may be a warning sign of a more serious ventricular dysrhythmia.

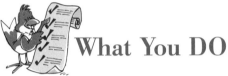 **What You DO**

Recognizing a PVC

The most distinguishing characteristic of the PVC is the wide and bizarre QRS that stands out in the midst of an otherwise mundane rhythm.

Characteristics

Rate: The underlying rate is normal, fast, or slow.
Rhythm: The underlying rhythm can be regular, but the PVC disrupts the regularity by firing prematurely.
P wave: None. May be directly before or after the PVC, yet unrelated to it.
QRS: Complex is wide (greater than 0.12 seconds), premature, bizarrely shaped.
ST segments and T waves: Both are sloped in opposite directions of the QRS.
Compensatory pause: Interval between the R waves of the normal beats surrounding the PVC (the one immediately before and after the PVC) should be equal to the intervals between three normal beats without a PVC.

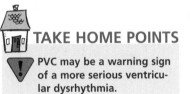 In the middle-aged adult, PVCs may need further follow-up for possible coronary artery disease. PVCs are more frequent in the older patient, especially those with long-standing pulmonary disease, cardiac disease, or both.

The QRS in the rhythm strip on the following page is 0.20 seconds in width. (Remember, the PVC ends at the J point.) In the PVCs in this strip, the ST segments are deep and the T waves are negative. Note that this is opposite to the upright T waves in the underlying rhythm.

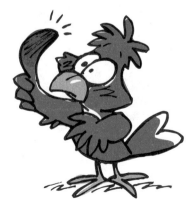 African-Americans have a higher incidence of coronary artery disease and sudden death; therefore they are more prone to PVCs.

A PVC sticks out like a sore thumb and is usually the easiest ectopic beat to recognize. If there is any doubt whether a beat is a PVC, it is sometimes helpful to look at it in a second lead.

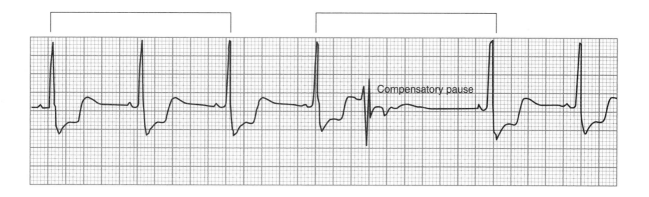

Compensatory pause

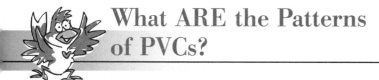

Do You UNDERSTAND?

DIRECTIONS: Circle all the possible characteristics of the PVC.

No P wave
P wave premature
PR greater than 0.20
No QRS
QRS wide

Compensatory pause
Flat ST segments
ST opposite of normal beats
T wave opposite of normal beats
QRS premature

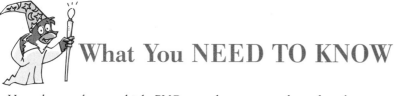

What ARE the Patterns of PVCs?

PVCs come in various forms depending on where they originate in the ventricle and the pattern in which they fire. Patterns of PVCs include unifocal, multifocal, couplets, bigeminy and trigeminy, and R-on-T phenomenon.

What You NEED TO KNOW

How do you know which PVCs are dangerous and need to be treated? Generally, occasional, unifocal, isolated PVCs are fairly common and harmless. All others should be closely evaluated because they may lead to more lethal dysrhythmias.

Answers: No P wave, QRS wide, Compensatory pause, QRS premature, ST opposite of normal beats, T wave opposite of normal beats.

Unifocal PVCs

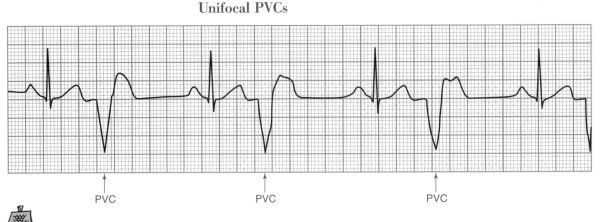

PVC   PVC   PVC

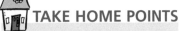

TAKE HOME POINTS

Uniform, isolated, infrequent PVCs are common and do not usually need to be treated. An increasing number of PVCs suggests increasing ventricular irritability and a need for closer attention.

Unifocal or uniform PVCs are premature ventricular beats that look the same (see above strip). They are caused by a single irritable focus in the ventricles. The PVC in the above strip is a simple, isolated, unifocal PVC.

Multifocal PVCs

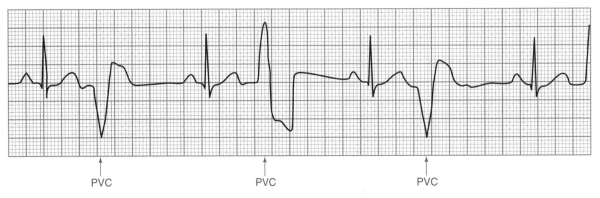

PVC   PVC   PVC

Multifocal PVCs indicate a more serious level of ventricular irritability than unifocal PVCs, and they are more likely to lead to more serious dysrhythmias.

Multifocal or multiform PVCs are those with different shapes—they do not all look alike because they are coming from different locations in the ventricles (see above strip). As you can imagine, multifocal PVCs indicate a more serious level of ventricular irritability than unifocal PVCs, and they are more likely to lead to more serious dysrhythmias (e.g., ventricular tachycardia or ventricular fibrillation).

Couplets

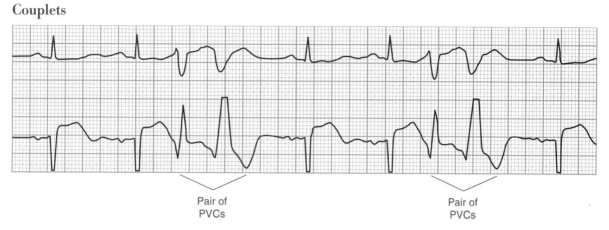

Pair of
PVCs

Pair of
PVCs

Couplets are paired PVCs or two PVCs in a row; they could be called "kissing cousins" (see above strip). They are usually unifocal (as in the following rhythm strip), but they may also be multifocal. Like multifocal PVCs, couplets are an indicator of advanced ventricular irritability.

Although couplets are not usually dangerous, they can suggest ventricular irritability and may eventually lead to ventricular tachycardia.

Ventricular Bigeminy and Trigeminy

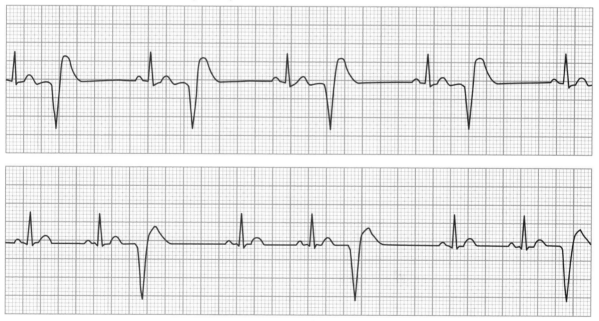

There are times when PVCs fall in a very regular and predictable pattern. (They have a "regular irregularity" about them.) Perhaps in palpating a patient's heartbeat, you have felt the pattern skip every other beat or skip a beat after two normal heartbeats. This pattern may be *ventricular bigeminy or ventricular trigeminy*.

Bigeminy occurs when every other beat is a PVC; in other words, there will be one normal beat and one PVC. Ventricular trigeminy is two normal beats and a PVC. Ventricular quadrigeminy is indicated by a PVC every fourth beat. These rhythms are not usually treated, but they are monitored closely.

R-on-T Phenomenon

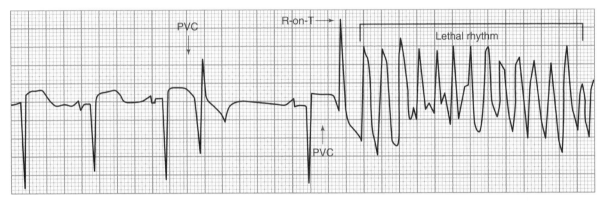

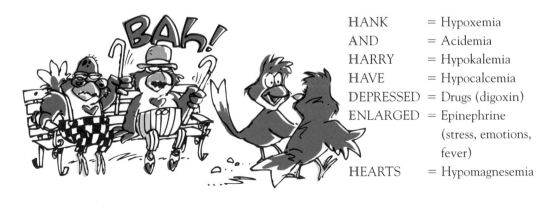

TAKE HOME POINTS

When PVCs become increasingly more frequent, multifocal, or coupled or when they fall close to the T wave, they should be taken more seriously as a sign that DANGEROUS, LIFE-THREATENING RHYTHMS, such as ventricular tachycardia and ventricular fibrillation, are possible. Therefore emergency drugs and a defibrillator should be immediately accessible.

The last type of PVC can be potentially dangerous to the patient. This danger does not have to do with the size or shape of the PVC; rather, it matters where it falls in the cardiac cycle. In R-on-T phenomenon, the R of the PVC is very close to or on the T wave (repolarization) of the previous beat. The last section of the T wave is considered the vulnerable (refractory) period of the heart's cycle. Any stimulus during this stage, when the electrolytes are trying to reorganize themselves, can set the heart into a run of life-threatening ventricular tachycardia.

Causes of PVCs (Acute)

Acute, treatable causes of PVCs include hypokalemia, hypoxemia, hypomagnesemia, hypocalcemia, acidemia, hypoxemia, stress, fever, and drugs. They may be remembered by the following pneumonic device:

HANK	= Hypoxemia
AND	= Acidemia
HARRY	= Hypokalemia
HAVE	= Hypocalcemia
DEPRESSED	= Drugs (digoxin)
ENLARGED	= Epinephrine (stress, emotions, fever)
HEARTS	= Hypomagnesemia

Chronic Causes of PVCs

There are certain chronic diseases of the heart in which PVCs are common and expected. Patients with these diseases may already be on oral antidysrhythmic drugs and are therefore not treated unless symptomatic. If treatment is indicated, lidocaine or amiodarone may be used.

CONDITION	CAUSE
Heart failure	Fluid build up in lungs; heart has to pump a heavier load and push against increased resistance
Myocarditis	Inflammation of the heart causes swelling and compression of chambers, thus decreasing filling
Arteriosclerotic heart disease	Hardening of cardiac arteries decreases blood supply to the heart
Ventricular aneurysm	Weakening of ventricular wall leads to weakening of the heart pump
Cardiomegaly	Enlarged heart will not contract as easily

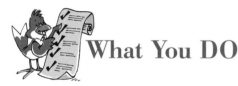 **What You DO**

When working with a patient with PVC, you should:

- Assess the patient for signs and symptoms of decreased cardiac output (e.g., hypotension, lightheadedness).
- PVCs are not always felt by the patient. The apical pulse may be greater than the radial because the PVCs may not perfuse as strongly or may be described as "skipped beats."
- Investigate the possibility of hypoxemia by monitoring pulse oximetry. Place patient on oxygen if necessary.
- Monitor serum electrolyte levels (potassium, magnesium, calcium), and supplement if necessary.
- Monitor digoxin level for toxicity and acid base level for acidosis.
- Assess sympathetic nervous system (SNS) causes (e.g., stress, pain, anger, fear, fever) and remove the cause if possible.
- Evaluate possibility of side effects from drugs such as caffeine, nicotine, aminophylline, dopamine, epinephrine.
- Assess chest pain to rule out acute coronary syndrome. (If indicated, obtain 12-lead ECG.)
- Document the presence and type of PVCs on a rhythm strip.
- Become familiar with your patient's history to know whether PVCs are commonly seen in the patient.

> **TAKE HOME POINTS**
>
> Some patients have chronic ventricular ectopy with which the health care provider may be perfectly comfortable and elect not to treat. Be sure to consult with the health care provider to determine whether the patient has preexisting ectopy, which does not need to be treated.

- Notify the health care provider if PVCs are a new finding.
- Lidocaine is the treatment of choice for PVCs if the patient is hemodynamically unstable or if there is a suggestion of acute coronary syndrome (see doses in table that follows). However, other drugs (e.g., nitrates, thrombolytic agents, platelet inhibitors, beta blockers, narcotics) may also be used.

TAKE HOME POINTS

⚠️ Advanced Cardiac Life Support (ACLS) protocols do not recommend that lidocaine (Xylocaine) be administered intravenous as routine treatment for PVCs. You should treat the cause of the ventricular irritability instead, and you should be more aggressive in PVCs associated with acute coronary syndrome. Prophylactic lidocaine is no longer recommended after myocardial infarction to prevent ventricular ectopy.

TREAT THE CAUSE BY:	WHY YOU DO:
O₂ by nasal cannula or mask	To counteract hypoxemia
Lidocaine 1.5 mg/kg IVP, followed by a continuous intravenous infusion at 2 to 4 mg/min (1 g/250 D5W)	To decrease ventricular irritability; may cause decreased contractility, seizures, neurologic problems, hypotension, and asystole
Procainamide 20 to 30 mg/min IVP, up to a total of 17 mg/kg; use only if lidocaine is ineffective	To decrease ventricular irritability but beware of hypotension, widened QRS

www.cpr-ecc.american-heart.org
www.usfca.edu/fac-staff/ritter/public_html/fourekg.htm
www.wices.com/icescardiac4.htm
www.ace.cr/newaclsguidelines.htm

Do You UNDERSTAND?

DIRECTIONS: Match the key words in Column A with the types of PVCs in Column B.

Column A

1. _____ All look the same
2. _____ One beat, one PVC
3. _____ All look different
4. _____ Four PVCs in a row
5. _____ Too close to the T wave
6. _____ Two beats, one PVC
7. _____ Low oxygen level
8. _____ Bronchodilating drug
9. _____ Rage
10. _____ pH of blood goes down
11. _____ Adrenaline
12. _____ May cause toxicity
13. _____ Elevated temperature
14. _____ Myocardial infarction
15. _____ Sympathetic stimulation

Column B

a. Couplets
b. Multifocal
c. Bigeminy
d. Unifocal
e. Ventricular tachycardia
f. R on T
g. Anger
h. Epinephrine
i. Stress
j. Digoxin
k. Hypoxemia
l. Acidemia
m. MI
n. Fever
o. Aminophylline

Answers: 1. d; 2. c; 3. b; 4. e; 5. f; 6. a; 7. k; 8. o; 9. g; 10. l; 11. h; 12. j; 13. n; 14. m; 15. i.

CHAPTER
12 Ventricular Tachycardia

What IS Ventricular Tachycardia?

Ventricular tachycardia (VT) is defined as three or more consecutive, premature ventricular contractions (PVCs) in a row and when the ventricular rate exceeds 100 beats per minute (bpm). It can occur without warning, or it may be preceded by some sign of ventricular irritability (e.g., PVCs).

What You NEED TO KNOW

VT can last from a short run of three PVCs (sometimes called a salvo) to a sustained, continuous rhythm. The two factors that determine how well the patient tolerates the rhythm are: (1) the ventricular rate, and (2) the presence or absence of myocardial dysfunction, such as ischemia or infarction.

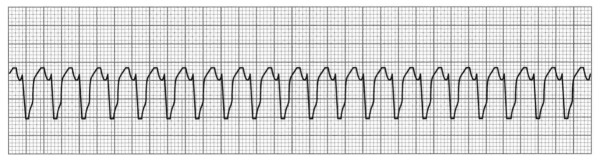

VT is one of the truly life-threatening heart rhythms.

The longer, more sustained and the faster the rhythm, the more dangerous it is. The more rapid the heart rate, the less time the ventricles have to fill with blood between beats, so the patient's cardiac output falls. A drop in cardiac output decreases blood supply to the vital organs.

The patient may or may not show a pulse, and the tachycardia rhythm can deteriorate into ventricular fibrillation (VF) and cardiac standstill. Therefore it must be recognized and treated immediately.

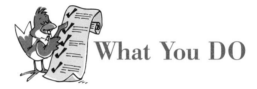 **What You DO**

The characteristics of VT are very striking. There are no normal-looking QRS complexes. The sole PVC that stood out in the midst of an otherwise mundane rhythm becomes a string of PVCs or a rhythm in itself.

To determine whether a rhythm is VT, you should observe for the following:
- **Rate:** Atrial rate is not usually countable. Ventricular rate is between 100 and 250 bpm.
- **Rhythm:** Ventricular rhythm is usually regular, but it can be slightly irregular.
- **P waves:** No consistent P waves associated with the QRS are evident, because the rhythm is not coming from the sinoatrial (SA) node. There may be *dissociated* P waves scattered throughout.
- **PR interval:** There are none.
- **QRS:** Complex is wide and bizarre shaped (>0.12 seconds).
- **QT:** QT intervals are within normal limits; T wave is in the opposite direction of the QRS.
- **Monomorphic VT:** Beats arise from the same focus.

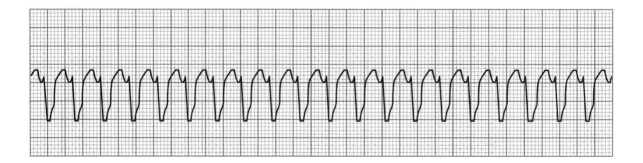

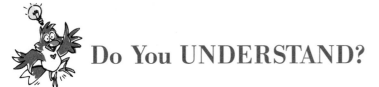

Do You UNDERSTAND?

DIRECTIONS: Place a check by the characteristics of VT.

1. _____ Atrial rate between 60 and 100 bpm
2. _____ Ventricular rate greater than 100 bpm
3. _____ PR interval within normal limits
4. _____ QRS between 0.06 and 0.10 seconds
5. _____ QRS greater than 0.12 seconds
6. _____ T wave opposite the normal QRS
7. _____ QT interval within normal limits
8. _____ QRS wide and bizarre

What You NEED TO KNOW

Proper treatment of monomorphic ventricular tachycardia is totally dependent upon the effect of the dysrhythmia on the patient. According to the American Heart Association's *Advanced Cardiac Life Support (ACLS)*, the following three possible scenarios and accompanying treatment algorithms may be present:

1. The patient has a pulse and is stable.
2. The patient has a pulse but is hemodynamically unstable.
3. The patient has no pulse.

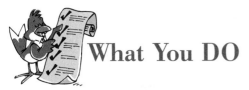

What You DO

The *universal algorithm* states that there are certain presumed actions taken in all patients being monitored. These include the initial assessment of the patient's airway, breathing, and circulation (ABCs), knowledge of a brief history of the patient's reason for being there, attachment to a cardiac monitor, the presence of a patent intravenous (IV) line, and supplemental oxygen (nasal cannula or nonrebreather mask), if needed.

Answers: 2, 5, 6, 7, 8.

When working with a patient with VT, you should remember:

- To document and quickly assess the rhythm strip. Because of the HR and QRS shape, the monitor will most likely alarm and run a strip automatically.
- To assess the patient's hemodynamic status (i.e., pulse, blood pressure, level of consciousness) and any other symptoms (e.g., chest pain, shortness of breath).
- To prepare to treat based on the patient's symptoms.

Treatment for Stable Ventricular Tachycardia

Short runs of VT are often well-tolerated and do not require treatment; however, they should be reported and documented. In some patients, even sustained VT may not cause symptoms—at least for short periods of time. The treatment of VT depends on how the rhythm affects the patient. If the patient has an adequate pulse and blood pressure and is alert and talking with no symptoms of chest pain, shortness of breath, or dizziness, he or she is considered stable.

Sustained VT in a stable patient is treated with medication. Lidocaine is the drug of choice; the patient is usually given 0.50 to 0.75 mg/kg in an IV bolus (pushed from the syringe straight into the IV line) or amiodarone 150 mg IV over 10 minutes as an alternative. If the VT resolves, an IV drip is hung (1 g in 250 cc) at 2 to 4 mg/min to maintain a therapeutic drug level.

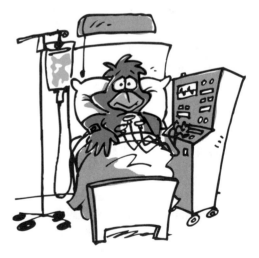

If the VT does not resolve, procainamide is the recommended second-line agent. Procainamide takes longer to work and has a greater potential for lowering blood pressure. Given as a steady infusion at 20 to 30 mg/min, the end points of procainamide administration are hypotension, a maximum of 17 mg/kg, greater than 50% widening of the QRS, or termination of the VT.

In other words, administration of procainamide will cause the VT rhythm to disappear or the patient's condition will worsen and threaten life. The drug should be administered until the patient either gets better or worse.

New ACLS guidelines incorporate amiodarone into the treatment protocol.

Treatment for Unstable Ventricular Tachycardia

If the patient has a pulse but is exhibiting chest pain, hypotension, decreased level of consciousness, shortness of breath or pulmonary edema, the VT is considered unstable. These symptoms are caused by decreased tissue perfusion secondary to decreased cardiac output, because the ventricles are beating so rapidly that there is not time for adequate ventricular filling between beats. The patient may appear pale, gray, or diaphoretic and may complain of nausea, dizziness, or palpitations.

The patient may lose consciousness because of lack of blood supply to the brain. As long as the pulse is still palpable, the following regimen of treatment is recommended:

- If the ventricular rate is greater than 150 bpm and the patient is unstable, the clinician should prepare for immediate cardioversion. Cardioversion is seldom needed for heart rates less than 150 bpm.
- To prepare for cardioversion, ensure that the patient has a patent IV.
- Connect the patient to a cardiac monitor, pulse oximetry, and a noninvasive blood pressure monitor.
- Ensure that a cardioverter/defibrillator, intubation equipment, and a suction device are available. If there is time and the patient is alert enough to feel the shock from the cardioversion, premedication should be administered with a sedative or analgesic.

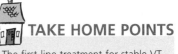

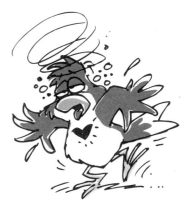

TAKE HOME POINTS

The first-line treatment for stable VT is to administer lidocaine or amiodarone.

Chest pain, hypotension, decreased level of consciousness, shortness of breath or pulmonary edema are symptoms of unstable VT.

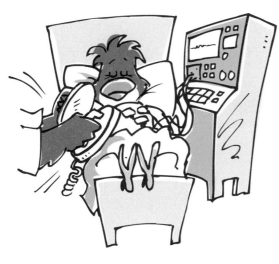

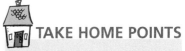

TAKE HOME POINTS

Usually, the faster the rate, the more decreased the cardiac output and the greater the symptoms.

Synchronized cardioversion is performed beginning at 100 joules. The shock is synchronized to avoid inadvertent striking of the shock on the T wave (relative refractory period), which could precipitate VF.

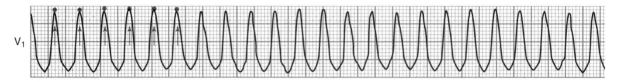

- If the first shock is unsuccessful, the cardioverter and defibrillator should be reset on "synchronize," and the charge should be increased to 200 joules. This process can continue with the next consecutive precordial shocks delivered at 300 joules and 360 joules, respectively.
- A brief trial of medications may be given as long as it does not cause a delay in preparing for cardioversion. Lidocaine 1.0 to 1.5 mg/kg IV push may be administered by one member of the resuscitation team while another prepares the defibrillator. Second-line drugs may include amiodarone, magnesium sulfate, procainamide, and propranolol.

Treatment for Pulseless Ventricular Tachycardia

If at any time during cardioversion, the patient becomes pulseless (either VT or VF), it is not necessary to synchronize the precordial shock; unsynchronized defibrillation is initiated. If the patient continues in sustained VT, this is likely to lead to VF and asystole.

The treatment of pulseless VT is exactly the same as that for VF (see Chapter 10).

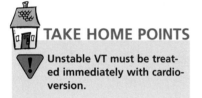

TAKE HOME POINTS

Unstable VT must be treated immediately with cardioversion.

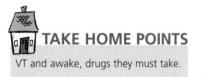

TAKE HOME POINTS

VT and awake, drugs they must take.

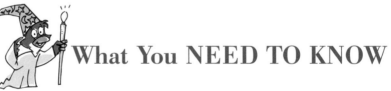

What You NEED TO KNOW

Polymorphic ventricular tachycardia (PMVT) is a variation of monomorphic VT in which there is more than one focus of irritability and therefore more than one shape of ventricular beat. The focus "wanders" and causes a "spindle-shaped" rhythm with some positive and negative complexes.

PMVT can result from the administration of drugs (e.g., amiodarone, procainamide, ibutilide), which prolongs the QT interval.

PMVT is also know as *torsades de pointes*, which is French for "twisting of the points.

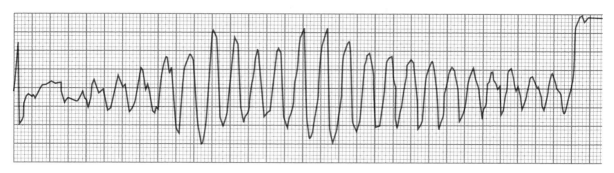

Treatment for Stable Polymorphic Ventricular Tachycardia

Treatment for stable PMVT with a prolonged QT interval is to correct abnormal electrolytes and administer magnesium or overdrive pacing. Alternatively, isoproterenol, phenytoin, or lidocaine can be administered to override the rate. Treatment for stable PMVT with normal QT intervals is to correct electrolyte imbalances, treat ischemia, and administer medications (e.g., beta blockers, lidocaine, amiodarone, procainamide). If these treatments fail, cardiac defibrillation at 200 joules (for adults) is started.

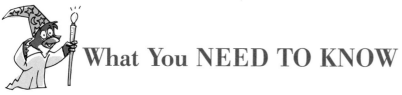

What You NEED TO KNOW

The same conditions that cause PVCs can cause VT. VT is primarily caused by ischemia of the heart. It occurs most frequently in patients with underlying heart disease.

Reperfusion after thrombolytic therapy is another cause of VT. In addition, illegal cardiac stimulants (cocaine) increase oxygen demand in the heart and can lead to VT (see Chapter 21). Certain medications, notoriously digoxin at toxic levels, can cause VT. An overdose of procainamide (Pronestyl) or quinidine (Cin-Quin) (the Class I-A antidysrhythmics) can lead to prolongation of the QT interval, which can precipitate polymorphic ventricular tachycardia.

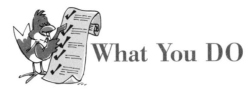

What You DO

VT is a wide QRS tachycardia; supraventricular tachycardia (SVT) is a narrow QRS tachycardia. It is imperative to differentiate whether the QRS is wide or narrow and therefore how the rhythm should be treated. However, there is a type of SVT that can have a wide QRS. This is called SVT with aberrant conduction. This rhythm originates above the ventricles and is treated differently than a rhythm coming from the ventricles themselves. Because a wide QRS tachycardia can be life threatening if it is ventricular, it is recommended that time must not be wasted trying to decipher whether the rhythm is ventricular or supraventricular. Because VT is more life threatening and less harm can be done by erroneously treating the rhythm as ventricular than by erroneously treating it as supraventricular, lidocaine is recommended as the first-line drug when there is any question about the origin of the rhythm.

Differentiating VT from SVT

Do not confuse SVT with VT. SVT is a narrow QRS tachycardia. If the QRS is wide, always consider it as ventricular and treat it as such.

It has been speculated that clinical criteria can help differentiate VT from SVT and that a patient with VT is more unstable than the patient with SVT. This premise has been disproved; some patients with VT may be more stable than those with SVT.

Electrocardiographic (ECG) criteria (especially QRS morphology in certain leads) are techniques that have been used to differentiate SVT with aberrant conduction from VT. This analysis may be a clinically useful strategy in the stable patient. However, if the patient with a wide QRS tachycardia is unstable, this time should be spent treating the patient, rather than analyzing the rhythm.

Severe hypotension may lead to the development of VF.

Administration of verapamil, one of the commonly used drugs for narrow QRS complex tachycardia, can be a lethal error in the treatment of VT, especially if the patient has atrial fibrillation with Wolff-Parkinson-White (WPW) syndrome. Severe hypotension may result, and it may lead to the development of VF.

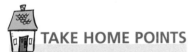

TAKE HOME POINTS

- It IS important to differentiate wide QRS tachycardia from narrow QRS tachycardia.
- In wide QRS tachycardia, it is NOT as important to differentiate VT from SVT. If there is any doubt as to whether a wide QRS tachycardia is ventricular or supraventricular, it should be treated as a VT until proven otherwise.

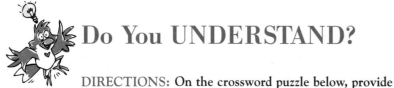

Do You UNDERSTAND?

DIRECTIONS: On the crossword puzzle below, provide the types of treatment for VT with its characteristics *(across)*. What is the treatment for unstable VT *(down)*?

1. Second-line drug for stable VT
2. First-line alternative to lidocaine in stable VT
3. A drug for stable VT
4. Can be lethal if given in VT
5. Treatment of choice for pulseless VT
6. Helps maintain O_2 saturation greater than 92%
7. What is the treatment of choice for unstable VT?

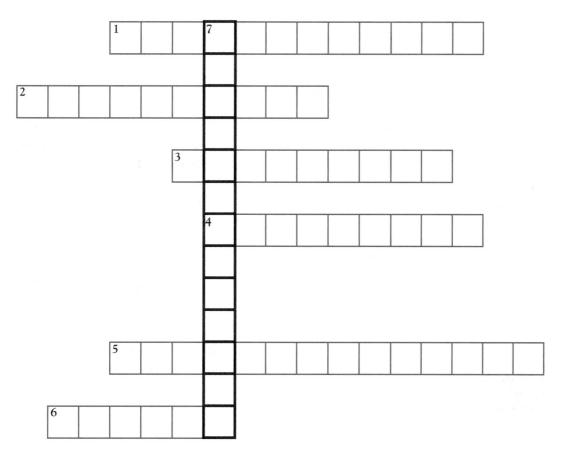

Answers: 1. procainamide; 2. amiodarone; 3. lidocaine; 4. verapamil; 5. defibrillation; 6. oxygen; 7. cardioversion.

13 Ventricular Fibrillation

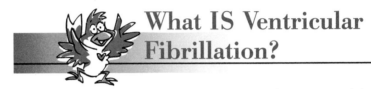

What IS Ventricular Fibrillation?

Ventricular fibrillation (VF) is the most frequent initial rhythm in sudden cardiac arrest. It is the single most important rhythm to recognize, because it is lethal and because it can be quickly reversed if a defibrillator is immediately available.

In ventricular fibrillation, multiple areas within the ventricles fire at random, asynchronous times, which produces a chaotic, completely disorganized rhythm, almost like a *seizure* of the heart. There is no effective contraction; the ventricles just quiver and twitch. As a result, there is no cardiac output, no pulse, and no blood pressure (BP). The patient is clinically dead and will become biologically dead unless the rhythm is swiftly terminated.

> ⚠ **In VF the patient is clinically dead and will become biologically dead unless the rhythm is swiftly terminated.**

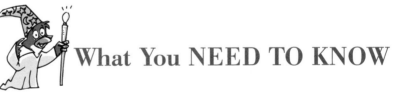

What You NEED TO KNOW

The electrical activity on the electrocardiographic (ECG) monitor is composed of coarse electrical waveforms that vary in size and shape. There are no measurable intervals; consequently the PR, QRS, and QT intervals are unobtainable. This rhythm is without pattern, and all of the normal characteristics are absent. VF rhythm may be mistaken for artifact at first glance.

> ⚠ **The VF rhythm has no countable atrial or ventricular rate.**

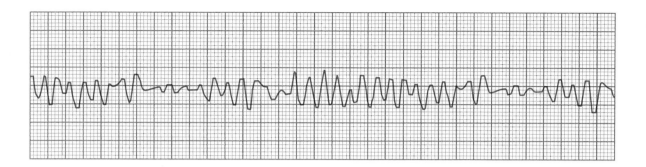

The VF rhythm on an ECG has these characteristics:

- *Rate:* Unobtainable and too fast to count (rapidly undulating waveforms)
- *Rhythm:* Grossly irregular
- *PR interval:* Unobtainable; absent P waves
- *QRS:* Unobtainable
- *QT:* Unobtainable

Patients that suddenly display VF rhythm often have significant heart disease. Many have had a history of myocardial infarction or heart failure. Patients at high risk for recurrent VF may have automatic implantable cardioverter defibrillators (AICDs) surgically implanted.

Causes of VF

Ventricular tachycardia (VT) may cause VF if not terminated. VF may also be caused by a strong stimulus at the wrong time in the vulnerable period of the cardiac cycle (i.e., middle of the T wave) or if the patient is inadvertently shocked at this point.

The same medications that cause premature ventricular contractions (PVCs) and VT can lead to VF. Hypoxia, acidosis, and electrolyte imbalances can also cause VF. In addition, VF can develop from electrical shock (e.g., shock from lightening strike or electrical devices).

Because VF must be treated immediately, automatic external defibrillators (AEDs) are now located in nonmedical, public places, such as airports and convention centers. They are intended for use by nonmedical personnel and require minimal training of updated basic life support certification (BLS) to use. AEDs sense the presence of VF and shock the patient only if indicated.

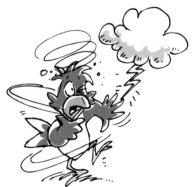

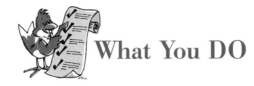

What You DO

When recognizing a VF pattern on a monitor, you should remember:

- To assess the patient's airway, breathing, and circulation (ABCs) quickly to rule out artifact (e.g., a loose electrode or movement) as the cause of the VF pattern. The patient with VF will be unresponsive, will have no pulse, and will not be breathing. There may also be accompanying seizures.
- To administer cardiopulmonary resuscitation (CPR) as soon as VF is confirmed, while waiting for the defibrillator. Electrical defibrillation is the definitive treatment for VF. A defibrillator must be obtained immediately.
- To never delay defibrillation while waiting for drugs, intravenous intubation, or CPR.
- To immediately defibrillate the patient. This step is the top priority.

⚠ Never delay defibrillation while waiting for drugs, intravenous intubation, or CPR.

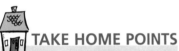

TAKE HOME POINTS

Defibrillation is an electrical charge applied externally to the heart from paddles or large electrode pads that are placed firmly on the chest. When discharged, a strong electrical shock fires all cardiac cells of the heart at one time. The cycle of the fibrillating heart must be broken so that the sinoatrial (SA) node may again take over as the normal pacemaker of the heart.

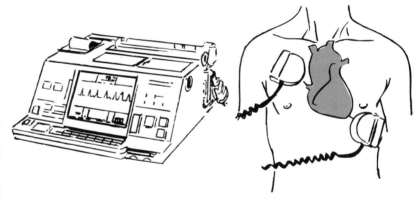

- Initially, a 200 joule (J) charge is delivered to the precordial surface. If this does not convert the rhythm, the charge is increased to 300 J. If this charge still does not convert the rhythm, the charge is increased to the maximal power of 360 J.
- If these first three shocks fail to convert the rhythm, CPR is begun and the patient is then intubated, an intravenous (IV) line is started, and a series of medications are given.

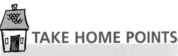

TAKE HOME POINTS

The **only** effective treatment for VF is defibrillation. The probability of successful defibrillation diminishes rapidly over time. VF tends to convert to asystole within a few minutes.

- Adrenaline (Epinephrine) is the first-line drug used to "jump start" the heart. Epinephrine is a pure catecholamine, which initiates the fight-or-flight response that causes the heart to beat faster and increases blood flow to the vital organs, especially to the brain. Epinephrine 1 mg IV push may be repeated every 3 to 5 minutes with no upper limit or maximal dosage.

- The American Heart Association's Advanced Cardiac Life Support (ACLS) guidelines suggest that vasopressin 40 units (U) IV push may be given as a single dose to replace epinephrine.

- Defibrillation at 360 J is then repeated. If VF is still present, a series of drugs should follow: amiodarone, then lidocaine, magnesium, and finally Pronestyl.

- The antidysrhythmic drugs are alternated with successive defibrillations at 360 J until the VF resolves. The goal is for the drug to help increase the fibrillation threshold, and the goal of the shock to break the cycle of the fibrillation. The sequence is drug-shock-drug-shock.

- If there is known preexisting metabolic acidosis, sodium bicarbonate may be administered to help the heart respond to the shock. In addition, as minutes go by and the heart becomes more hypoxic and acidotic, coarse VF will become finer and less likely to respond to defibrillation. Oxygen and epinephrine help make fine VF coarser so that it will more likely respond to the shock.

- If an IV cannot be obtained, emergency drugs may be administered with endotracheal (ET) intubation. **N**arcan, **A**tropine, **V**asopressin, **E**pinephrine, and **L**idocaine (NAVEL) can all be administered by this route. The dose is doubled and is squirted down the ET tube followed by 10 cc normal saline and dispersed by manually ventilating the patient. Lidocaine and epinephrine are indicated in VF. Vasopressin may be administered to replace epinephrine. Atropine is used in asystole and bradycardia, and Narcan is used to reverse narcotic overdose.

- Secondary assessment is now indicated for ABCs: **A**irway (ET tube, laryngeal mask airway, or Combi tube), **B**reathing (assess by an end carbon dioxide monitor), and **C**irculation (monitor pulse and secure IV access).

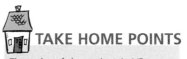

TAKE HOME POINTS

The order of drugs given in VF include:
- Epinephrine
- Amiodarone
- Lidocaine
- Magnesium
- Pronestyl

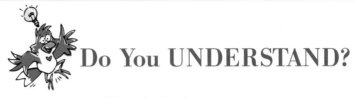

Do You UNDERSTAND?

DIRECTIONS: Fill in the blanks.

1. Name four characteristics of VF.

_____

_____

_____

_____

DIRECTIONS: Indicate in the spaces provided whether the following statements are *true* or *false*.

2. _____ Lightning can cause VF.

3. _____ The PR interval in VF is greater than 0.12 seconds.

4. _____ During VF the patient is biologically dead.

5. _____ Hypokalemia, hypomagnesemia, and hypocalcemia can cause VF.

6. _____ VF is associated with sudden cardiac death.

DIRECTIONS: Fill in the blanks.

7. Emergency stopping of all heart activity with an unsynchronized electrical charge is called _____.

8. The correct amount of joules for shocking VF are _____, _____, and _____,

9. _____

"jump starts" the heart when administered during VF.

Answers: 1. No P waves, no QRSs, no rates to count, no regular rhythm, chaotic and disorganized, no conduction intervals to count; 2. true; 3. false; 4. false; 5. true; 6. true; 7. defibrillation; 8. 200, 300, and 360; 9. Epinephrine.

10. The order of drugs administered during VF might include:

_____,

_____,

_____,

_____,

and _____.

11. _____ _____

is given in metabolic acidosis (either known preexisting or confirmed

by arterial blood gases).

14 Asystole or Ventricular Standstill

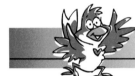

What IS Ventricular Standstill?

Ventricular standstill is the absence of any cardiac rhythm. It is also known as asystole. Asystole is more of a confirmation of death than a rhythm to be treated. Recovery is rare unless the cause of the asystole can be quickly reversed. As with ventricular fibrillation (VF), the patient has no cardiac output, no pulse, and no blood pressure. The pupils soon dilate and may become fixed because of the absence of blood supply to brain cells.

What You NEED TO KNOW

Patients rarely go directly from sinus rhythm to asystole. The heart will usually show some gradual slowing before stopping. There may be an occasional QRS complex or irregular P wave preceding ventricular standstill, which is known as an *agonal rhythm* (the rhythm of a dying heart). Within minutes, however, as hypoxia and acidosis are imminent, the rhythm will become a flat line.

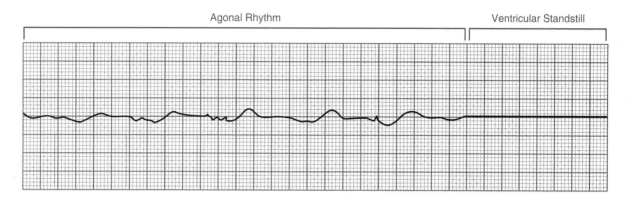

Agonal Rhythm   Ventricular Standstill

Because the prognosis in asystole is very poor, the goal is to prevent the conditions that can cause asystole in the first place. When asystole does occur, the goal is to identify quickly and treat the conditions that may have caused the asystole.

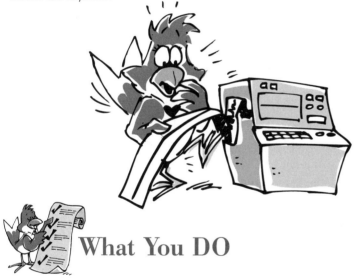

What You DO

When recognizing the pattern of asystole on the cardiac monitor, you should remember the following:

- Identify ventricular standstill:
  Rate: None (perhaps some P waves)
  Rhythm: None
  P waves: None on a consistent basis
  PR: None
  QRS: None
  QT: None
- Confirm asystole in more than one lead before treatment.

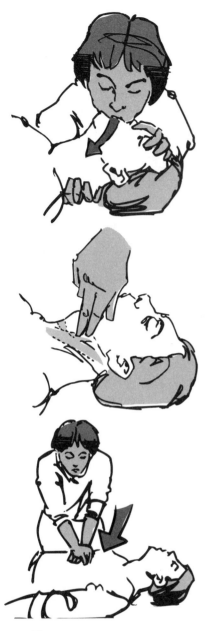

- What appears like asystole could be fine VF that may have a chance of converting with defibrillation. A fine VF pattern continues to have some irregular twitching or deflections on the electrocardiographic (ECG) strip. In contrast, asystole is a flat baseline on the monitor, regardless of the lead.
- A straight line may also appear if there is a technical problem with the equipment. Check to see that the leads are securely attached and that the correct lead is selected on the monitor.
- Once asystole is confirmed, cardiopulmonary resuscitation (CPR) is initiated immediately. Endotracheal (ET) intubation is performed as soon as possible and intravenous (IV) access is established (if not already present).
- The causes of asystole are assessed. The only hope of recovery in asystole is to reverse the causes. They can be remembered by the following acronym: **Hubert H. Hoover HAD asystole.**

Hubert	Hypoxia
H	Hyperkalemia
Hoover	Hypokalemia
H	Hypothermia
A	Acidosis
D	Drug overdose

- A transcutaneous pacer may be applied to the precordium to provide an artificial pacing stimulus. To have any chance of capturing the myocarduim, pacing must be performed early and accompanied by appropriate drug administration.
- Epinephrine 1 mg rapid IV push is the first line drug of choice in asystole. Its action is to "jump-start" the heart and preferentially route blood to the vital organs. It may be repeated every 3 to 5 minutes.
- Atropine 1 mg IV push is the other drug used in asystole. It blocks vagal stimulation so that the sympathetic nervous system can take over and the HR can increase, once the epinephrine gets it started. Atropine may be administered every 3 to 5 minutes up to a total of 0.04 mg/kg.
- If all efforts to resuscitate have failed, consider termination of efforts.

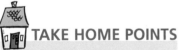

TAKE HOME POINTS

Compression rate for CPR is 100 compressions per minute for adults, children, and infants, and 120 per minute for neonates.

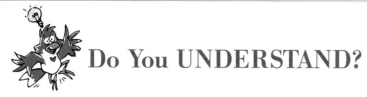

Do You UNDERSTAND?

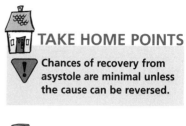

TAKE HOME POINTS

Chances of recovery from asystole are minimal unless the cause can be reversed.

DIRECTIONS: **Place a checkmark by the treatment for ventricular standstill.**

1. _____ Atropine
2. _____ Epinephrine
3. _____ Defibrillation
4. _____ Cardioversion
5. _____ CPR
6. _____ Pacemaker
7. _____ Lidocaine
8. _____ Adenosine

 www.circulationaha.org

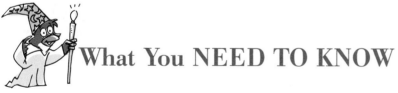

What IS Pulseless Electrical Activity

Pulseless electrical activity (PEA) is a mechanism in which there is electrical activity observed on the heart monitor, but there is no pulse in the patient. It *appears* that the patient has a pulse, but there is none. What makes the rhythm but no pulse? It is therefore treated much like asystole, except a pacemaker is not indicated since the electrical stimulation of the heart is already present.

What You NEED TO KNOW

Recognition

The rhythm of PEA cannot be recognized by specific waveform criteria because the electrocardiographic (ECG) pattern can appear as any number of rhythms. The following are a few examples of how PEA may appear. What makes it PEA is that there is no pulse associated with the rhythm.

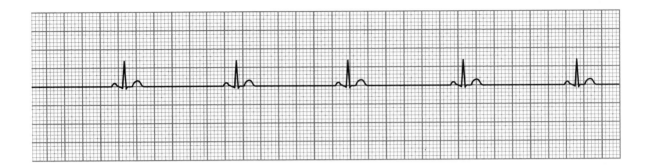

The above strip *appears* to be sinus bradycardia, but if there is no pulse, it is PEA.

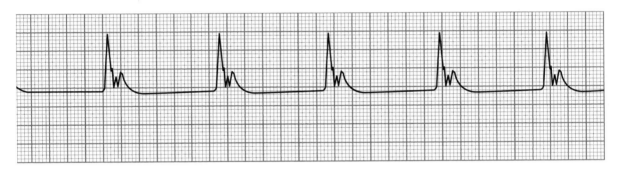

The above strip *appears* to be idioventricular rhythm, but if there is no pulse, it is PEA.

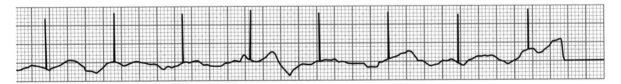

The strip above *appears* to be a paced rhythm, but there is no capture of the myocardium and therefore no pulse, so it is also PEA.

PEA can appear like any rhythm. So do not be fooled by the monitor—ALWAYS CHECK THE PATIENT. The key to recognition is that it is pulseless. Does this mean that you have to insert an arterial line in every patient to know whether his or her rhythm is a true rhythm or PEA? No. PEA is usually discovered in a cardiac arrest situation. However, knowing your patient's diagnosis will help ensure the timely treatment of PEA, once discovered.

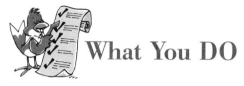

What You DO

- Check ABCs.
- Initiate CPR.
- Obtain an airway.
- Administer epinephrine to "jump-start" the heart.

If the heart rate on the monitor is less than 60 beats per minute (bpm), atropine may also be given. As in asystole, very little hope of recovery exists unless the cause is reversed. The causes of PEA and their possible treatments are listed in the following table.

PEA: Causes and Possible Treatments

CAUSE	TREATMENT
Hypoxia	Administer 100% oxygen and fluids.
Hypovolemia	Administer 100% oxygen and fluids.
Acidosis	Hyperventilate and administer sodium bicarbonate.
Potassium (too high or low)	Administer potassium, insulin, and sodium to drive potassium back into cell and calcium gluconate to counteract negative inotropic effects on the myocardium.
Drug toxicity	Administer specific antidote.
Tension pneumothorax	Initiate chest decompression with a needle or chest tube.
Tamponade (cardiac)	Initiate needle pericardiocentesis.
Myocardial infarction	Not immediately treatable because it is not easily recognizable.
Temperature (too low)	Warm the patient.
Pulmonary embolus	Not immediately treatable because it is not easily recognizable.

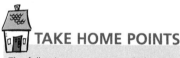

TAKE HOME POINTS

The following acronym may help with the memory of the causes to consider: for **H**ealthy **H**earts **A**nd **P**arts, **D**on't **T**reat **T**he **M**onitor, **T**reat the **P**atient!

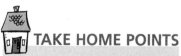

TAKE HOME POINTS

An easy way to remember the treatment for PEA is to use the initials of the name itself:

P = possible causes

E = epinephrine

A = atropine.

15 Atrioventricular Blocks

What IS Atrioventricular Block?

Atrioventricular (AV) *block* is defined as a delay or interruption in conduction between the atria and ventricles. It is sometimes simply called *heart block* (HB).

AV block is not just one block; it is a series of blocks that represent a progression in severity. These blocks range from simple prolonging of the AV conduction time (first-degree AV block) to complete lack of electrical transmission between the atria and ventricles (third-degree AV block).

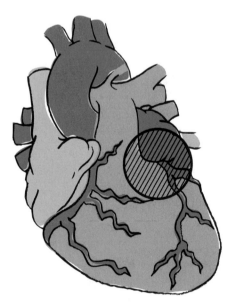

HBs may be caused by ischemia, necrosis, or fibrosis along the conduction pathway, or they may be caused by an increase in the refractory period of a portion of the conduction pathway, such as that caused by digoxin.

If the ventricular rate decreases and therefore the blood supply to the brain and body decreases, the patient may have symptoms resulting from hypoxemia. Symptoms of hypoxemia may range from lightheadedness and dizziness to temporary loss of consciousness (syncope).

AV blocks range from first to third degree. The following is a list of the least to most severe forms of AV block:

- First-degree AV block
- Second-degree AV block, type I (Mobitz type I or Wenckebach)
- Second-degree AV block, type II (Mobitz type II)
- Third-degree AV block (complete HB)

What IS First-Degree AV Block?

A *first-degree AV block* occurs when the conduction between the atrium and ventricle is prolonged beyond 0.2 seconds. Think of this as driving to work or school. You know how long it normally takes; however, if you run into an unexpected traffic delay it will take you longer to go the same route.

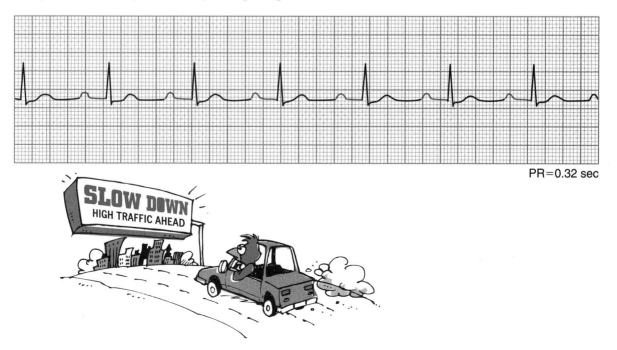

PR=0.32 sec

SLOW DOWN
HIGH TRAFFIC AHEAD

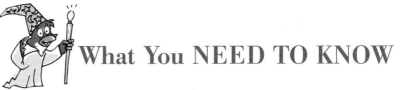

What You NEED TO KNOW

In first-degree AV block, the length of time it takes for the electrical impulse to get from the atria to the ventricles is longer than normal. Therefore the PR interval is consistently longer than normal (greater than 0.2 seconds). Everything else in the rhythm strip is normal. In fact, if you do not look closely and measure the PR interval, you may see only a normal sinus rhythm (NSR) and overlook the first-degree AV block.

A first-degree AV block can be temporary or permanent. There are several possible causes. For example, ischemia secondary to swelling could cause a temporary HB after open-heart surgery or myocardial infarction (MI). AV HBs tend to occur after injury to the right coronary artery. Digoxin (Lanoxin), even at normal therapeutic doses, can cause a prolonged PR interval (first-degree AV block). Calcium channel blockers, such as nifedipine (Procardia), and beta-blockers, such as metoprolol (Lopressor), can cause HBs. If medication is thought to be the cause of an AV block, it should be held.

Age-Related Specifics

HB increases in frequency in older adults. As people age they lose pacemaker cells. Ventricular septal defects (VSDs) in young children and the surgical procedures to correct these abnormalities can cause edema and HB.

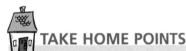

TAKE HOME POINTS

- **ECG criterion:** First-degree AV block
- **Atrial and ventricular rates:** Greater than 60 bpm but less than 100 bpm
- **Rhythm:** Regular
- **P waves:** Present and countable
- **PR interval:** Greater than 0.2 seconds
- **QRS:** Normal (one for every P wave)
- **QT:** Normal

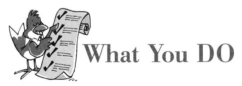

What You DO

First-degree AV block usually does not cause symptoms, so treatment is not necessary. However, this rhythm can be a clear warning that more severe blocks are "soon to come." Therefore you should monitor the patient for further advanced levels of HB. You should also review the medication record; medications that can cause first-degree HB should be held, and the prescribing health care provider should be notified.

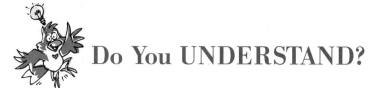

Do You UNDERSTAND?

DIRECTIONS: **Place a check next to the characteristics of first-degree AV block.**

1. _____ Atrial rate below 60 bpm
2. _____ Irregular atrial and ventricular rhythms
3. _____ PR interval between 0.12 and 0.2 seconds
4. _____ PR interval greater than 0.2 seconds
5. _____ Wide and bizarre QRS complex
6. _____ QT interval within normal limits

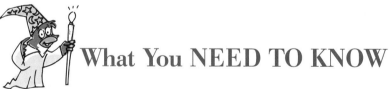

What IS Second-Degree AV Block?

Second-degree HB is a more severe type of AV block that comes in two varieties: (1) type I (often called Mobitz I or Wenckebach) and (2) type II (called Mobitz II). Although they have different characteristics, communication to the ventricles is not always complete with every beat in both types. In other words, there are more Ps than QRS complex; some Ps are not conducted.

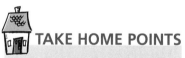

What You NEED TO KNOW

Type I Second-Degree Block (Mobitz I)

Type I second-degree block (Mobitz type I) is characterized by a PR interval that may be initially normal; however, with each successive beat, the PR interval gets longer and longer until there is a P wave that sits alone.

TAKE HOME POINTS

When treating the patient with type I second-degree (Mobitz, type I) AV block, you should look for the following:

- **Atrial rate:** Faster than ventricular rate.
- **PR interval:** Grows progressively longer until the P wave is not conducted. (In our example, the PR interval goes from 0.24 to 0.32 to 0.36 seconds; then a P wave sits by itself.) After the nonconducted P wave, the cycle starts again with a short PR interval and then each consecutive PR interval progressively lengthening until a beat is dropped again.

Answers: 4 and 6 are characteristics of first-degree AV block.

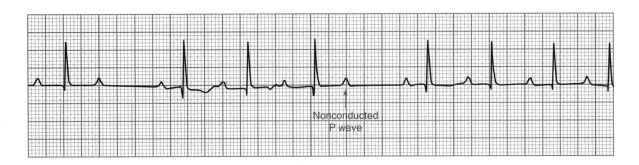

Nonconducted
P wave

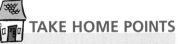

TAKE HOME POINTS

When treating the patient with type I second-degree (Wenckebach) AV block, you should look for the following:

- **Atrial rate:** Faster than ventricular rate
- **Atrial rhythm:** Regular
- **Ventricular rhythm:** Irregular at the dropped QRS
- **P waves:** Appear the same (like sinus P)
- **PR interval:** Gradual increase in length until a beat is dropped
- **QRS complex:** Absent after the nonconducted P wave; normal configuration
- **QT interval:** Not affected, normal

When treating the patient with type II second-degree (Mobitz II) AV block, you should look for the following:

- **Rate:** Normal atrial rate; slower ventricular rate
- **Rhythm:** Regular atrial rhythm; ventricular is irregular ventricular rhythm at the dropped beat
- **P wave:** Normal (each with a QRS, except those that are blocked)
- **PR interval:** May be normal or prolonged but remains constant
- **QRS complex:** Usually within normal limits; may be greater than 0.10 seconds and less than 0.12 seconds if the block is closer to the ventricles
- **QT interval:** Duration is usually greater than 0.44 seconds

Because this beat never makes it to the ventricles, this characteristic is often called a nonconducted P wave. The cycle after the dropped P wave starts over with a normal PR that gradually gets longer until it drops again; then the cycle repeats itself.

Type I Second-Degree Block (Wenckebach)

Type I second-degree block (Wenckebach) is not difficult to recognize, but you must be looking for it to find it. The recognition of "grouped beatings" at first glance should alert you to look for it. Wenckebach is often caused by an increase in parasympathetic tone or drug effect (digoxin, propranolol, verapamil). It is usually transient and its prognosis is good.

The QRS complex and QT interval are not affected because the problem is above the ventricles. Second-degree type I HB is relatively benign. It is the least serious of the second-degree blocks and rarely progresses to third-degree HB. The patient's symptoms are related to how slowly the ventricles are beating.

Type II Second-Degree Block (Mobitz II)

Type II second-degree block (Mobitz II) is more advanced and severe than Wenckebach. In Mobitz II the AV node refuses to allow certain beats through to the ventricles in a fixed ratio (every second or third beat may be dropped). The PR interval for the conducted beats remains constant.

The PR interval is what differentiates Mobitz type II from type I Wenckebach. In Wenckebach, a clear warning is given by PR interval lengthening. In second-degree type II the PR interval remains constant, but the QRS complex is dropped without warning.

In second-degree type II AV block, the atrial rate may be two, three, or even four times the ventricular rate. The following example demonstrates a 2:1 block; that is, there are two P waves for every QRS complex.

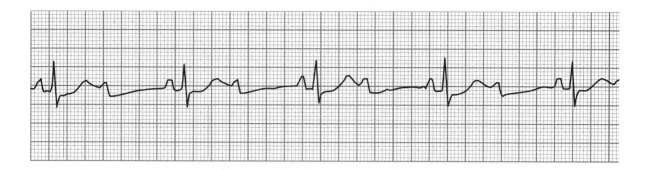

The rhythms of the atria and ventricles can be regular or irregular. The PR interval is consistent and usually within normal limits; it does not lengthen before a dropped beat as with Wenckebach. The QRS complexes are normal; they may be up to 0.12 seconds. The QT interval may be longer than normal because this rhythm is generally a bradycardia. Even if the patient is not symptomatic, this rhythm is dangerous because it is more likely to evolve into third-degree HB. Second-degree type II AV block is rarely the result of increased parasympathetic tone or drug effect. It is due to more serious causes, such as ischemia.

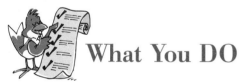

What You DO

When working with a patient with second-degree HB, you should remember the following:

1. Identify underlying causes, if possible.
2. No treatment is needed if the ventricular rate is normal and the patient does not have symptoms.
3. If the patient has symptoms such as lightheadedness or dizziness or is hypotensive, remember the following:
   - Start an intravenous (IV) line and administer atropine 0.5 to 1.0 mg intravenous push (IVP).
   - Prepare a temporary transcutaneous pacemaker, which stimulates the heart through the chest wall via electrodes attached to an external machine.
   - A temporary transvenous pacemaker may be inserted at the bedside.
   - If a permanent pacemaker is needed, it is generally inserted in the operating room or cardiac catheterization laboratory.

- If the patient has just had open heart surgery, the temporary epicardial wires attached to the external generator box are on standby. This pacemaker may be turned on to the operational mode.

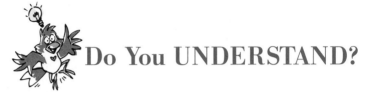

Do You UNDERSTAND?

DIRECTIONS: **Fill in the blanks with the appropriate characteristics for the rhythm.**

1. First-degree AV block
   a. Rate _____
   b. Rhythm _____
   c. P wave _____
   d. PR interval _____
   e. QRS complex _____
   f. QT interval _____

2. Second-degree AV block, type I
   a. Rate _____
   b. Rhythm _____
   c. P wave _____
   d. PR interval _____
   e. QRS complex _____
   f. QT interval _____

3. Second-degree AV block, type II
   a. Rate _____
   b. Rhythm _____
   c. P wave _____
   d. PR interval _____
   e. QRS complex _____
   f. QT interval _____

Answers: 1. a. >60 <100, b. regular, c. normal, d. >0.2, e. normal, f. normal; 2. a. atrial>ventricular, b. irregular, c. normal, d. gets longer, e. normal, f. normal; 3. a. atrial>ventricular, b. regular or irregular, c. normal, d. usually <0.2 and consistent, e. normal when present, f. long.

What IS a Complete (Third-Degree) HB?

A *third-degree HB*, or *complete HB* (CHB), occurs when there is no communication between the heart's atrial and ventricular conduction systems (i.e., there is complete dissociation between the two parts of the heart). The effective teamwork that makes the heart pump efficiently is gone.

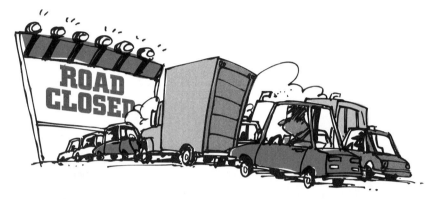

CHB is the most severe form of AV block. The underlying *escape* rhythm (the rhythm responsible for stimulating the ventricles) either comes from the AV node or the ventricles themselves. If it were not for an escape rhythm, there would be ventricular standstill or asystole, because none of the P waves make it past the AV node to stimulate the ventricles. The following example demonstrates a ventricular escape rhythm.

CHB with a nodal escape rhythm may be caused by increased parasympathetic tone associated with inferior MI, toxic drug effect, or damage to the

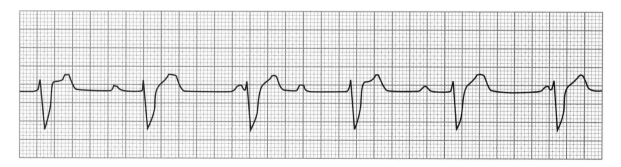

AV node. This type of HB is likely to be transient and associated with a more favorable prognosis. CHB with a ventricular escape rhythm indicates the presence of extensive conductive system disease involving both bundle branches. It is more serious and more permanent, requiring a transvenous pacemaker insertion.

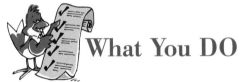

What You NEED TO KNOW

- In CHB the atria beat at their own rate in a regular manner, and the ventricles do the same. However, both follow their inherent pacemaker rates, that is, the atria beat between 60 and 100 bpm and the ventricles fire at 20 to 40 bpm, if ventricular escape, or 40 to 60 bpm if nodal escape.
- The rhythm of each chamber of the heart is regular with itself (both the P-to-P interval and the R-to-R interval are regular).
- The PR intervals are inconsistent because the P waves are unrelated to the QRS complex.
- If the escape rhythm comes from the ventricles, the QRS complex will be wide (less than 0.12 seconds) and slow (20 to 40 bpm).
- If the escape rhythm comes from the AV node, the QRS complex may be less than 0.12 seconds and the rate will be between 40 and 60 bpm.
- The QT interval is usually long with a bradydysrhythmia.

What You DO

CHB is almost always a cause of severe symptoms in the patient because of the slow heart rate. Complaints of severe fatigue and increasing dyspnea are common. There may be a marked change in the level of consciousness. The patient may be hypotensive. These symptoms are treated similarly to type II second-degree AV block.

When working with patients with CHB, you should remember:

- To start an IV.
- To give the patient oxygen to elevate SaO_2 levels.
- That you may give atropine 0.5 to 1.0 mg IVP while the pacer is being obtained.
- To initiate transcutaneous pacing.
- To prepare for insertion of a transvenous pacemaker.

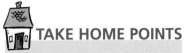

TAKE HOME POINTS

When treating the patient with CHB, you should look for the following:

- **Rate:** Atrial normal (60 to 100 bpm); ventricular between 20 and 40 bpm if ventricular escape; 40 to 60 if nodal escape
- **Rhythm:** Regular
- **P wave:** All appear the same (sinus rhythm) in origin
- **PR interval:** Varying because there is no relationship
- **QRS complex:** May be normal (if nodal escape) or wide (if ventricular escape)
- **QT:** Longer than normal

If atropine is ineffective, catecholamine infusion of dopamine or epinephrine may be started to treat CHB. Isuprel is rarely used because of the increased oxygen demand on the heart.

TAKE HOME POINTS

Do not treat ventricular escape beats with lidocaine. Even though they are ventricular beats, they are not PVCs. The mechanism is different; they are the ventricles' attempt to help out a failing heart. To suppress them is to erase the only ventricular stimulation there is, and this will lead to asystole.

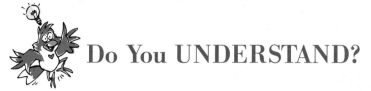

Do You UNDERSTAND?

DIRECTIONS: Fill in the words in the crossword puzzle.

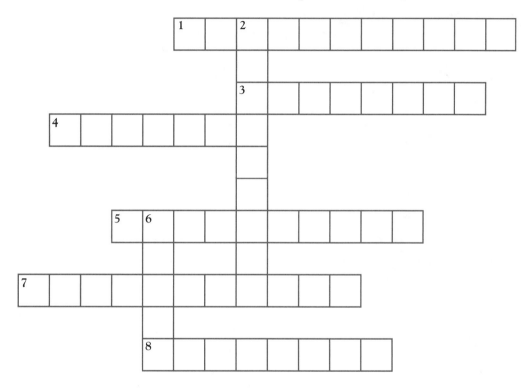

Across

1. Low blood pressure
3. Third degree or _____ HB
4. Fainting
5. Mobitz I
7. Catecholamine infusion
8. Drug of choice in bradycardia

Down

2. Makes a spike before the QRS complex
6. Swelling

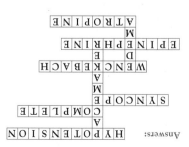

Answers:

16 Cardiac Noninvasive Diagnostic Tests

Several different noninvasive cardiac diagnostic tests are discussed in this chapter, including the echocardiogram (ECHO), Holter monitor, signal-averaged electrocardiogram (SAECG), and stress test.

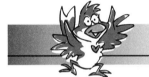

What IS an ECHO?

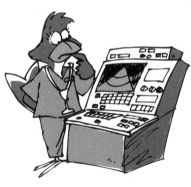

A traditional transthoracic *ECHO* is a noninvasive acoustic-imaging procedure that examines the size and shape of the heart, as well as the position, thickness, and movement of the heart valves and chambers. An ultrasonic beam is deflected off the heart structures and received back into an oscilloscope that creates a two-dimensional (2-D) image.

A transthoracic ECHO has four components:

1. **M-mode.** Provides an "ice-pick" view of the heart and a black-white and gray printout on the strip chart recorder.
2. **2-D ECHO.** Provides a real-time, high-resolution view of the heart and great vessels. It can detect a pericardial effusion as little as 20 to 30 cc. Its most common use is to measure chamber size and wall thickness.
3. **Doppler echo.** Provides measurement of gradients in stenotic or regurgitant heart valves and intracardiac shunts. It also detects atherosclerosis by evaluating blood flow through the carotid arteries. Ultrasound waves are reflected off of the red blood cells (RBCs), and the frequency of these waves is altered according to the blood flow velocity. (Blood flowing through the carotid arteries produces the characteristic "swooshing" sound of each heartbeat.) When Doppler echo is combined with 2-D echo, the echo may be called a duplex Doppler. *Color-flow Doppler* integrates the structural information provided by 2-D echo with pulsed

2-D ECHO is the most common technique and is used to detect valvular problems, cardiac birth abnormalities in newborns, heart enlargement, cardiac tumor, and abnormalities in left ventricular motion.

Doppler color-coded flow maps that depict the direction, velocity, and turbulence of blood flow through the cardiac chambers and great vessels. This information is used to estimate intracardiac pressure, valve gradients, and intracardiac shunting. It is sometimes called a noninvasive angiogram. Color-flow Doppler is particularly valuable when attempting to assess the degree of valvular dysfunction noninvasively (especially mitral regurgitation). Calculations are made through computerized instrumentation, and the studies are recorded onto a videotape.

Transesophageal echocardiogram (TEE) is a special ultrasound test that uses a transmitter to generate high-frequency sound waves to take pictures of the back of the heart. Intravenous (IV) conscious sedation is given, the throat is anesthetized, and an ultrasound probe attached to a flexible gastroscope is inserted into the posterior pharynx and advanced into the esophagus. TEE shows a clear picture because the esophagus is against the back of the heart and is parallel to the aorta. This is especially useful in obese patients or patients with chronic obstructive pulmonary disease (COPD), whose transthoracic echo images are obscured by the lungs, rib cage, or both. TEE can pinpoint the site of a suspected aortic dissection, rule out the heart as a source of clots in patients who have had strokes, visualize valve defects, assess prosthetic valve function, and ensure that the left atrium is free from clots before mitral valvuloplasty is performed. Patients with atrial fibrillation of greater than 2 days duration have traditionally required several weeks of anticoagulation before and after electrical cardioversion because of the high incidence of thromboembolic events. TEE can identify whether a thrombus is present in the left atrium and therefore prevent the need for anticoagulation before cardioversion.

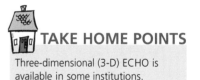 Better resolution for ECHOs occurs in children because they are thinner and the chest wall is less dense.

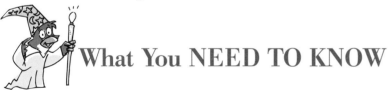

What You NEED TO KNOW

- A transthoracic echo can be performed at the bedside and takes about 30 to 60 minutes.
- There is no special preparation required.
- Conductive gel is placed over the third through fifth intercostal spaces to the left of the sternum, where the transducer is placed and angled.
- The patient will be asked to turn onto his or her side, with the left arm above the head to minimize the distance between the heart and the transducer (for better visualization).
- The patient must ingest nothing by mouth (NPO) for several hours before a transesophageal ECHO is performed.

TAKE HOME POINTS

Three-dimensional (3-D) ECHO is available in some institutions.

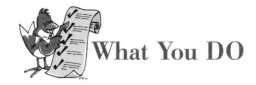

What You DO

When treating patients who need an ECHO, you should:
- Tell them that they must lie still unless asked to move during the procedure.
- Explain that there should be no discomfort or side effects from the procedure. The patient should notify the nurse if the rare complications of hemoptysis or dyspnea occur.
- Withhold fluids and food after a TEE until the patient's swallowing and gag reflexes are restored.
- Tell the patient that a sore throat is common after the TEE procedure.

Do You UNDERSTAND?

DIRECTIONS: **Place a check mark next to the terms and statements that apply to 2-D echocardiography.**

1. a. _____ Invasive test
   b. _____ Patient must be NPO
   c. _____ Conductive gel
   d. _____ Test tubes
   e. _____ Images the size of heart
   f. _____ TEE
   g. _____ Detects pericardial effusions
   h. _____ Six-dimensional picture

DIRECTIONS: **Indicate in the spaces provided whether the following statements are *true* or *false*.**

2. _____ A TEE may provide better visualization than a transthoracic ECHO in obese persons.
3. _____ ECHOs have better resolution in children than adults.
4. _____ ECHOs are useful in determining pacemaker failure.
5. _____ Frequent movement by the patient is necessary to improve resolution of an ECHO.

Answers: 1. c, e, f, g; 2. true; 3. true; 4. false; 5. false.

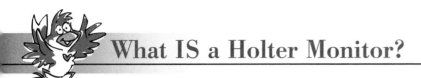

What IS a Holter Monitor?

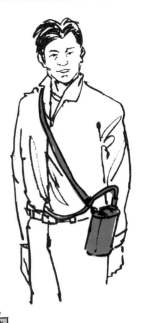

A *Holter monitor* is a small, portable, electrocardiogram (ECG) recorder that the patient wears while engaging in normal activities for a specified period of time, usually 24 hours. It is commonly used to detect cardiac dysrhythmias, evaluate effectiveness of dysrhythmic therapy, and to detect the ST segment and T wave changes of myocardial ischemia.

Most systems provide at least two-lead recording, which permits ready differentiation of ventricular versus supraventricular dysrhythmias and easier detection of artifact.

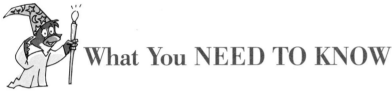

What You NEED TO KNOW

The Holter monitor is used to record continuous electrical heart activity, usually for periods of 24 hours. It can detect cardiac ischemia, dysrhythmias, pacemaker dysfunction, and conduction disturbances with sleep apnea syndrome. These may be signs of cardiomyopathy, coronary artery disease (CAD), cerebral ischemia, or mitral valve prolapse, which may explain episodes of syncope.

The patient records all activity and symptoms experienced at all times within the 24-hour period on a small, diary-type book pad. The ECG from the Holter monitor is correlated to the documented activity and symptoms to help diagnose or rule out abnormalities.

Electronic Holter monitor scanners can record more than 100,000 heartbeats in a 24-hour period. Holter findings correlate with symptoms in 25% to 50% of patients tested.

Patients must keep electrodes dry and in place. Therefore they should avoid swimming and bathing during the time the Holter monitor is worn.

TAKE HOME POINTS

Common symptoms of cardiac dysrhythmias are palpitations, dizziness, syncope, angina, and shortness of breath. These are also the signs of pacemaker failure.

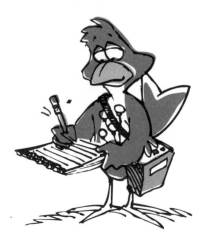

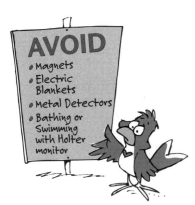

AVOID
- Magnets
- Electric Blankets
- Metal Detectors
- Bathing or Swimming with Holter monitor

⚠ **You should instruct patients to avoid bathing (except for sponge bath) and swimming for the time they are hooked up to the monitor so the electrodes remain intact.**

⚠ **You should instruct patient to avoid magnets, metal detectors, and electrical blankets because they interfere with monitor recordings.**

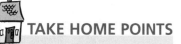

TAKE HOME POINTS

Symptoms of dysrhythmias or pacemaker dysfunction include dizziness and syncope, palpitations, shortness of breath, or chest tightness.

What You DO

When treating patients who are wearing Holter monitors, you should remember:

- Lead placement will depend on the system used for monitoring. Commonly, modified versions of lead II (RA/LL) and lead VI (fourth intercostal space [ICS] at right sternal border) are used so that the inferior and anterior surfaces of the heart may be monitored simultaneously.
- Three to seven electrodes are applied to the skin that is free of hair (you should clip hair if necessary) and that has been cleansed with acetone. Electrodes are taped securely to minimize artifact.
- Check to see that the monitor has a full supply of paper (for the printed readout) and that the batteries are fully charged.
- Instruct patients to engage in normal activities.
- Explain (if appropriate) how the patient can connect the Holter monitor to the telephone to send the ECG reading over the telephone line to be printed out at the doctor's office or hospital.
- Instruct the patient when and where to return the Holter monitor.
- Holter monitors are used for detection of ectopic beats, bradydysrhythmia and tachydysrhythmia identification, and the evaluation of antidysrhythmic drug therapy.

Do You UNDERSTAND?

DIRECTIONS: **Connect the activities and things that a person wearing a Holter monitor should avoid. Then explain what ECG waveform results from connecting the Xs?**

1.

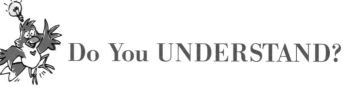

sponge bath	walking	electrical blanket	apples	reading
X	X	X	X	X
X	X	X	X	X
magnet	showering	eating	metal detector	swimming

Answers: 1. magnet, showering, electrical blanket, metal detector, swimming (a P wave or a T wave results from connecting the Xs).

DIRECTIONS: **For each patient description, state a nursing intervention for a Holter monitor.**

2. Hairy body

_____

_____

3. To wear Holter monitor for 72 hours

_____

_____

4. Monitor brought back by one patient and now needed for another

_____

_____

What IS an SAECG?

SAECG is a noninvasive ECG that is sensitive to detecting very low-amplitude, high-frequency electrical activity in the terminal QRS complex. The presence of the activity suggests that certain factors (e.g., PVCs, ischemia, electrolyte abnormalities) may more easily trigger ventricular tachycardia. In SAECG, the ECG is recorded at high speed and high sensitivity. The signals are then filtered for the baseline noises that obscure late potentials from being seen on the standard 12 lead. The inability to detect low-frequency potentials in the SAECG correlates with a low risk for sustained malignant ventricular dysrhythmias. If SAECG is positive for late potentials, electrophysiologic testing is warranted because malignant dysrhythmias, such as ventricular tachycardia (VT), are likely.

What You NEED TO KNOW

SAECG monitoring cannot be performed with a standard ECG machine unless it is specially programmed. Lead placement varies by the SAECG manufacturer, but basically, bipolar leads are placed on the anterior and posterior torso.

Ectopic beats and artifact are NOT included in the averaging of the cardiac cycles. Therefore it will take longer to complete this test in patients who have a lot of ectopy or artifact.

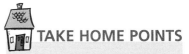

The procedure takes about 20 minutes because the cardiac cycles are averaged over time to give an ECG reading.

TAKE HOME POINTS

- SAECG is useful in determining risk for developing life-threatening dysrhythmias in high-risk patients.
- Because the cardiac cycles are averaged over time, the test takes longer in persons who are bradycardic (less than 60 bpm) and shorter in persons who are tachycardic (greater than 100 bpm).
- SAECGs are NOT useful in atrial dysrhythmias and rhythms with wide QRS complexes (bundle branch block).

Answers: 2. Clip where electrodes are to be placed; 3. Check amount of paper on roll and replace if needed; 4. Replace battery.

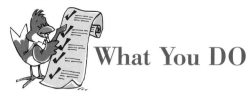

What You DO

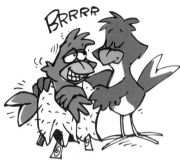

- Avoid patient shivering and provide calm environment for test or artifact will occur, resulting in increased testing time.
- Remove all electrical interference (i.e., put IV pumps on battery [not electricity], turn off hypothermia machines, televisions, and radios) so artifact does not result.
- Position patient supine or head of bed elevated at 15-degree angle.
- Clip hair from potential lead placement sites; then cleanse with an alcohol wipe.
- Teach patients to lie very still and try to relax their muscles during the test.

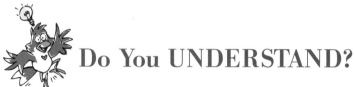

Do You UNDERSTAND?

DIRECTIONS: Place a check next to each high-risk history that indicates the patient that will require an SAECG

1. a. _____ Cardiac arrest
   b. _____ High blood pressure
   c. _____ Ventricular fibrillation
   d. _____ Gastrointestinal upset
   e. _____ Bradycardia
   f. _____ Bundle branch block

DIRECTIONS: Write the nursing interventions for someone undergoing an SAECG.

2. Electrical IV pump with fluids running

   _____

   _____

3. Electrical hypothermia blanket on

   _____

   _____

4. Patient wearing radio headphone

   _____

   _____

Answers: 1. a, c, e; 2. Run on battery; 3. Turn blanket off; 4. Turn off and remove (to keep patient from moving head to the beat of the music).

DIRECTIONS: **Place a check next to the requirement(s) NOT necessary for someone undergoing an SAECG.**

5. a. _____ Alcohol wipe
   b. _____ Chest leads
   c. _____ Scissors or razor
   d. _____ Lying still
   e. _____ Calm environment
   f. _____ Watching television

What IS a Stress Test?

A *stress test* is a noninvasive procedure that involves the monitoring of the cardiac electrical and mechanical response to continuous, progressively strenuous exercise. The exercise acts as a stress or "workload challenge" to the heart to determine its work capacity. Stress testing is used mainly to detect and evaluate the functional effect of CAD. Because physical stress causes an increase in myocardial oxygen demand, if CAD is present, this demand will exceed the supply and ischemia will result.

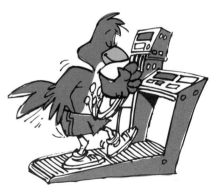

The stress can be induced by exercising on a stationary bicycle, stair stepper, or treadmill, or it can be induced by medications (dobutamine, adenosine, dipyridamole) to increase heart rate and blood pressure. The exercise stress test identifies individuals prone to cardiac ischemia during activity but not at rest, and the pharmacologic stress test identifies those with known CAD or those who are unable to perform satisfactory exercise (older adults, patients with joint or respiratory problems). Patients are monitored continuously during a stress test.

Stress tests are often combined with myocardial perfusion imaging, which compares any specific areas of ischemia before and after exercising. Single photon emission computed tomography (SPECT) is the gold standard of myocardial perfusion imaging. The patient is taken to nuclear medicine for a baseline scan to determine perfusion at rest. During peak exercise, a radioisotope (thallium = 201 or technetium sestamibi tagged to Cardiolite) is IV injected and the patient is rescanned. This test helps differentiate viable myocardium from nonviable myocardium. For many patients with CAD and left ventricle dysfunction, the data obtained will determine whether the patient will benefit from coronary artery bypass grafting (CABG).

Answer: 5. f.

A *dobutamine stress ECHO* is an alternative to thallium imaging to determine the efficiency of the heart and the reversibility of dysfunctional myocardium. Dobutamine causes an increase in myocardial oxygen demand by stimulating beta-2 receptors, which is similar to the response in exercise. Images are recorded at rest and during an infusion of dobutamine at 5 to 10 mcg/kg/min. Functional improvement of poorly moving ventricular walls at rest (in response to low-dose dobutamine) is highly predictive of viability and improvement of function. The test may also be used to diagnose ischemia.

What You NEED TO KNOW

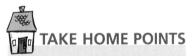 **Do not perform a stress test on patients with active unstable angina, ethanol intoxication, chest pain, myocarditis or pericarditis, congestive heart failure, digitalis toxicity, recent pulmonary embolism, or uncontrolled dysrhythmias.**

- Stress tests must be performed by health care practitioners certified in advanced cardiac life support (ACLS), exercise physiologists, physical therapists, or physicians.
- Instruct the patient to wear comfortable walking shoes and clothes if scheduled for exercise-induced stress test, because the test takes about 1 hour. If nuclear imaging is performed, the test will take several hours.
- Ask the patient to refrain from food, fluids, nicotine, and caffeine (tea, coffee, soda) for at least 2 hours before the test.
- In most cases, patients may take their regular medications, but you should check with the physician to see if any should be withheld.
- Explain that the patient will be asked to lie on a table with arms over the head for 20 to 25 minutes during nuclear scanning.
- Dobutamine may cause some mild side effects, which include chest tightness, dyspnea, flushing, nausea, headache, paresthesias, chills, palpitations, and anxiety. You should inform the patient that these side effects will only last a few minutes. (The half-life of dobutamine is only 2 minutes.)

TAKE HOME POINTS

Electrolyte imbalances and lung diseases can affect conditions to perform a stress test.

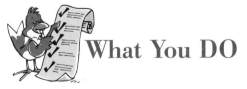 # What You DO

- Gradually discontinue beta blocker medications before the test per prescribing health care provider's order (see table on the following page).
- Have an emergency crash cart available at all times.
- Attach appropriate ECG leads to hair-free areas and a blood pressure cuff to the patient's arm.

Beta-Blocker Medications

GENERIC NAME	TRADE NAME
acebutolol	Sectral
atenolol	Tenormin
betaxolol	Betoptic
esmolol	Brevibloc
metoprolol	Lopressor
nadolol	Corgard
penbutolol	Levotol
propranolol	Inderal
sotalol	Betapace
timolol	Timoptic

- For the pharmacologic-induced stress test only, establish IV access and administer dobutamine by infusion pump at an initial rate of 5 to 10 mcg/kg/min; double the rate every 3 minutes until a maximum of 40 mcg/kg/min or until symptoms or signs appear.
- Check medication order. Remind the patient that the medication injection during the pharmacologic-induced stress test may cause temporary discomfort, but it will only last a few minutes.
- For exercise stress test, instruct patient to begin exercising.
- Run a baseline ECG.
- Terminate testing if you notice signs of ischemia (ST segment depression on the ECG of greater than 1 to 2 mm) or if maximal effort is achieved, as evidenced by dyspnea or systolic blood pressure greater than 250 mm Hg, or if the maximal heart rate for patient's age is obtained. You should also stop the test if dysrhythmias, chest pain, faintness, dizziness, or extreme fatigue occur.

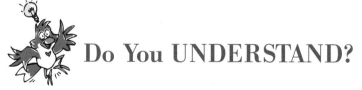

Do You UNDERSTAND?

DIRECTIONS: Select the best stress test for the following patients. Place an *E* if an exercise-induced stress test is the best or a *P* if the pharmacologic-induced stress test is indicated:

1. _____ Patient with CAD
2. _____ Athlete's annual physical examination
3. _____ 102-year-old patient
4. _____ 56-year-old patient with "bad" knees

Answers: 1. P; 2. E; 3. P; 4. P.

DIRECTIONS: **Fill in the blanks.**

5. What certification is required by a health care provider to be able to implement a stress test?

_____

6. State four types of equipment necessary for a pharmacologic-induced stress test.

_____

_____

_____

_____

DIRECTIONS: **Your patient is scheduled to have an exercise stress test in 5 hours and calls you from home to ask some questions. Place a check in the "yes" or "no" column to indicate the answer to each question.**

	yes	no
7. Can I take my morning potassium pill?	_____	_____
8. Can I have a cup of coffee?	_____	_____
9. Should I bring new shoes to wear on the treadmill?	_____	_____

CHAPTER

17 Myocardial Infarction

A heart attack, or myocardial infarction (MI), is the death of heart tissue. MI is usually caused by a complete blockage from a blood clot of a coronary artery narrowed by atherosclerosis. Atherosclerosis is the development of plaque from fattylike substances that collect in the intima of the coronary artery. This narrowing of the arteries is a process that occurs over years to decades.

The area of infarction upsets the normal electrical conduction patterns and leaves a telltale electrical sign. The electrical sign from the infarction changes the electrocardiogram (ECG) dramatically.

In this chapter, the 12-lead ECG and the identification of ischemia, injury, and infarction are examined. In addition, we discuss the diagnosis of an infarction from a 12-lead ECG.

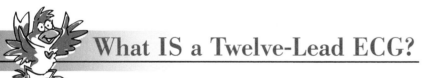

What IS a Twelve-Lead ECG?

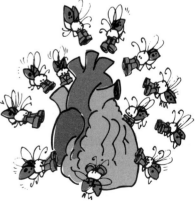

The basic components of heart monitoring and the differentiation between continuous monitoring and a 12-lead ECG are discussed in Chapter 7. We examined two of the leads. In this chapter, additional leads are described.

The *12-lead* ECG examines the heart from 12 different views and provides information about what is happening in the heart. The 12-lead ECG is made up of three sections: (1) limb leads, (2) augmented leads, and (3) precordial or chest leads.

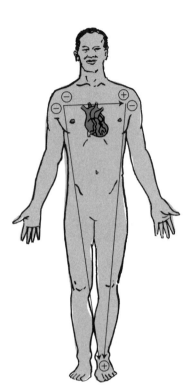

What You NEED TO KNOW

Limb Leads

There are several limb leads with which you should be familiar:

- Lead I measures the current of energy from the right arm (negative pole) to the left arm (positive pole); it looks at the lateral surface of the left ventricle.

- Lead II measures the current of energy from the right arm (negative) to the left leg (positive). You should have become familiar with this lead (primary monitoring lead) in previous chapters. Lead II looks at the inferior surface of the left ventricle.

- Lead III has its negative pole at the left arm and the positive pole at the right leg. This lead (along with leads II and avF) looks at the inferior surface of the left ventricle. Think of the positive pole as a smiling, clever lovebird that is looking at events coming toward it. Also, note this clever bird (positive pole) looks at events occurring in the inferior surface of the heart in leads II and III. The following strips show what normal events are recorded in leads I, II and III. Note that the R wave is prominent in these three leads. These form a triangle with the heart at the center (Einthoven's triangle). These leads are also in the frontal plane or the up-and-down, superior-to-inferior look at the heart.

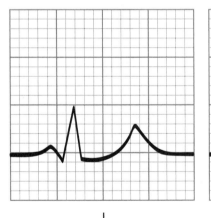
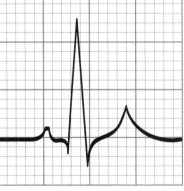
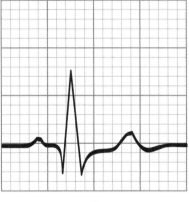

I   II   III

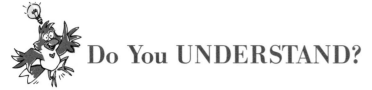

Do You UNDERSTAND?

DIRECTIONS: On the following figure, draw leads I, II, and III of a
12-lead ECG and use a positive (+) or negative (−)
sign to indicate the appropriate poles.

1.

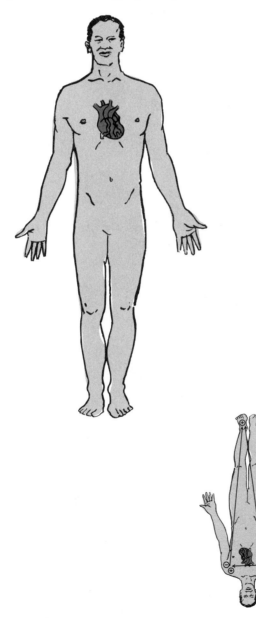

Answer:

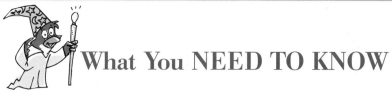

What You NEED TO KNOW

Augmented Leads

The next three leads are also on the frontal surface of the heart. They are called augmented leads and labeled with a small *a*, because the stimulus has to be increased in power to record information from these leads. Augmented leads are also called *unipolar*, because they measure the action of one lead and a body limb.

The last letter in the lead in this system tells you where the positive electrode is placed:

- aVR records activity from the heart (−) to the right shoulder (+)
- aVL records activity from the heart (−) to the left shoulder (+)
- aVF records activity from the heart (−) to the left foot (+)

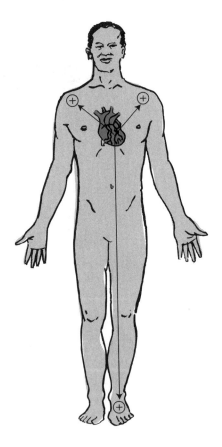

The following strips show the normal electrical activity recorded in these leads. Again, the smiling lovebird will see events at the bottom of the heart or inferior surface in aVF, because the positive electrode is looking up from the foot.

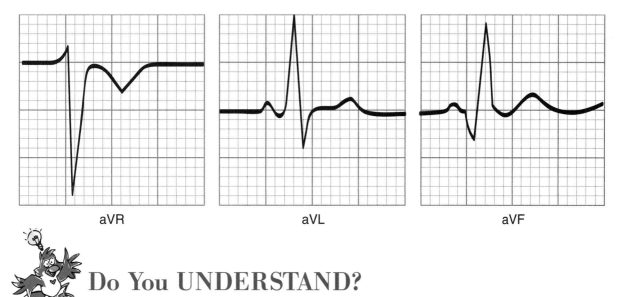

aVR aVL aVF

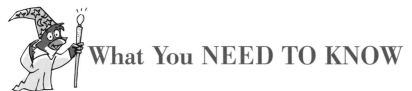

Do You UNDERSTAND?

DIRECTIONS: **Fill-in the blanks for the positive poles of the augmented leads.**

Positive electrode placement

1. aVR   _____

2. aVL   _____

3. aVF   _____

What You NEED TO KNOW

Precordial Leads

The last six leads of a 12-lead ECG look at events in the horizontal plane or surface from the front of the heart toward the patient's back. These are called the precordial or chest leads; they are unipolar leads.

Answers: 1. right arm, 2. left arm, 3. foot.

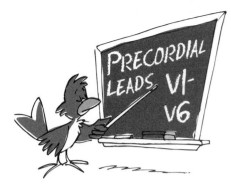

The positive electrode is always in front of the heart, and the negative electrode is the left shoulder. These leads are labeled V1 through V6 and are placed across the chest from the right of the sternum to the left axilla.

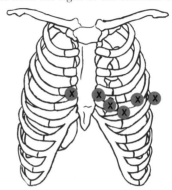

The leads should become progressively more positive as they advance from V1 through V6. The first chest lead is V1, and it is located on the fourth intercostal space (ICS) to the right of the sternum. The second chest lead, V2, is located next to V1 but to the left of the sternum. Next, we skip V3 and locate V4. V4 is found at the fifth ICS at the midclavicular line or at the point of maximal impulse (PMI). V3 is found easily now, because it is half way between V2 and V4 leads.

V1 through V4 are placed so that they look at events occurring in the anterior portion of the left ventricle. V6 is located next and is found in the left midaxillary line (sixth ICS). V5 is found half way between V4 and V6. Both V5 and V6 look at the lateral surface of the left ventricle.

Placement of the precordial leads in the exact location is essential. If they are not correctly placed, important changes in heart activity may be missed.

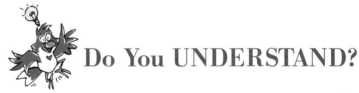

Do You UNDERSTAND?

DIRECTIONS: Match the V lead in Column A to the definition of its location in Column B.

Column A	Column B
1. _____ V1	a. Midaxillary line, fifth ICS
2. _____ V2	b. Fifth ICS, midclavicular line (MCL)
3. _____ V3	c. Half way between V2 and V4
4. _____ V4	d. Fourth ICS, right of the sternum
5. _____ V5	e. Fourth ICS, left of the sternum
6. _____ V6	f. Half way between V4 and V6

Answers: 1. d; 2. e; 3. c; 4. b; 5. f; 6. a.

What IS a Transmural Infarction?

Now that you can label the leads of a 12-lead ECG, we discuss what you should look for in these areas. In a *transmural infarction*, there are three zones to examine. These areas are sometimes called the current of injury of an infarction. The areas of ischemia, injury, and infarction involve T wave, ST segment, and Q wave changes of the cardiac cycle.

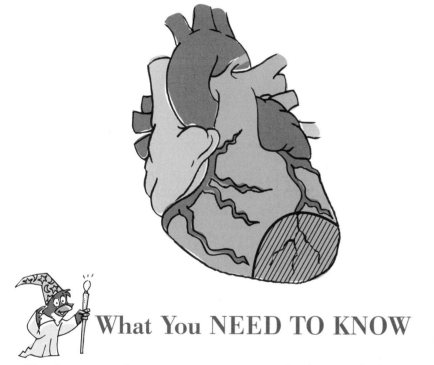

What You NEED TO KNOW

The three zones of injury may not occur immediately. Instead, they may evolve over time. The first zone is the outermost area. This is the area of ischemia and is usually the first to change.

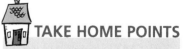

TAKE HOME POINTS

The first zone is an area of reversible ischemia, but if the damage continues, the next zone occurs.

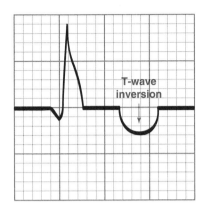

The T waves usually invert or flip over because of a lack of oxygen and potassium leaking from the damaged heart muscle cells. Remember, normal T waves are upright, larger than P waves, and slightly asymmetrical.

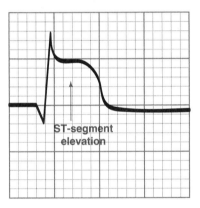

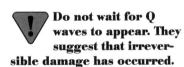 If some action is not taken by this second change, an infarction can occur.

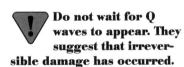 Do not wait for Q waves to appear. They suggest that irreversible damage has occurred.

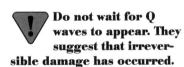 MIs are diagnosed in conjunction with signs and symptoms, cardiac enzymes, cardiac echocardiography, and cardiac catheterization. The ECG should NEVER be used as the sole basis of diagnosis.

- The second change to occur is elevation of the ST segment. ST segments are usually isoelectric and need to be greater than 1 mm high to be considered elevated.
- Elevated ST segments indicate prolonged, severe injury to the myocardial cells.
- The ST segments may be elevated so high that the T wave may not be seen until several days later.
- Elevated ST segments indicate acute injury. This is the point at which intervention must take place. They are the first to recede to normal within several days postinfarction.
- If there are Q waves and flipped T waves without ST segment elevations, the MI is not acute but has happened recently. However, if some action is not taken by this second change, an infarction can occur.

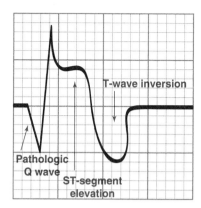

T-wave inversion

Pathologic
Q wave

ST-segment
elevation

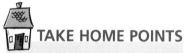
Women wait longer to seek medical attention for symptoms of infarction. Women also have more complications and death with hospitalization, because they are usually older and sicker. Many have other underlying conditions like diabetes and heart failure. Women with high serum uric acid levels after an MI have a poorer prognosis.

- The last change to occur is the Q wave. Taken together, flipped T waves, ST segment elevation, and Q waves are a reliable signs (along with cardiac enzymes) that irreversible myocardial necrosis or death has occurred.
- The R wave in the lead disappears and a Q wave develops. The Q wave must be greater than 0.04 seconds in width and greater than 25% of the height of the R wave to be pathologic change.
- Treat while there is still some myocardium viable—during ST segment elevation!

Diabetes and hypertension, two leading risk factors for MI, occur more frequently in African-Americans. Obesity is more common in African-American women and is a risk factor for coronary atherosclerosis.

Non–Q Wave MI

Occasionally, a patient may show symptoms of an MI with elevated enzymes but a depressed ST segment and no Q waves. This patient may have infarcted the inner part of the muscle wall, the subendocardial surface.

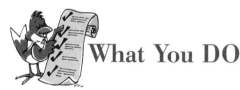

What You DO

If you suspect the patient is having a MI, you should remember to:
- Follow the ABCs of airway, breathing, and circulation.
- If the ABCs are present, reassure the patient and ensure that he or she maintains bedrest.
- Administer oxygen to keep the SaO_2 greater than 93%.
- Administer sublingual nitroglycerine.
- Give morphine sulfate at 2 mg intravenously (IV) if three successive sublingual nitroglycerine do not abate the patient's chest pain or symptoms.

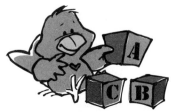

TAKE HOME POINTS

In a transmural infarction, the following characteristics are seen:
- **Rate and rhythm:** Can be anything. Rhythm may degrade to ventricular tachycardia (VT) and ventricular fibrillation (VF) if untreated.
- **PR interval:** Intervals are normal.
- **QRS complex:** Q waves present in leads looking at the infarction. Qs are greater than 0.04 seconds wide and one fourth the height of the R wave.
- **ST segment:** Segments are elevated greater than 1 mm.
- **QT interval:** Intervals are normal
- **T wave:** Waves are usually inverted in leads looking at infarcted area.
- **Other:** Because of ventricular irritability, PVCs may be present.

You must closely observe the patients who show symptoms of an MI with elevated enzymes and ST and T wave changes but no Q waves, because almost half of them extend their infarct damage into the transmural wall.

- Administer aspirin and beta blockers to the patient. Aspirin has been shown to be effective in decreasing clot formation in patients experiencing MI. Beta blockers help reduce the heart rate and decrease oxygen demand on the heart. Bradycardia and hypotension must be ruled out before administering beta blockers.
- Administer (via IV) nitroglycerine and heparin. Heparin prevents further clot formation and nitroglycerine helps dilate coronary arteries and decrease the workload of the heart by vasodilatation.
- Institute thrombolytic therapy to lyse the clot obstructing the coronary artery. Tissue plasminogen activator (TPA) or its newest version, tenectaplase (TNK) (an enzyme derivative of TPA), may be used, especially if there will be a delay in more definitive therapy.

Ongoing assessments for the signs and symptoms of heart failure, dysrhythmias, and shock are important.

The health care provider should anticipate further diagnostic studies to be prescribed. Stat cardiac markers or enzymes, electrolytes, and ECG should be requested, and the patient may be prepared for emergency cardiac catheterization, angioplasty, or open-heart surgery for coronary artery bypass grafting (CABG).

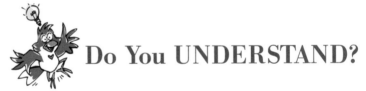

Do You UNDERSTAND?

DIRECTIONS: **Fill in the blanks.**

1. The areas of ischemia, injury, and infarction respectively involve

   _____, _____,

   and Q wave changes of the cardiac cycle.

2. The first zone or _____ area is usually the

   first to change and the area of ischemia; _____ waves invert

   or flip over because of lack of _____ and

   _____. Three

   zones of injury may not occur immediately but evolve over time.

3. If there are Q waves and flipped T waves without ST segment elevations, the MI is not acute but has occurred

   _____.

Answers: 1. T wave, ST segment; 2. outermost, T, oxygen, potassium leaking from the damaged heart muscle cells; 3. recently.

4. MIs are diagnosed in conjunction with signs and symptoms, cardiac _____, cardiac echocardiography, and cardiac _____.

5. If the health care provider suspects the patient is having an MI, he or she should first check _____, _____, and _____.

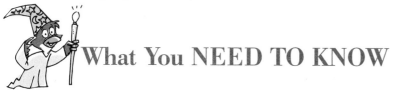

What ARE the Types of Infarction?

Now that you are familiar with all 12 leads and the current treatment of injury for an MI, it is time to discuss the infarction locations and where they can be found. Types of infarction include anterior, inferior, lateral, and posterior, which all refer to the *left ventricle*, because we are primarily concerned with the booster pump to the body.

What You NEED TO KNOW

The size of an MI is determined by how proximal the occlusion is. An anterior infarction is usually the most lethal for the patient, mainly because there is more muscle to lose. In an anterior infarction, the blood supply via the left anterior descending artery has been stopped before reaching the anterior wall of the ventricle. If the left main coronary artery becomes occluded, there is little chance that the patient will survive.

Studies show that a woman's susceptibility to anterior infarction leading to mortality rises after menopause.

The leads that look at the left ventricle's anterior surface are V1 through V4. If this wall of the ventricle has infarcted, you will see Q waves, ST segment elevation, and flipped T waves in the first four V leads.

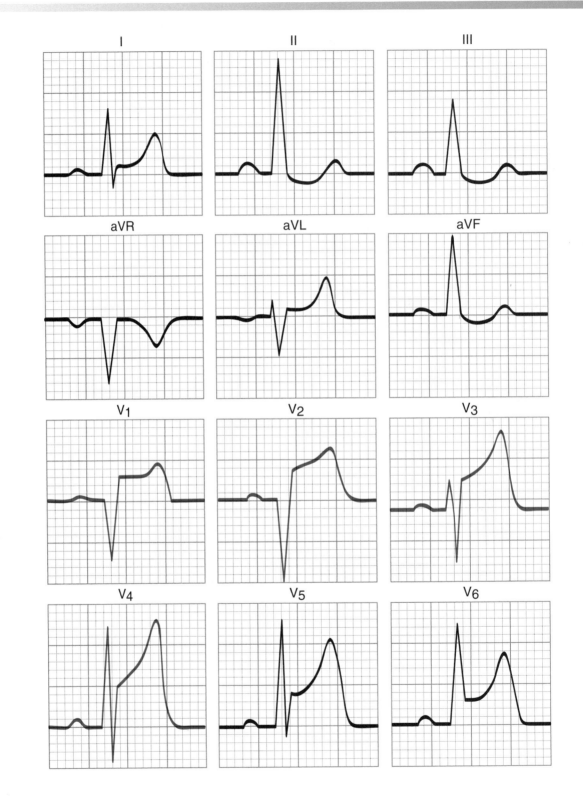

An inferior MI involves the bottom or diaphragmatic surface of the left ventricle. ECGs suggesting that the patient has suffered an MI would have three changes in leads II, III and aVF. Inferior wall MIs are caused by a blockage in the right coronary artery (RCA). Often patients suffering from inferior MIs have heart blocks because the RCA supplies the sinoatrial (SA) and atrioventricular (AV) nodes in a large percentage of the population.

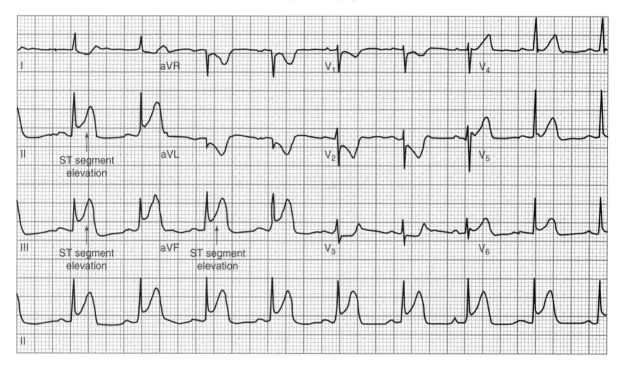

A lateral wall infarction of the left ventricle is confirmed by looking in lead I, aVL, V5, and V6. The circumflex artery supplies the lateral wall of the ventricle.

Isolated posterior wall MIs are very rare. Additional electrodes can be added to the 12 leads on the patient's back at V7 (posterior axillary line), V8 (midscapular line), and V9 (3 cm from the spinal column). In addition, reciprocal (opposite) changes in the chest leads can be examined. In V1 and V2, the R wave is usually at its lowest voltage. Reciprocal changes in these leads suggest a posterior wall MI, indicated by tall R waves in V1 and V2 (opposite of deep Qs), ST segment depression, and high, peaked T waves.

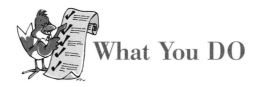

What You DO

When checking for the 12-lead ECG for evidence of an infarction, you should:

- Look in the V leads first (these are the most dangerous).
- Look in the inferior leads next (II, III, aVF).
- Look in the lateral leads next (I, aVL, V5, V6).
- Examine V1 and V2 for tall R waves, ST segment depression, and tall T waves.

To summarize which leads look at what surfaces, examine the following table:

 www.ajn.org/continuing/ce

LEADS	SURFACES OF THE HEART AFFECTED	VESSEL
I, aVL, V5, V6	Left lateral surface	Circumflex
II, III, aVF	Inferior or diaphragmatic	RCA
V1 to V4	Anterior surface	Left anterior
V1 to V2	Posterior	Distal circumflex

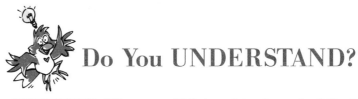

Do You UNDERSTAND?

DIRECTIONS: **What type of MI does the strip on the following page represent?**

1. _____

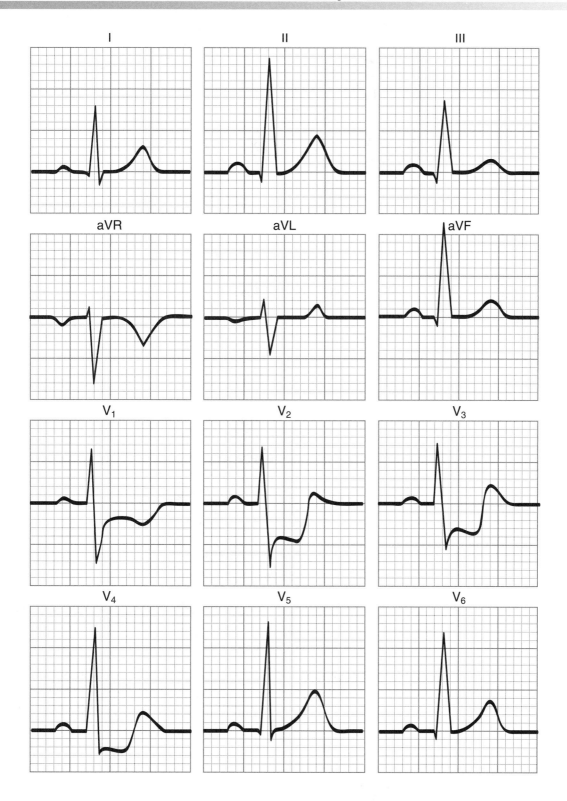

Pericarditis and Cardiac Tamponade

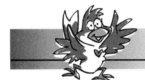

What ARE Pericarditis and Cardiac Tamponade?

Pericarditis is an inflammation of the heart sac (pericardium). The pericardium is a double-layered membrane lining the heart. The outer layer is called the *pericardium*, and the inner layer is called the *epicardium*. The potential space between the two layers contains 30 to 50 cc of serous, lubricating fluid.

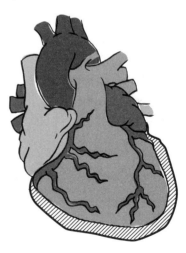

Viral infections (e.g., coxsackievirus, varicella, influenza, human immunodeficiency virus [HIV]) and bacterial infections (e.g., tuberculosis [TB]) are the most common causes of this inflammation. Uremia, renal failure, rheumatic fever, posttraumatic pericarditis and connective tissue diseases (systemic lupus erythematosus, scleroderma, and rheumatoid arthritis) may also cause pericarditis.

Pericarditis can also be caused by medications such as procainamide and hydralazine; radiation treatment for Hodgkin's disease, breast cancer, leukemia, or lymphoma; tumor metastasis to the heart from lung cancer, breast cancer, leukemia, or lymphoma; and by cardiac trauma related to surgery, blunt trauma, or penetrating trauma (see Chapter 21).

Sometimes pericarditis is the result of a myocardial infarction (MI) across all muscle layers of the heart (transmural infarction). The dead and ischemic tissues in an MI stimulate the body's immune response to send white cells and fibrin deposits to the area of injury. The fluid from this injured area can grow large enough to lead to compression of the heart, causing a decrease in cardiac output. This emergent condition is called *cardiac tamponade*.

As intrapericardial pressure rises during cardiac tamponade (more fluid builds up in the sac), right ventricular filling decreases and less blood is delivered to the lungs. Ultimately this decreased blood flow leads to less blood going to the left ventricle, which decreases stroke volume. As a result, the pericardial heart sac stretches to accommodate the increased fluid. This causes increased heart rate, peripheral constriction, and sodium and water retention. Should these compensatory mechanisms fail, the patient experiences an increase in intravascular volume, which increases pericardial pressure and leads to a severe decrease in stroke volume and circulatory collapse. The end result is hypoperfusion of all organs.

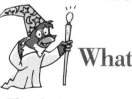

What You NEED TO KNOW

The classic presentation of pericarditis is chest pain, which worsens on inspiration (pleuritic pain) or when lying down. This pain is described as sharp with abrupt onset. The pain lessens when the patient sits up and leans forward.

When listening to the heart, a scratchy sound is also present. This is called a friction rub and is caused by the roughened surfaces of the heart rubbing over one another. The heart sounds may become distant if enough fluid is present.

Classic signs of cardiac tamponade include elevated central venous pressure (CVP), distant heart sounds, arterial hypotension, dyspnea, tachycardia, pulsus paradoxus (pulse becomes weaker during inspiration), and electrical alternans on the electrocardiogram (ECG) (the height of the QRS complex changes with each successive beat, or it is alternately increased and then decreased).

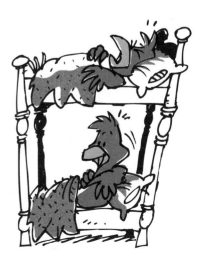

A 12-lead ECG may show the following during pericarditis and cardiac tamponade:

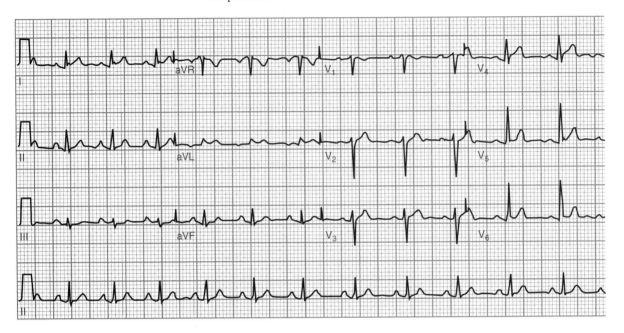

- Sinus rhythm or sinus tachycardia is normal.
- PR interval of the ECG may be depressed but of normal duration.
- Voltage of the QRS complex may be low.
- QRS complexes may alternate voltage with each beat in a large-small pattern. In other words, one complex is taller, the next is smaller, the next is taller, and so on. This is known as electrical alternans and may indicate that large amounts of fluid are compressing the heart's blood inflow (cardiac tamponade).
- ST segment is elevated as with an MI; however, it is elevated throughout the leads of the ECG. Unlike an MI, pericarditis involves the whole heart, not different locations of the heart.
- Q waves do not occur.
- ST segment has a saggy or concave appearance.
- QT interval time is not affected by pericarditis; however, the T wave is upright initially.
- In the recovery phase, the T wave inverts.

The following table shows the differences between ECG changes in an MI versus pericarditis.

Insulin Pump Problems and Solutions

	MI	PERICARDITIS
PR interval	Can prolong block	Unchanged into heart
QRS complex	Q waves	No Q waves
ST segment	Elevated in leads looking at the MI	Elevated with concave ST segment in all leads
QT interval	Longer in inferior MI	Unchanged
T wave	Inverted in leads looking at the infarction	Upright in all leads, then inverted in all

MI, Myocardial infarction.

Differences in laboratory values in MI versus pericarditis include:

- Elevated erythrocyte sedimentation rate (ESR) caused by inflammation process in pericarditis.
- Pericardial fluid analysis reveals lower fibrinogen and hematocrit values than the peripheral blood values in pericarditis.

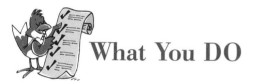

What You DO

When treating patients with pericarditis, you should:

- Position the patient in semi-Fowler's position.
- Auscultate the left lower sternal border where the pericardium lies and where you can best hear a pericardial friction rub (high-pitched scratchy sound heard at the end of inspiration).
- Anticipate possible performance of an echocardiogram (ECHO) to confirm the diagnosis of pericarditis. An ECHO is a noninvasive test performed at the bedside that uses Doppler technology to check the heart and underlying structures.
- Position the patient who has precordial pain in a comfortable position, which is usually sitting upright or leaning forward over the bedside table.
- Assess for increased CVP via a central or pulmonary artery catheter line.
- Assess for pulsus paradoxus, dyspnea, and low urine output.
- Administer oxygen if the SaO2 is less than 93%.
- Administer prescribed drugs. Analgesics, such as salicylates and codeine and nonsteroidal antiinflammatory drugs (NSAIDs) are commonly used to decrease pain and inflammation. Prednisone can be prescribed for severe acute pericarditis but not if the cause is TB, because prednisone exacerbates TB.

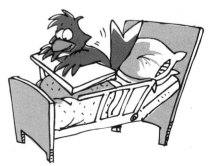

TAKE HOME POINTS

The following are general characteristics of pericarditis:

- **PR interval:** Normal time may be depressed from baseline
- **QRS complex:** Low voltage; may have electrical alternans
- **ST segment:** Elevated with concave appearance in all leads
- **QT interval:** Normal duration
- **T wave:** Elevated in acute phase, inverted later

⚠ Immediately notify the health care provider and prepare for a pericardiocentesis (insertion of a needle under the xyphoid process into the pericardial sac to withdraw the fluid) if the patient develops muffled heart sounds, distended neck veins, and a rapidly decreasing blood pressure (Beck's triad).

- Target treatment toward the underlying cause of the pericarditis, such as antibiotics for bacterial infections.
- Remember that most patients recover within a few weeks.

If you must assist with a pericardiocentesis, you should have an ECG machine on standby. The needle used to remove the fluid from the pericardial sac is attached to the ECG machine with a special clamp. The needle then becomes the electrode. The health care provider pulls the needle back when the ECG shows ST segment elevation, indicating the needle is in the myocardium. Aspiration is then performed.

If the pericardiocentesis is successful, the results to the patient are generally immediate and dramatic. The patient's heart sounds become clearer, the blood pressure (BP) rises, and the neck veins become flat. Sometimes a small chest catheter or chest tube is inserted and left in place, especially if it is thought that fluid will build up again. Sometimes a sclerosing agent (bleomycin, cisplatin, tetracycline) is instilled into the pericardial space to produce an inflammatory response that closes up the space.

In addition, surgery (a pericardial window) can be performed to remove a small piece (a few centimeters) of pericardium to allow the fluid to drain out.

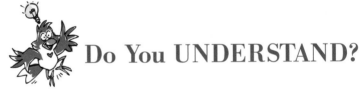

Do You UNDERSTAND?

DIRECTIONS: **List the causes of pericarditis.**

1. Viral causes

_____
_____
_____
_____

2. Other causes

_____
_____
_____
_____
_____
_____
_____
_____
_____
_____

Answers: 1. coxsackievirus, human immunodeficiency virus (HIV), varicella, influenza; 2. uremia, renal failure, rheumatic fever, post-traumatic pericarditis, systemic lupus erythematosus, scleroderma, rheumatoid arthritis, MI, medications, radiation therapy, cancer metastasis to the heart, cardiac trauma, bacterial infections.

DIRECTIONS: Place a check mark in front of the signs and symptoms of pericarditis.

3. a. _____ Dull, achy pain

   b. _____ Sharp, stabbing pain

   c. _____ Pain worsening on expiration

   d. _____ Pain eases with leaning forward

   e. _____ Distant muffled heart sounds

   f. _____ Heart friction rub

DIRECTION: Fill in the blanks.

4. The classic sign of cardiac tamponade is when the patient's pulse becomes weaker during inspiration; it is called

   _____ _____ .

5. The noninvasive test that will tell if the patient has pericarditis is

   _____ .

6. The position of comfort to decrease pain from pericarditis is

   _____ .

7. Two drugs given to decrease inflammation from pericarditis are

   _____ and _____ .

8. If the SaO_2 is less than 93%, _____ is administered.

9. Three signs and symptoms (Beck's triad) that signal a pericarditis may be changing into cardiac tamponade are

   _____ ,

   _____ ,

   and _____ .

10. Auscultation of the pericardium is best at what anatomic location?

    _____

11. Prednisone should not be administered to patient's with pericarditis who have what other disease?

    _____

Answers: 3. b, d, e, f; 4. pulsus paradoxus; 5. ECHO; 6. leaning forward; 7. NSAIDs and salicylates; 8. oxygen; 9. muffled heart sounds, rapidly decreasing blood pressure, distended neck veins; 10. left lower sternal border; 11. tuberculosis (TB).

Drug Effects, Toxicities, and Electrolytes

Drugs can have a striking effect on the waveforms of an electrocardiogram (ECG). Some medications (digoxin, Pronestyl, quinidine) can alter normal patterns. In addition, changes on the ECG can help determine whether patients are developing toxicity from their medications. Serum electrolyte level changes can also show up on the ECG; occasionally, the health care provider can observe changes before serum level reports are back. Therefore it is important for you to know how drugs and electrolytes cause ECG changes.

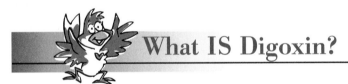

What IS Digoxin?

Digoxin (Lanoxin, Lanoxicaps) is a widely used drug that slows the transportation of sodium and potassium across the heart cell membrane. Digoxin is in a class of drugs called the cardiac glycosides; it slows the influx of sodium and allows an influx of calcium that helps the cardiac muscles to contract. This leads to greater contracting strength of the myocardial cells (positive inotropy). Because the heart is a more efficient pump, it causes an increase in cardiac output.

Digoxin also slows the heart rate (negative chronotropic effect) and atrioventricular (AV) conduction (negative dromotropic effect). This effect can be beneficial in slowing fast rhythms; however, if the heart rate slows too much, low cardiac output results.

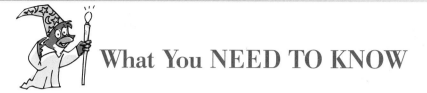

What You NEED TO KNOW

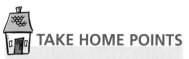

TAKE HOME POINTS

Digoxin is used to increase cardiac contractility; it is often used in heart failure to improve cardiac output. Digoxin can be used to slow down fast cardiac rhythms, such as atrial fibrillation and flutter. It does this by slowing down AV conduction. Digoxin can cause a slurring or scooping of the ST segment. Sometimes the T wave will be lost in this scooping effect.

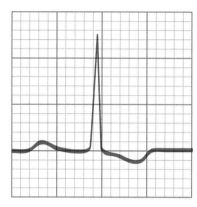

Digoxin can have a depressive effect that causes bradycardia and heart block. Excessive digitalis can result in any type of abnormal heart rhythm, including those with slower heart rates (junctional rhythms, heart blocks) or those with faster atrial rates (atrial tachycardia with block). Other signs of digoxin's affect on the heart that you can see on the ECG strip include:

- **PR interval:** May be prolonged (>0.20 seconds)
- **ST segment:** May have a scooped effect
- **QT interval:** May be shortened
- **T wave:** May fuse into the ST segment

Digitalis can cause the QT interval to shorten and the PR interval to prolong. Dysrhythmias thought to be caused by digitalis toxicity or excess are diagnosed clinically and not strictly from the ECG. The following conditions can increase the chance of developing higher than normal digoxin levels:

CONDITIONS THAT INCREASE DIGOXIN TOXICITY	
Hypokalemia	Hypercalcemia
Renal impairment	Advanced age
Acute hypoxia	Hypothyroidism
Quinidine	

TAKE HOME POINTS

Digoxin has a very narrow therapeutic margin of 0.5 to 1.5 mg/dL, and it is excreted from the body slowly.

Serum digoxin levels need to be monitored, especially in older patients.

Hypokalemia is a common culprit that causes digitoxicity even if the digoxin level is normal. Therefore you should monitor the patients' potassium level and watch for signs of weakness.

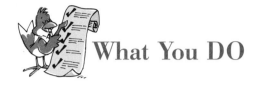

What You DO

> **Toxicity can cause a variety of undesirable disturbances. PVCs, heart blocks, and ventricular tachycardia can be digoxin induced.**

> **Do not give digoxin to patients with heart blocks, sick sinus syndrome, or Wolff-Parkinson-White syndrome with atrial fibrillation or flutter. The treatment of patients with accessory AV pathways and paroxysmal supraventricular tachycardia (PSVT) is usually direct-current cardioversion.**

> **Quinidine can double digoxin levels. Consult the prescribing health care provider if both drugs are ordered. The digitalis dose may be cut in half.**

When treating patients who are receiving digitalis, you should perform the following:

- Monitor serum digoxin levels or remind the health care provider to order a digitalis level.
- Withhold the digoxin dose if digitalis toxicity is suspected and report to the health care provider.
- Monitor for signs of toxicity that include abnormal heart rhythms, visual disturbances (green or yellow halos around objects), and gastrointestinal symptoms (nausea, vomiting, diarrhea).
- Monitor for conditions that increase toxicity.
- Administer lidocaine and phenytoin (Dilantin) to counteract abnormal ventricular rhythms caused by digoxin.
- Administer digoxin immune FAB (Digibind) to reverse life-threatening digitoxicity. However, Digibind is expensive. If the patient has normal kidney function and the dysrhythmias associated with the digitoxicity are not life threatening, the digitalis can be eliminated without medication.

Do You UNDERSTAND?

DIRECTIONS: **Complete the following exercises.**

1. List two ways that digoxin improves the pumping action of the heart.

_____

_____

2. What are the potentially negative effects of digoxin?

_____

_____

DIRECTIONS: **Fill in the blanks.**

3. The normal therapeutic range for serum digoxin is _____ to _____ mg/dL.

4. Digoxin has a _____ effect on the ST segment.

Answers: 1. increases contractility, slows conduction in fast-heart rhythms; 2. If a patient on digoxin already has a slow heart rate, low cardiac output can result; 3. 0.5, 1.5; 4. scooping.

5. Electrolyte imbalances that can cause digitalis toxicity include
_____ and _____.

6. _____, _____,
and _____
cardiac rhythms can be caused by too much digoxin.

7. Do not give digoxin to patients with _____,
_____ and _____
heart rhythms.

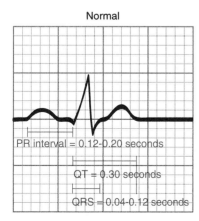

What IS a Class IA Antidysrhythmic?

Class IA antidysrhythmics are a group of drugs that include procainamide (Pronestyl-SR, Procan SR), quinidine (Quinalan, Quinaglute) and disopyramide (e.g., Norpace). These drugs slow entrance of sodium into the cardiac cell and thus decrease the rate of depolarization. These medications depress ectopic areas in both atria and ventricles.

What You NEED TO KNOW

Class IA antidysrhythmic drugs slow down both atrial and ventricular rates. They do not affect rhythm but will prolong AV conduction. When patients receive antidysrhythmic drugs, the ECG may show a slight widening of the QRS complex and a lengthening of the QT interval.

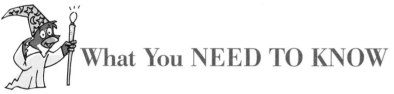

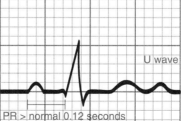

Normal	Class IA Antidysrhythmics
	U wave
PR interval = 0.12-0.20 seconds	PR > normal 0.12 seconds
QT = 0.30 seconds	QT > 0.44 seconds
QRS = 0.04-0.12 seconds	QRS = 0.12 seconds

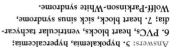

Answers: 5. hypokalemia, hypercalcemia;
6. PVCs, heart blocks, ventricular tachycardia; 7. heart block, sick sinus syndrome,
Wolff-Parkinson-White syndrome.

If the QT interval prolongs more than one half the preceding R-to-R time, the patient may develop Torsade de pointes.

In toxicity, heart block can develop and the QT interval can prolong even further. The rate may become so slow that sometimes another small, positive, upright wave (U wave) occurs after the T wave. A U wave is thought to be caused by repolarization of the Purkinje fibers.

Torsade de pointes is a variant type of ventricular tachycardia (VT); the wide QRS in this rhythm twists and turns above and below the baseline (see Chapter 12).

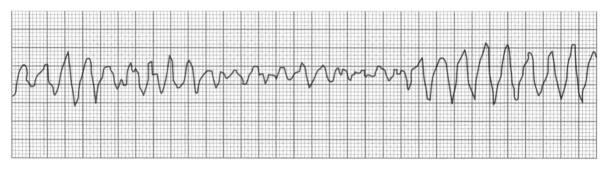

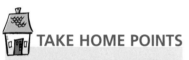 **TAKE HOME POINTS**

Class IA antidysrhythmics may affect the ECG in the following ways:

- **Rate:** Decreased atrial and ventricular rates
- **Rhythm:** No effect
- **PR interval:** Longer than normal
- **QRS complex:** May widen (usually around 0.12 seconds)
- **QT interval:** Longer than normal (greater than 0.44 seconds)
- **Other:** Development of a U wave

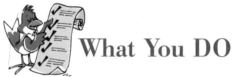 **What You DO**

- Be prepared to administer magnesium and institute cardiac pacing to override this abnormal stimulus electronically and slow down the heart rate if torsades de pointes occurs.
- Observe the patient's ECG closely for excessive prolongation of the PR interval, QRS complex, and QT and RR intervals.
- Hold the drug and notify the health care provider if the QT prolongs more than one half the RR.
- Monitor for signs and symptoms of gastrointestinal effects, such as nausea, vomiting, and diarrhea.

Monitor the patient who is taking Pronestyl for lupuslike syndromes, which may start as rash, fatigue, and swollen achy joints. Also, watch for bleeding.

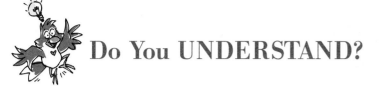

Do You UNDERSTAND?

DIRECTIONS: Indicate in the spaces provided whether the following
statements are *true* or *false*.

1. _____ Class 1A antidysrhythmics block the renin and angiotension
cycle.
2. _____ Class 1A antidysrhythmics do not affect the rhythm, but they
will prolong conduction.
3. _____ In toxic doses, Class 1A antidysrhythmics can cause prolongation of the QT interval and heart block.
4. _____ Class 1A antidysrhythmics may cause a U wave to occur.
5. _____ The U wave is thought to be stimulation of the His bundle.

DIRECTIONS: Match the term in Column A with the definition in
Column B.

Column A

6. _____ U wave
7. _____ Torsade de pointes
8. _____ Lupus
9. _____ PR interval
10. _____ Magnesium
11. _____ Cardiac pacing
12. _____ QT interval

Column B

a. Pronestyl, quinidine, and Norpace
b. Trouble if prolongs more than one
half the R-R
c. Longer than 0.20 seconds
d. Positive deflection between T and P
waves
e. Rash; fatigue; and swollen, achy joints
f. Treatment for torsade de pointes
g. Greater than 0.44 seconds
h. Twisting of the QRS around the baseline

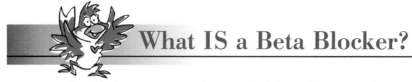

What IS a Beta Blocker?

Beta blockers are commonly prescribed drugs that are used to control blood pressure (BP) and to slow down the heart rate in fast rhythms. Beta blockers work by blocking the action of the sympathetic nervous system (SNS); that is, they block the fight-or-flight response of circulating catecholamines. The desired effect is decreased oxygen demand on the heart. These drugs belong to the class II antidysrhythmic drugs. Commonly used drugs in this class are metoprolol (Lopressor), acebutolol (Sectral), esmolol (Brevibloc) and sotalol (Betapace).

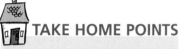

TAKE HOME POINTS

Generic beta blockers may be distinguished by other drug classes by name; most of the generic names end in *olol*.

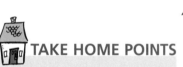

TAKE HOME POINTS

Beta blockers may affect the ECG in the following ways:

- **Rates:** Slows the heart rate.
- **Rhythm:** May cause heart blocks.
- **PR interval:** May prolong PR interval.
- **QRS complex:** If widening of greater than 25% occurs, the dose should be decreased.
- **QT interval:** Shortens the QT interval.

What You NEED TO KNOW

Beta blockers work by slowing down the sinoatrial (SA) node rate. They also slow down conduction. The PR interval may be slightly prolonged, and the QT interval may be shortened.

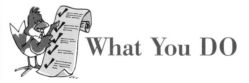

What You DO

When treating patients receiving beta blockers, you should:

- Monitor the patient's heart rate, BP, and ECG.
- Pay particular attention to the duration of the QRS; hold the drug and notify the health care provider if the QRS expands 25% (when compared with previous width).

- Monitor serum electrolytes and correct any imbalances before starting beta blockers.
- Remember that symptoms of asthma or bronchospasm can occur in some patients, because drugs in this class have pulmonary effects.
- Avoid this medication if the patient is bradycardic, in heart block, or is hypotensive.
- Remember that beta blockers decrease contractility and are not used in heart failure, with the exception of carvedilol (Coreg), which is a combination alpha 1 and beta blocker.
- Observe the patient for signs and symptoms of heart failure, especially when used in combination with other drugs (digoxin) that also slow the heart rate.

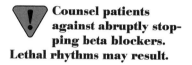

Counsel patients against abruptly stopping beta blockers. Lethal rhythms may result.

Do You UNDERSTAND?

DIRECTIONS: Indicate in the spaces provided whether the following statements are *true* or *false*.

1. _____ Before starting therapy with beta blockers, serum electrolytes should be corrected.
2. _____ You should monitor the patient for signs of heart failure when they are taking beta blockers.
3. _____ Beta blockers work by slowing down the amount of calcium entering the cardiac cells.
4. _____ Beta blockers shorten the PR and QT intervals.
5. _____ A widening of the QRS complex of more than 25% is an expected outcome of beta-blocker therapy.

What IS a Calcium Channel Blocker?

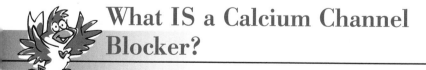

Calcium channel blockers are drugs given to lower the BP in patients with hypertension. They also slow down the heart rate in fast rhythms (e.g., atrial tachycardia, atrial flutter, atrial fibrillation).

Answers: 1. true; 2. true; 3. false; 4. false; 5. false.

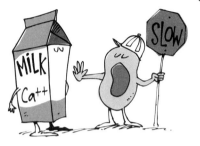

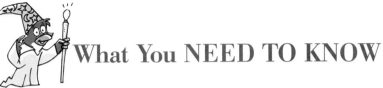

What You NEED TO KNOW

Calcium channel blockers work by slowing down the influx of calcium into the cardiac cell, thus decreasing the contractility of the cell. They are in a class of drugs known as class IV antidysrhythmics. Some of the drugs in this class are verapamil (Calan), nifedipine (Procardia), and diltiazem (Cardizem).

Calcium channel blockers are most commonly used for supraventricular tachycardias (SVTs) because of their ability to slow AV nodal conduction time and prolong AV nodal refractory time.

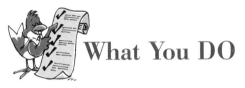

What You DO

⚠ Calcium channel blockers should never be given to patients with bradycardia, sick sinus syndrome, or heart blocks.

When treating patients who are receiving calcium channel blockers, you should:

- Monitor the patient's heart rate, BP, and ECG when starting calcium channel blockers.
- Advise the patient to rise slowly from a resting position. Calcium channel blockers can cause postural hypotension.
- Consult the health care provider if dizziness or postural hypotension continues. The dose may need to be changed.

⚠ The patient can have adverse effects to calcium channel blockers that include bradycardia, heart failure, and hypotension.

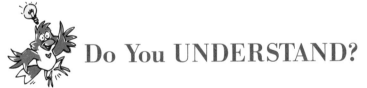

Do You UNDERSTAND?

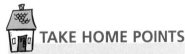

TAKE HOME POINTS

Calcium channel blockers can cause the following ECG changes:

- **Rates:** Slowed from previous rate
- **PR interval:** May be prolonged
- **QT interval:** May be prolonged

DIRECTIONS: **Fill in the blanks.**

1. Calcium channel blockers work by _____ down the influx of calcium into the cardiac cell, thus _____ the contractility of the cell.

2. The patient can experience adverse effects from calcium channel blockers that include _____, _____, and _____.

ELECTROLYTE EFFECTS

Serum and tissue electrolyte imbalances most frequently associated with ECG changes include abnormal potassium, calcium, and magnesium levels (see *Real World Nursing Survival Guide: Fluids & Electrolytes*, Chapters 5, 7, and 8). Normal electrolytes values vary; therefore it is important to check the "normals" for the institution. In general, blood levels of these electrolytes are:

- Potassium = 3.5 to 5.2 mEq/L
- Calcium = 8.5 to 11 mg/dL
- Magnesium 5 1.5 to 2 mEq/L

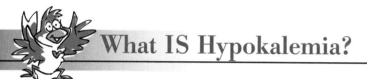

What IS Hypokalemia?

Hypokalemia is a potassium level of below 3.5 mEq/L. The loss of potassium can lead to PVCs, VT, and ventricular fibrillation (VF).

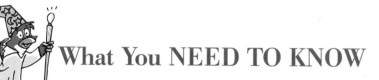

What You NEED TO KNOW

Hypokalemia can be caused by conditions that remove potassium from the body. Although many drugs can do this, the most common culprits are digoxin (Lanoxin); potassium-wasting diuretics, such as furosemide (Lasix), and corticosteroids (Solu-Cortef).

Potassium can also be lost from the urine in patients with elevated blood glucose levels.

Hypokalemia can also be created by conditions that decrease potassium from coming into the body. Dieting, decreased dietary ingestion of potassium, and vomiting can lead to this condition. Serum potassium levels can also be decreased by diarrhea and gastric suctioning.

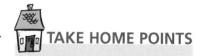

TAKE HOME POINTS

The most common cause of hypokalemia is potassium-wasting diuretics.

Untreated hypokalemia can lead to PVCs, VT, and VF. These are life-threatening dysrhythmias!

The diagnosis of hypokalemia is never made on ECG changes alone. It must always be confirmed with a serum potassium level before treatment. A potassium below 3.5 can cause the following ECG changes to the normal waveform (see below):

- ST segment: Depressed
- OT interval: Prolonged
- T wave: Decreased amplitude
- U waves: Present (if a U wave is present, the QT interval is measured to the end of the U wave and is sometimes called the QU interval.)

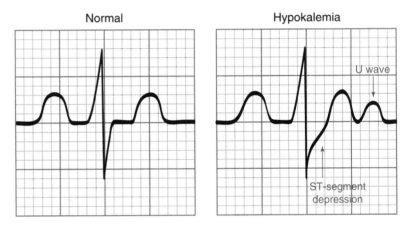

Normal   Hypokalemia

U wave

ST-segment depression

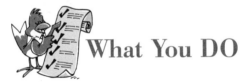

What You DO

When treating patients with hypokalemia, you should remember to:

- Monitor the ECG for ventricular irritability. Potassium replacement therapy may be necessary, particularly if the patient is taking potassium-wasting diuretics.
- Monitor the patient for signs and symptoms of hypokalemia (weakness, fatigue), and teach the patient energy-conserving measures.
- Increase dietary intake of potassium with foods high in potassium, and prescribe supplemental potassium. Foods high in potassium include bananas and dried fruits.
- Administer an antiemetic such as prochlorperazine (Compazine) if hypokalemia is a result of losses through nausea and vomiting; it can be given rectally or by injection.

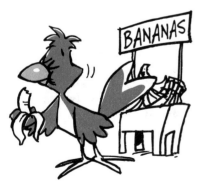

BANANAS

- Use potassium-sparing diuretics, such as spironolactone (Aldactone), as an alternative to potassium-wasting diuretics, such as Lasix (furosemide).
- Once laboratory results have confirmed a low potassium level, administer potassium either orally or intravenously (IV). It is essential to follow institutional protocols for potassium administration, because potassium given IV can cause vein irritation. It is always diluted when given orally or IV.

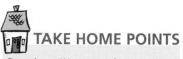

TAKE HOME POINTS

Potassium: "No matter the route, always dilute!"

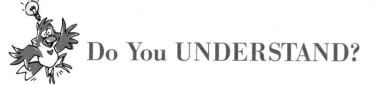

Do You UNDERSTAND?

If potassium is given via IV too rapidly, it can cause cardiac arrest.

DIRECTIONS: **Fill in the blanks.**

1. Name three ways the body can lose potassium.

   _____

   _____

   _____

2. Normal serum potassium level is _____ to _____ mEq/L.

3. An untreated, low potassium can lead to what?

   _____

   _____

   _____

4. If potassium is administered too rapidly via IV, it can cause what?

   _____

Answers: 1. decreased ingestion; potassium-wasting drugs; vomiting, diarrhea, high serum glucose levels, and gastric suctioning; 2. 3.5, 5.2; 3. PVCs, VT, VF; 4. cardiac arrest

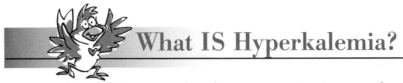

What IS Hyperkalemia?

Hyperkalemia occurs when the serum potassium is greater than 5.2 mEq/L. High levels of potassium cause heart complexes to become wider until they merge into a sine wave. A *sine wave* or *pattern* is a very wide QRS-ST-T pattern that appears like someone taking the PQRST and pulling it from the P to the T, trying to pull it apart.

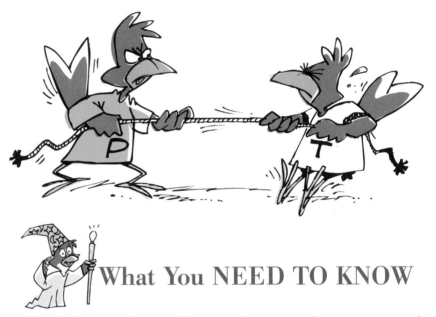

What You NEED TO KNOW

Hyperkalemia can be caused by impaired excretion of potassium as a result of renal disease. Too rapid administration of potassium can cause hyperkalemia. Most of the body's potassium is found inside the cells. Massive tissue injuries, such as crush injuries, myocardial infarction, and burns, can liberate potassium from the cells into the serum.

Laboratory values that reflect a sudden high level of potassium could be the result of poor phlebotomy technique. Using a small needle can destroy red blood cells, causing potassium to be falsely high in the collected specimen. Additionally, removing blood samples from lines that infuse potassium can cause higher levels.

When drawing blood samples from multiple lumen catheters (MLC) or peripheral inserted central catheters (PICCs), the potassium in the IV must be temporarily turned off and a small sample should be discarded. Otherwise, the patient's potassium may be inappropriately high on the laboratory report, which could lead to inappropriate treatment.

Watch for conditions that cause potassium to shift from the tissues into the bloodstream, such as high-level glucose or acidosis.

Signs and symptoms of hyperkalemia include nausea, vomiting, diarrhea, drowsiness, and metal confusion. Neuromuscular changes, such as weakness or paresthesias, may also occur.

Characteristics of hyperkalemia evident on the ECG include small or low voltage P waves. T waves become very tall and peaked. The monitor may double-count the heart rate if the T becomes as tall as the R wave.

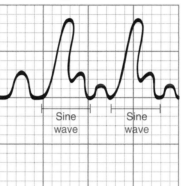

Normal   Hyperkalemia

> ! **Serum potassium levels should be monitored in patients whose pH is reduced (as caused by respiratory or metabolic acidosis) and in those with increased glucose (as caused by diabetic ketoacidosis).**

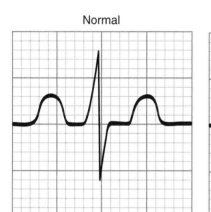

TAKE HOME POINTS

Hyperkalemia can cause the following ECG changes:

- **Rates and rhythm:** Often a bradycardia or heart block; may result in arrest
- **PR interval:** Small, flattened P waves
- **QRS complex:** Widened
- **QT interval:** Prolonged
- **T waves:** Very tall and peaked
- **Other:** Sine wave or arrest if potassium level is very high

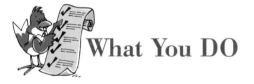

What You DO

When treating patients with hypokalemia, removing potassium from the serum or driving it back into the cell is the goal. You should remember to:

- Administer nonpotassium-sparing diuretics such as furosemide (Lasix) to treat those with mild cases.
- Administer Kayexalate with sorbitol to treat those with moderate cases. Kayexalate binds with potassium in the bowel and eliminates potassium from the body through the feces.
- Administer calcium gluconate to treat those with dangerously high levels of potassium. Calcium gluconate counteracts the negative inotropic effects on the heart.
- Regular insulin and sodium bicarbonate can be added to IVs to drive potassium into the cell when acidosis causes a high level of serum potassium.

- Eliminate all foods, medications, and IVs that contain potassium.
- Consider hemodialysis to decrease serum potassium levels in patients with renal failure or those with severe hyperkalemia.

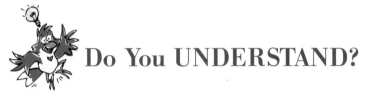

Do You UNDERSTAND?

DIRECTIONS: Determine the serum potassium level, ECG signs, and treatment for hypokalemia and hyperkalemia.

Hypokalemia

1. Serum level: _____

2. ECG signs: _____

    _____

    _____

3. Treatment: _____

Hyperkalemia

4. Serum level: _____

5. ECG signs: _____

    _____

    _____

6. Treatment: _____

Answers: 1. Less than 3.5mEq/L; 2. prolonged PR intervals, U wave, PVCs can lead to ventricular tachycardia; 3. K+ replacement oral or IৢV; 4. greater than 5.2 mEq/L; 5. small P wave, tall peaked T wave, prolonged QRS, bradycardias, cardiac arrest; 6. diuretics, calcium, HCO_3, and insulin, Kayexalate, hemodialysis.

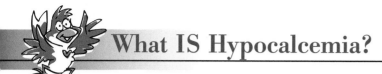

What IS Hypocalcemia?

Calcium is important for cellular excitability, smooth muscle contractility, and transmission of nerve impulses. Most of the body's calcium is stored in the bone, and only approximately 1% is found in the serum. One half of serum calcium is free or ionized, which is the active form of calcium. The other half is bound to albumin, which is a serum protein.

With normal levels of serum albumin, those with ionized calcium levels below 8.5 mg/dL are considered to have *hypocalcemia*. Calcium is needed by the cardiac cells to help with contraction. When calcium is low, the heart does not beat as strongly as it should.

What You NEED TO KNOW

Causes of low calcium include hypomagnesemia or hypoparathyroidism. A decreased dietary intake of calcium, as well as diarrhea, can cause calcium loss. Since one half of the serum calcium is bound to serum proteins (albumin), a low level of blood proteins will also lower the level of serum calcium. Prolonged bedrest with limited vitamin D and exposure to sunlight can cause hypocalcemia in critically or chronically ill patients. Surgical removal of the parathyroid can also result in hypocalcemia. As the level of serum phosphorus increases, calcium decreases. Calcium can be lost in burn fluid, peritonitis, and infection. A calcium below 8.5 mg/dL can cause the QT interval to prolong. The T waves may become flatter. A low serum calcium level can cause ventricular dysrhythmias.

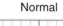

TAKE HOME POINTS

Magnesium and calcium deficiencies are often found together. Monitor the magnesium level as well.

Normal

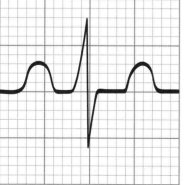

Hypocalcemia

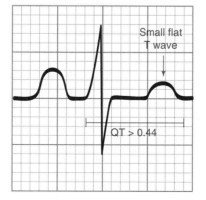

Small flat T wave

QT > 0.44

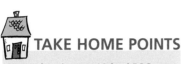

TAKE HOME POINTS

Hypocalcemia on a 12-lead ECG can cause the following changes:

Rate: May be anything

Rhythm: Possible regular, ventricular dysrhythmias

PR interval: Can prolong

QRS complex: Lengthened

ST segment and T wave: Flattened

QT interval: Prolongs

The patient may exhibit signs or symptoms of decreased cardiac contractility. Cardio-vascular effects can include decreased cardiac output and congestive heart failure, which can lead to cardiac arrest.

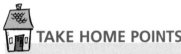

TAKE HOME POINTS

Low levels of calcium are treated with the oral administration of calcium, IV push, or IV infusion of calcium gluconate chloride.

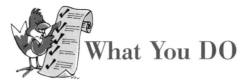

What You DO

When treating patients with hypocalcemia, you should remember to:

- Observe and monitor calcium levels and report any abnormal levels to the health care provider.
- Assess the patient for signs and symptoms of a low level of calcium. Chvostek's sign (facial twitching after a finger tap on the supramandibular portion of the parotid gland) and Trousseau's sign (carpopedal spasm after inflation of blood pressure cuff to upper arm) are indicators of the neuromuscular irritability that accompanies hypocalcemia.
- Be prepared for emergency airway management, which may include endotracheal intubation or tracheostomy. Patients with low levels of calcium can have laryngeal spasms, resulting in airway obstruction.

Do You UNDERSTAND?

DIRECTIONS: Provide answers to the following questions.

1. Hypocalcemia may have what electrophysiologic effects?

    _____
    _____
    _____

2. What neuromuscular signs does hypocalcemia include?

    _____
    _____
    _____
    _____
    _____

3. A true medical emergency of hypocalcemia includes what?
    (*Give at least two symptoms.*)

    _____
    _____
    _____
    _____

Answers: 1. QTs get longer, T waves may flatten, ventricular dysrhythmias are possible; 2. neuromuscular irritability, numbness, tingling, Chvostek's sign, Trousseau's sign; 3. Seizures, airway obstruction, heart failure, cardiac arrest.

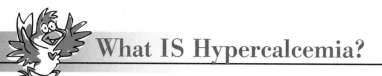

What IS Hypercalcemia?

Hypercalcemia is a calcium blood level of above 11 mg/dL. High levels of calcium affect the heart by reducing threshold potential and decreasing excitability.

What You NEED TO KNOW

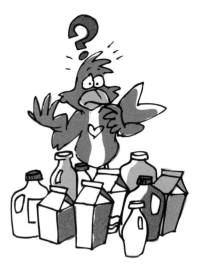

Hypercalcemia is caused by excessive bone reabsorption of calcium, which is often the result of an increase in parathyroid hormone or metastatic cancers. The body usually increases renal excretion of calcium when there is either greater dietary consumption or ingestion of calcium supplements. Hypercalcemia can also occur if there is ingestion of increased calcium in the presence of kidney failure.

ECG changes from hypercalcemia may include a shortened ST segment and QT interval and a prolonged PR interval and QRS complex. In severe hypercalcemia, AV blocks may occur.

Women who are taking calcium supplements to prevent the effects of osteoporosis should be taught the correct dose and the importance of hydration to prevent the formation of kidney stones.

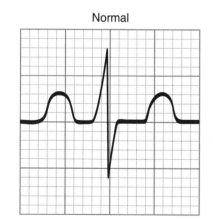

Normal

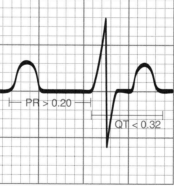

Hypercalcemia

PR > 0.20
QT < 0.32

TAKE HOME POINTS

High calcium can cause the following ECG changes:

Rate: Slow
Rhythm: May be variable
PR interval: Normal
QRS complex: Progressive widening
QT segment: Shortened

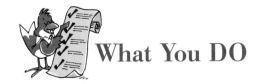

What You DO

When treating patients with hypercalcemia, you should remember to:
- Monitor calcium levels and the neurologic status of the patient. Fatigue, loss of deep tendon reflexes (DTRs), thirst, constipation, and kidney stones may be present.
- Administer large amounts of IV saline to dilute the calcium and help it pass from the body.
- Administer loop diuretics, if prescribed.
- Administer IV phosphate, if prescribed. Phosphate and calcium work in opposition. As the phosphate levels rise, calcium levels decrease.
- Eliminate foods containing calcium from the patient's diet.
- Include cytoxic antibiotics (e.g., Mithracin) and hormones (e.g., calcitonin) that block bone release of calcium as a treatment of extreme hypercalcemia.

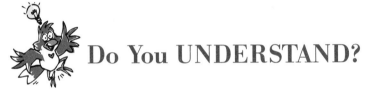

Do You UNDERSTAND?

DIRECTIONS: **Provide four risks for hypercalcemia?**

1. _____
2. _____
3. _____
4. _____

DIRECTIONS: **Describe three ECG changes observed with hypercalcemia.**

5. _____
6. _____
7. _____

Answers: 1. prolonged bedrest; 2. renal failure; 3. hyperparathyroidism; 4. cancer may be at risk for hypercalcemia; 5. short or absent ST segment; 6. decreased QT interval; 7. prolonged PR and QRS.

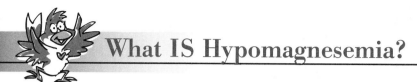

What IS Hypomagnesemia?

Magnesium is primarily found in the cells and bones. It is important for maintaining neuromuscular activities, blood clotting, and normal cardiac-action potentials. A low level of magnesium places patients at risk for developing a lethal form of VT, known as torsades de points. *Hypomagnesemia* is a condition in which the magnesium level falls below 1.5 mEq/L.

A decrease in the level of magnesium slows the release of an enzyme called acetylcholine. Acetylcholine helps stimulate the parasympathetic nervous system. Therefore a low level of magnesium will increase the fight-or-flight response.

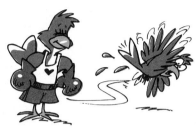

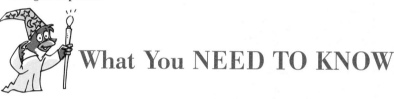

What You NEED TO KNOW

A low level of magnesium has the same effects as hypocalcemia, and it has the same causes. Review the discussion of hypocalcemia on pages 223-224 in this chapter.

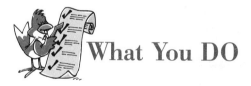

What You DO

When treating patients with hypomagnesemia, you should remember to:
- Identify low levels of magnesium and determine the causes.
- Assess for signs of neuromuscular irritability and institute seizure precautions.
- Consider prescribing calcium or magnesium supplements. Magnesium sulfate may be given as a continuous or intermittent infusion. A typical dose is 2 to 6 g IV over several minutes.
- Watch for potassium depletion, which may also occur with hypomagnesemia.

When administering magnesium sulfate, the patient's heart rate, blood pressure, respirations, SaO$_2$, ECG, and neurologic changes must be monitored. Deep tendon reflexes and the level of consciousness must be evaluated, because an increased magnesium can also lead to cardiac arrest as a result of inadequate heart stimulation.

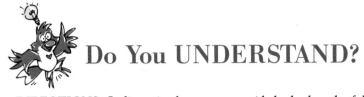

Do You UNDERSTAND?

DIRECTIONS: **Indicate in the spaces provided whether the following statements are *true* or *false*.**

1. _____ Dose is 3.5 to 5.2 mEq/kg.
2. _____ Dose is always given diluted.
3. _____ Dose is 2 to 6 g IV push
4. _____ Calcium supplements may also be given
5. _____ Can be mixed in an IV bag and administered via drip

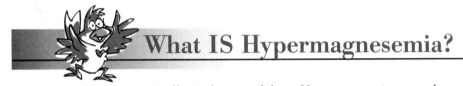

What IS Hypermagnesemia?

Magnesium is a cell membrane stabilizer. *Hypermagnesemia* is an elevated level of magnesium, and it causes the cells to be less sensitive to stimuli. If the levels are high, the cells may not respond to *any* stimulus. The clinical presentation of a high level of magnesium includes muscle weakness, confusion, and respiratory paralysis. At levels greater than 6 mEq/L, the patient may develop bradycardia, hypotension, increased PR intervals, widened QRS complexes, and elevated T waves.

A high level of magnesium is similar to a high level of calcium. Review the section on hypercalcemia on pages 225-226 in the chapter.

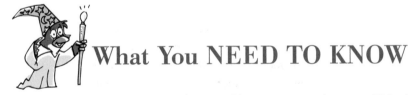

What You NEED TO KNOW

High levels of magnesium can be caused by increases in the rate of IV solutions that contain magnesium, such as parenteral nutrition or hyperalimentation solutions. Antacids that contain magnesium include aluminum hydroxide (Maalox) and simethicone (Mylanta). Overuse of antacids can cause the magnesium levels to rise. In addition, overuse of laxatives such magnesium hydroxide (Milk of Magnesia) can cause hypermagnesemia.

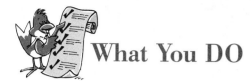

What You DO

When treating patients with hypercalcemia, you should remember to:

- Monitor serum magnesium levels.
- Observe for the early signs of hypermagnesemia.
- Assess the use of over-the-counter medications for the potential effects of hypermagnesemia.
- If prescribed, administer calcium gluconate to treat the cardiac effects of hypermagnesemia.
- If prescribed, administer diuretics to increase magnesium loss.
- Monitor vital signs and cardiac status.

> **!** **Diuretics should be administered only to patients with normal renal function.**

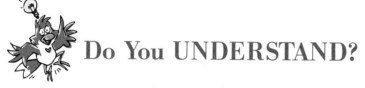

Do You UNDERSTAND?

> **!** **Observe the patient for signs of respiratory depression. Resuscitation equipment should be readily available.**

DIRECTIONS: **Place a check next to the features associated with hypermagnesemia.**

1. _____ Magnesium level < 1.5 mEq/L
2. _____ Magnesium level > 2 mEq/L
3. _____ Shortened QT interval
4. _____ Administer magnesium sulfate
5. _____ Administer diuretics/saline infusions

20 Conduction Defects and Accessory Pathways

This chapter covers special conduction syndromes that may occur in your patients. Two of the more common conduction system defects, (1) Lown-Ganong-Levine (LGL) syndrome and (2) Wolff-Parkinson-White (WPW) syndrome, and the accessory pathways associated with them are discussed.

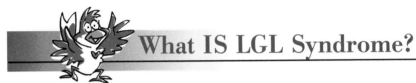

What IS LGL Syndrome?

LGL syndrome is a rhythm caused by the presence of an alternative conduction pathway that bridges the atria and ventricles by avoiding the atrioventricular (AV) node and entering the upper end of the bundle of His. The accessory pathway is referred to as James fibers.

This disorder was first described by the American physicians Lown and Levine and by physiologist Ganong. It is characterized by a stimulus bypassing the AV node and exciting the ventricles earlier than normal. Patients with this syndrome, which is difficult to detect, may complain of intermittent palpitations and experience supraventricular tachydysrhythmias.

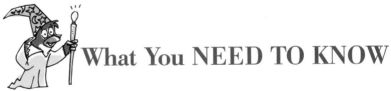

What You NEED TO KNOW

When a stimulus bypasses the AV node in LGL, the PR interval is shortened, because the impulse is not delayed at the AV node. There is no preexcitation of the ventricular muscle; therefore there is no aberrant ventricular conduction. For this reason, LGL syndrome is sometimes called the short PR normal QRS syndrome.

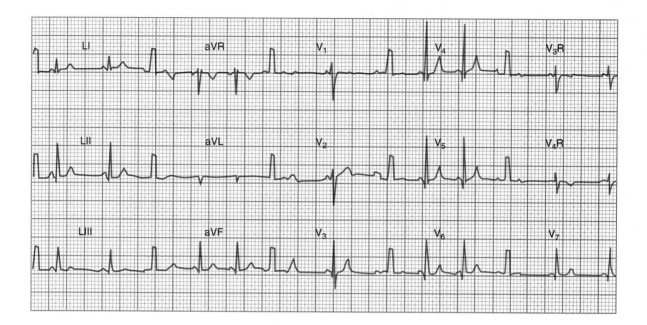

Supraventricular tachycardia (SVT) is also one of the distinguishing features of LGL syndrome. The tachycardias in LGL syndrome are thought to be from an AV-reciprocating mechanism that causes a marked difference in conduction times between retrograde conduction up the fast (bypass) pathway and slow conduction down the regular nodal pathway, providing opportunity for reentry (reactivation of a tissue for the second time by the same impulse).

What IS WPW Syndrome?

WPW syndrome is an abnormal condition in which the ventricles are stimulated by an early impulse traveling down an alternative conduction pathway that bridges the atria and ventricles either anteriorly or posteriorly. This conduction pathway is called *Kent's bundle*. Because of the presence of the Kent's bundle, descending atrial impulses have two routes between the atria and ventricles. The accessory pathway has a greater conduction velocity than the normal conduction pathway because it bypasses the delay at the AV node.

TAKE HOME POINTS

The characteristics of LGL syndrome include:

- **PR interval:** Short (less than .12 seconds)
- **QRS complex:** Normal width (less than 0.12 seconds)
- **Rhythms:** Fast supraventricular rhythms
- **Other:** Holter monitoring may be used for 24-hour observation

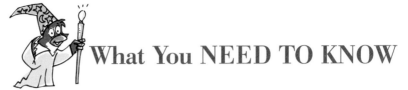

What You NEED TO KNOW

In WPW syndrome, a depolarization wave from the SA node may reach the AV node and the accessory pathway at the same time; the impulses traversing the two pathways may reach the ventricular cells at different times.

The characteristics of WPW syndrome include:

- PR interval is short (less than 0.12 seconds). Unlike the PR interval in LGL syndrome, the PR interval in WPW syndrome has a delta wave. A delta wave is a slurring of the QRS complex, resulting from impulses traveling to the ventricles by different conduction pathways and depolarizing the ventricular myocardium from different directions at the same time.
- QRS complex is 0.12 seconds wide or wider. Aberrant ventricular conduction is present.

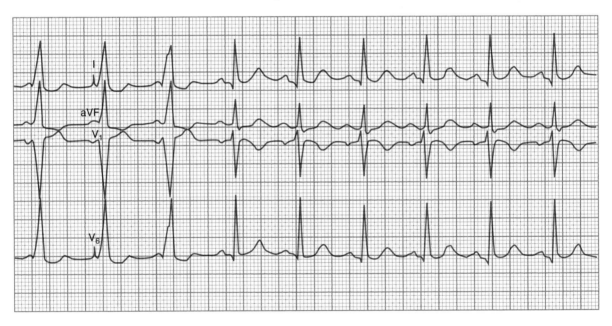

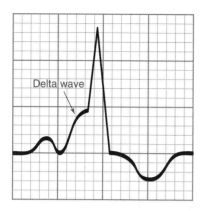

Delta wave

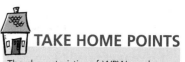

TAKE HOME POINTS

The characteristics of WPW syndrome include:

- **PR interval:** Short (less than 0.12 seconds).
- **QRS complex:** Aberrant ventricular conduction; 0.12 seconds wide or wider
- **Rate:** Normal or fast

- Rate can be normal or fast. Patients with WPW may experience dysrhythmias, such as SVT, atrial flutter, and atrial fibrillation. Supraventricular tachydysrhythmias in WPW may result from a reentry circuit using the accessory pathway and the AV node. If the patient develops atrial fibrillation, the ventricular rate may become so rapid that the rhythm will deteriorate to ventricular fibrillation.

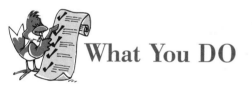

What You DO

The treatments for LGL and WPW are very similar. In patients with LGL, electrical physiologic studies (EPSs) may be performed to determine the location of the abnormal conduction pathway. EPSs are invasive tests that determine more about the abnormal conduction in the heart and the specific, effective therapy for the conduction disturbance.

Surgical interruption or radio frequency ablation of the abnormal AV pathway may be indicated in patients with LGL syndrome. Complications of radio frequency ablation may include postprocedure heart blocks.

When working with patients with WPW syndrome, you should first administer adenosine (Adenocard) to block fast tachydysrhythmias. However, this may not work if the patient is in atrial fibrillation or flutter.

If the QRS complex becomes wide during the tachycardia, do not give verapamil to the patient unless the tachycardia is known with certainty to be supraventricular in origin. Verapamil can accelerate the heart rate and decrease the blood pressure. The recommendation from the 1992 National Conference on CPR and ECC is to use lidocaine as the first agent in ventricular tachycardia (VT) and any wide complex tachycardia of unknown origin.

If either LGL or WPW is apparent, you should remember to perform the following:

- Observe for fast, tachydysrhythmias. If the patient experiences signs and symptoms, such as hypotension, chest pain, shortness of breath, or any change in level of consciousness, you should contact the health care provider and be prepared for intervention following the institution's accepted protocols.
- Treat the patient with SVT, which is aimed at interrupting the fast rhythm. If the patient is hemodynamically unstable, synchronized cardioversion is indicated.
- In the stable patient, practice vagal maneuvers and administer antidysrhythmic drugs (adenosine, verapamil). Vagal maneuvers may slow the heart rate and help you determine the underlying rhythm.
- Overdrive pacing may be successful in terminating the rhythm.

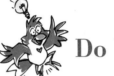 Do You UNDERSTAND?

DIRECTIONS: **Fill in the blanks.**

1. List three characteristics of LGL syndrome:

_____

_____

_____

DIRECTIONS: **Place a check in the spaces under each conduction syndrome (LGL or WPW) if the symptom is associated with the syndrome(s).**

	LGL	WPW	Symptom
2.	_____	_____	Short PR interval
3.	_____	_____	Long QRS
4.	_____	_____	Delta wave
5.	_____	_____	Normal QRS
6.	_____	_____	Tachydysrythmias
7.	_____	_____	Long QT interval

Answers: 1. Short PR interval (less than 0.12 seconds), normal width QRS complex (less than 0.12 seconds), fast supraventricular rhythms; 2. LGL, WPW; 3. WPW; 4. WPW; 5. LGL; 6. LGL, WPW; 7. WPW.

DIRECTIONS: **Place a check in the spaces under each conduction syn-**
drome (LGL or WPW) if the drug is treatment for the
syndrome(s).

LGL	WPW	Symptom
8. _____	_____	Digoxin
9. _____	_____	Beta-blockers, such as propranolol (Inderal)
10. _____	_____	Adenosine
11. _____	_____	Verapamil (Calan)
12. _____	_____	Pronestyl

DIRECTIONS: **Complete the crossword puzzle.**

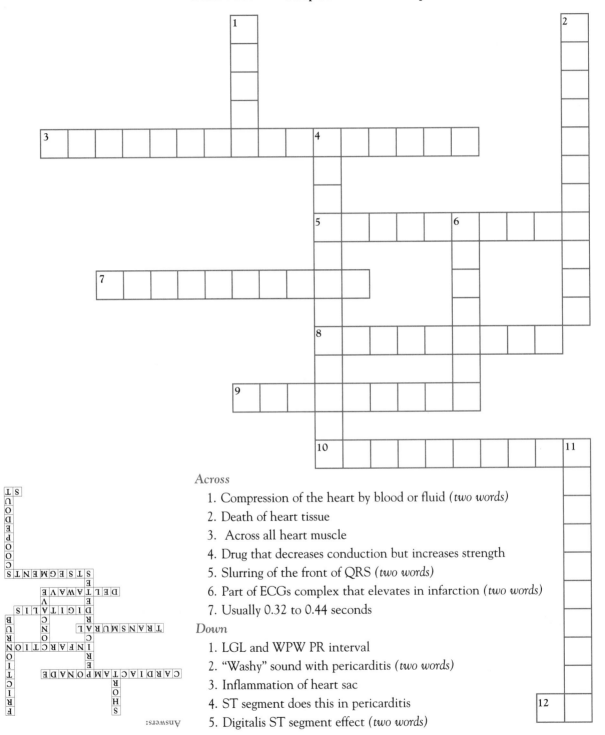

Across

1. Compression of the heart by blood or fluid (*two words*)
2. Death of heart tissue
3. Across all heart muscle
4. Drug that decreases conduction but increases strength
5. Slurring of the front of QRS (*two words*)
6. Part of ECGs complex that elevates in infarction (*two words*)
7. Usually 0.32 to 0.44 seconds

Down

1. LGL and WPW PR interval
2. "Washy" sound with pericarditis (*two words*)
3. Inflammation of heart sac
4. ST segment does this in pericarditis
5. Digitalis ST segment effect (*two words*)

Answers:

21 Special Considerations

This chapter provides a synopsis of major cardiac events that have special considerations for electrocardiogram (ECG) monitoring. Four distinct areas provide reference for ECG considerations pertaining to electrical cardiac therapy, drug abuse, surgical therapy, and cardiac trauma.

ELECTRICAL CARDIAC THERAPY

Sudden cardiac death (SCD) is the result of an electrical malfunction of the heart that leads to a dangerous heart rhythm. In some situations (drug toxicity, electrolyte imbalance, myocardial infarction [MI]), the triggering event can be remedied and the life-threatening rhythm can be resolved. Although some patients respond favorably to antiarrhythmic medications, when the cause of the malfunction is not identified or if pharmacologic treatments are ineffective or poorly tolerated, dangerous heart rhythms are sometimes treated with electrical therapy delivered by an implantable cardioverter defibrillator (ICD). Since their introduction, ICD use has reduced the recurrence rate of SCD from 25% to 2%.

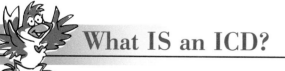

What IS an ICD?

An *ICD* is designed to detect and treat life-threatening dysrhythmias, such as ventricular tachycardia (VT) and ventricular fibrillation (VF). It is also used to treat less-threatening conditions, such as atrial fibrillation. When a

⚠ **Electromagnetic interference from electronic antitheft surveillance devices (often used in stores and libraries) can cause complete AV block. Should this happen, you should move the patient away from the antitheft equipment immediately.**

⚠ **Transcutaneous nerve stimulators (TENS) used for pain control can create electrical artifact, leading to inappropriate ICD delivery.**

⚠ **Magnet mode is very important during acute resuscitation efforts, because the functioning of the ICD may interfere with emergency treatment.**

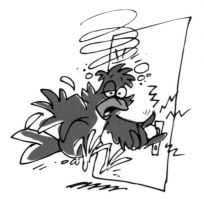

dangerous rhythm is recognized, the ICD provides a shock (electrical stimulation) directly to the heart muscle to stop dysrhythmias and allow the heart to resume its normal electrical pattern. The device consists of one or more thin, insulated wires (leads) that are in contact with the heart muscle and connected to an implanted pulse generator. Rapid technologic advancements in electrophysiology have produced sophisticated ICDs that can be programmed to deliver a variety of patterns and intensities of electrical therapy in response to abnormal rhythms. The sensation experienced by the individual when the device discharges varies with the pattern and intensity of the therapy. The individual's body may go limp and fall, a tingling sensation may be noted, or in some instances, an individual may not even be aware that the device has discharged.

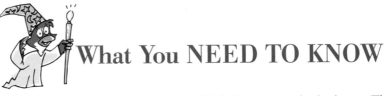

What You NEED TO KNOW

ICDs use electrical impulses to control life-threatening dysrhythmias. These devices are programmed to recognize certain rhythms and deliver specified electrical therapy.

ICDs are implanted in a procedure very similar to pacemaker implantation. The surgeon guides the lead placement through a major vein via fluoroscopy, and the generator is implanted in a superficial skin pocket in the abdomen or upper chest.

A standard pacemaker magnet placed over the ICD pulse generator activates the *magnet mode* feature. Although the magnet mode feature varies among manufacturers; it is generally used to *suppress* ICD therapy.

Symptoms of a malfunctioning ICD may include:

- Dizziness
- Syncope
- Palpitations
- Inappropriate "shocks"

If you suspect that a patient's ICD is suspected of malfunctioning, you must continuously monitor the ECG for VT or VF.

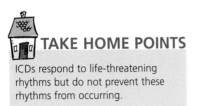

🏠 TAKE HOME POINTS

ICDs respond to life-threatening rhythms but do not prevent these rhythms from occurring.

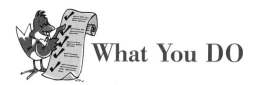

What You DO

When treating patients with ICDs, you should remember the following:

- During the admission assessment, obtain as much information as possible regarding the device used by the patient. Ask if the patient was given an "ICD information and identification card" and when the device was implanted. If no card is available, determine the approximate date of implantation. Generally, newer devices are more sophisticated than those implanted years ago.
- Keep resuscitation equipment handy if the device is suspected of malfunctioning.
- Continuously monitor the ECG of a symptomatic patient. Watch for signs of VT and VF.
- Have a pacemaker magnet available to deactivate the ICD if necessary. It may be necessary to deactivate the ICD with a pacemaker magnet to prevent interference with resuscitation efforts.
- If you are unfamiliar with the functions of the particular device, call for assistance before placing a magnet near the ICD generator.
- If dangerous rhythms (VT, VF) occur despite the presence of an ICD, resuscitate the patient per ACLS guidelines.
- Advise patients to stay away from antitheft electronic devices found in stores or libraries to avoid atrioventricular (AV) block.

Signs of VT

- *Rate:* Rapid in the patient with supraventricular tachycardia (SVT) or VT
- *Rhythm:* Usually not possible to determine the atrial rhythm; regular ventricular rhythm
- *P-waves:* Usually not visible; obscured by the QRS complexes
- *QRS complex:* Wide (greater than 0.14 seconds)

 TAKE HOME POINTS

Cellular telephones only interfere with ICDs during telemetric transmission and programming. Otherwise they are safe for use by patients with ICDs.

Do not use a TENS unit on someone with an ICD, because it will create artifact leading to ICD delivery.

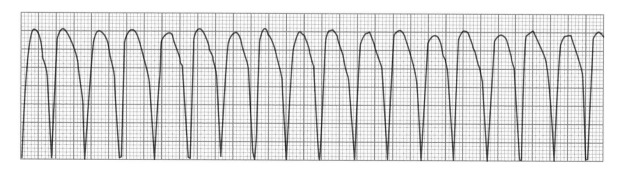

Signs of VF

VF is rapidly fatal if left untreated.

- *Rate:* Not measurable
- *Rhythm:* Irregular, chaotic
- *P waves:* Not visible
- *QRS complex:* No identifiable complexes

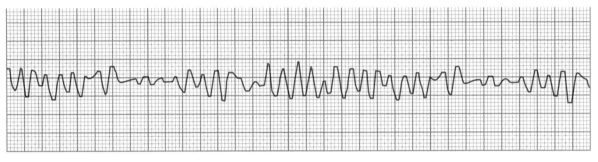

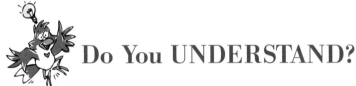

Do You UNDERSTAND?

DIRECTIONS: **Indicate in the spaces provided whether the following statements are *true* or *false*.**

1. _____ ICD devices are one of the **initial** techniques used to treating rhythm disturbances.
2. _____ ICDs detect potentially lethal dysrhythmias.
3. _____ Placement of an ICD requires an open thoracostomy procedure.
4. _____ A patient who has a potentially lethal arrhythmia despite the presence of an ICD should be resuscitated according to ACLS guidelines.
5. _____ The ICD device consists of one or more insulated metal leads in contact with the myocardial tissue and connected to a pulse generator.

Answers: 1. false; 2. true; 3. false; 4. true; 5. true.

DIRECTIONS: Unscramble the letters in the word jumble to fill in the blanks. When all words in the jumble have been unscrambled and entered into the blanks, the circled letters form one last jumbled word. What is it?

6. __ ◯◯ __ __ __ __ SIPLUME

7. __ __ ◯ __ __ __ __ __ __ __ __ VERANTUSSNO

8. __ ◯ __ ◯ __ ◯ __ __ __ TEERGARON

9. __ __ __ ◯ __ ◯ __ __ __ LETILCAER

10. __ __ __ __ ◯ OKCHS

11. ◯◯◯◯◯◯◯◯

DIRECTIONS: Answer the following questions.

12. What potential danger could occur if a patient with an ICD stands near the generator of a department store's alarm system?

13. Your patient has an ICD and asks you if he or she can use his cellular telephone. What is your response?

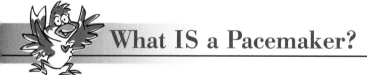

What IS a Pacemaker?

Heart muscle contracts when it is stimulated by an electrical impulse. This electrical impulse normally originates in the sinoatrial (SA) node of the right ventricle and travels along a specific pathway to the ventricles. This specialized function has earned the SA node the title of "the heart's natural pacemaker." Deviations from the usual electrical impulse pattern cause changes in heart rhythm. The heart may beat too fast or slow. Perhaps the designated pathway is blocked preventing impulses from reaching their destination. When the heart's natural pacemaker falters, an artificial pacemaker is used to restore a healthy electrical impulse pattern.

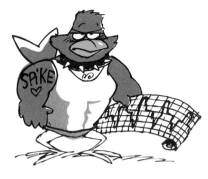

A *pacemaker* is a programmable, battery-operated device that delivers a precisely timed electrical impulse to the heart muscle. The electrical impulse comes from the pacemaker generator and is delivered through thin insulated wires called *leads*. The electrical stimulus is seen on the ECG as a pacemaker *spike*. If depolarization occurs, it will be observed as a P wave (atrial depolarization) or QRS complex (ventricular depolarization). The term *capture* indicates that the electrical stimulus has successfully depolarized the heart muscle and now controls the chamber.

Most pacemakers *sense* the heart's naturally occurring rhythm and deliver the battery-generated impulse only when necessary; this is called *demand pacing*. In certain emergency situations (when a patient is asystolic or extremely bradycardic), *fixed rate pacing* delivers the electrical stimulus, regardless of the patient's own heart rhythm.

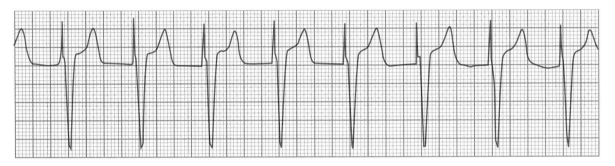

Temporary Versus Permanent Pacemakers

Temporary pacemakers are used in emergency situations and for short-term therapy. Leads for a temporary pacing system may be placed directly into the heart muscle and exit through the skin of the chest (epicardial leads). This type of pacing commonly occurs with postoperative cardiac surgery patients. Temporary leads might also be threaded into place through a large vessel and emerge through the skin in the subclavian area. The temporary leads are attached to a generator box that remains outside the body where the settings can be adjusted manually, if necessary. Exposed transvenous or epicardial pacing wires should be insulated to prevent delivery of unintentional *microshocks* to the heart muscle. Because the wires are in direct contact with the heart muscle, even weak static-generated electrical impulses can be problematic. In emergency situations, temporary pacing is sometimes accomplished via electrode patches placed on the chest wall. This is called *transcutaneous pacing* and is used until a temporary or permanent transvenous pacer can be inserted.

Leads for a *permanent pacemaker* are usually guided to the inner heart wall through a large vein using radiographic images (fluoroscopy or transvenous placement). The leads are tunneled beneath the skin, connecting the heart muscle to the pacemaker. Permanent pacemakers are about the size of a silver dollar and weigh approximately 1 ounce.

Modern, implanted pacemakers are true wonders of technology. The feature that makes them so useful in the treatment of dysrhythmias is their ability to be *programmed* transdermally to meet the needs of the individual. The programmer is a device that uses radio waves to communicate with the pacemaker's pulse generator. The pacemaker generator can be reprogrammed without surgery because the radio frequencies are detected through the skin.

Pacemaker *check-ups* can take place over the telephone. Information about the individual's rhythm, the status of the pulse generator's battery, and the pacemaker's pacing capability are delivered to the medical facility by a transmitting unit over telephone lines.

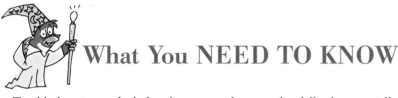

What You NEED TO KNOW

Troubleshooting a dual-chamber pacemaker may be difficult, especially if you are unsure how it is programmed. The general rule is to notify the health care provider if the patient is symptomatic or there is any suggestion of pacer malfunction. Symptoms of *malfunctioning* pacemaker may include:

- Dizziness
- Fainting spells (syncope)
- Change in mental status
- Difficulty breathing
- Prolonged weakness or fatigue
- Prolonged hiccups
  Vital signs may reveal:
- Decreased heart rate (less than preset low limit)
- Increased heart rate (greater than 100 bpm)
- Irregular heart rhythm
- Decreased blood pressure
- Increased respiratory rate

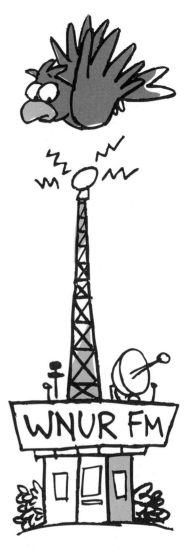

Pacemakers are unaffected by common household appliances. Arc welding or powerful magnets (including those used in magnetic resonance imaging) can affect pacemaker function.

A discharging pacemaker is visible on a monitor or ECG strip. The electrical stimulus causes a *spike* or pacemaker artifact, followed by depolarization. If no pacer spike is observed and the rhythm is not dangerous, it may indicate that the patient's own rhythm is being sensed and stimulation is unnecessary. However, a symptomatic individual with a pacemaker should always receive continuous monitoring.

Single-chamber pacemakers sense and pace in either the right ventricle or the right atrium.

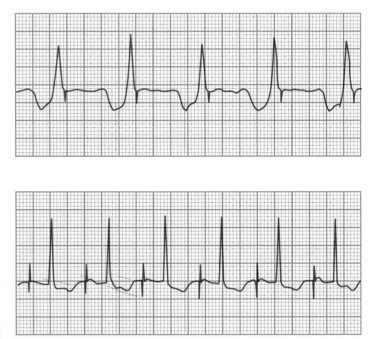

Dual-chamber pacemakers sense and pace both the right atrium and the right ventricle in a precisely timed pattern.

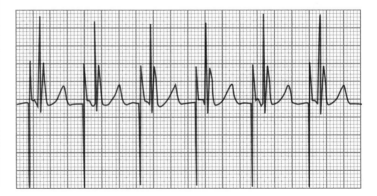

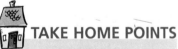

TAKE HOME POINTS

Look at the **individual.** How is the rhythm being tolerated?

- **Rate:** Because parameters are set during programming, a very fast or slow rhythm may indicate a malfunctioning pacemaker.

- **Rhythm:** Rhythm is regular, if the pacemaker is functioning appropriately.

- **P waves:** P waves are present if an atrium is being paced; they are not present if only a ventricle is being paced.

- **QRS complex:** Indicates ventricular depolarization; it should be regular in response to pacemaker stimuli. A wide QRS complex is a normal finding in paced rhythms.

- **QT interval:** It is within normal limits.

Pacemakers are sophisticated, programmable devices that are designed to compensate for a failing electrical conduction system in the heart. They cannot compensate for failing heart muscle or structural damage.

Evidence of pacemaker function is visible on ECG and on monitoring (pacemaker *spike* followed by evidence of depolarization). *Capture* occurs when an electrical stimulus has successfully depolarized the heart muscle and taken control of the heart chamber. A QRS will be seen.

Follow Advanced Cardiac Life Support (ACLS) guidelines when treating the individual who has a life-threatening rhythm.

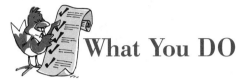

What You DO

When treating patients with pacemakers, you should perform the following:

- Assess airway, breathing, circulation (ABCs).
- Continually monitor the symptomatic individual with a pacemaker. Assess the patient for capture, sensing, and pacing of pacemaker.
- Observe, document, and report changes in vital signs.
- Assess for chest pain, indigestion, changes in level of consciousness.
- Assess heart and lung sounds.
- Make available a pacemaker magnet in acute care situations. Although magnet mode varies from manufacturer to manufacturer, the magnet may be needed to temporarily disrupt pacemaker function.
- Assess for swelling of feet and ankles, jugular vein distention, and pulmonary edema.
- Teach patients to carry pacemaker identification cards and to become familiar with the settings and capabilities of implanted pacemakers.

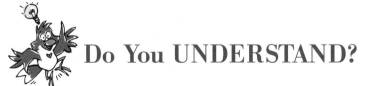

Do You UNDERSTAND?

DIRECTIONS: Fill in the blanks.

1. Heart muscle contracts in response to _____ stimuli.
2. Temporary pacemakers are used in cases of _____ and _____.

Answers: 1. electrical; 2. emergency, short-term therapy situations.

3. Leads that are placed directly into the cardiac muscle through an opening in the chest are called _____ leads.

4. Leads that are placed on the inner heart wall after being threaded through a large vein are called _____ leads.

5. Most modern pacemakers can be reprogrammed using _____ and do not require additional surgery.

6. Common household appliances are safe for use by individuals with pacemakers. Powerful _____ and _____ can affect pacemaker function.

7. The pacemaker artifact seen on an ECG or a monitor is also called a _____.

8. _____ pacemakers sense and pace in both the right atrium and the right ventricle.

9. Pacemakers are designed to compensate for a failing electrical conduction system in the heart. They cannot compensate for _____ or _____.

10. Symptoms of pacemaker failure may include:

_____

_____

_____

_____

_____

_____

Answers: 3. epicardial; 4. transvenous; 5. radio frequency; 6. magnets, arc welding; 7. spike; 8. Dual chamber; 9. failing heart muscle, structural damage; 10. Dizziness, syncope, change in mental status, difficulty breathing, weakness and fatigue, prolonged hiccups.

DRUG ABUSE

What ARE the Effects of Drug Abuse on the Heart?

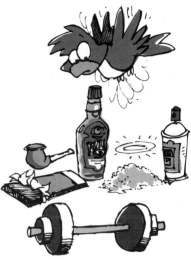

The heart can be affected by the overuse and abuse of authorized and illicit drugs. These drugs include alcohol, cocaine, amphetamines, phencyclidine (PCP), inhalants, caffeine, and anabolic steroids. Some substances of abuse do not cause cardiac effects that will affect the conduction system beyond tachycardia or bradycardia. These drugs include marijuana, sedative hypnotics, opioids, and tricyclic antidepressants. They affect the central nervous system and do not usually cause dysrhythmias. However, other drugs, such as cocaine, heroin, and PCP, as well as caffeine, can produce profound and long-term effects.

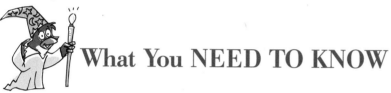

What You NEED TO KNOW

Many people abuse drugs, and some die after just one episode of substance abuse. Drug abuse can affect the cardiac, pulmonary, central nervous, and metabolic systems. Drug abusers may seek health care only for an event that they perceive to be a major threat to life. Thorough assessments during routine health care check-ups can help identify patients at risk for experimentation with illicit drugs. Assessments should include ECG analysis and further questioning about current or past substance abuse.

Acute crises may require immediate stabilization with cardiac drugs, depending on the dysrhythmia or situation. Long-term drug abuse can result in chronic cardiac problems, including cardiomyopathy, congestive heart failure, and conduction problems. Many substance abusers develop significant cognitive problems from their abuse that impairs their understanding of their condition and compliance with the necessary life-style changes and medications.

TAKE HOME POINTS

- Assessment should include ECG analysis and further questioning about current or past substance abuse.
- Substance abuse can have short- and long-term cardiac consequences, depending on the substances abused.

Cocaine and Crack

Cocaine stimulates the sympathetic nervous system and is a powerful euphoric. Catecholamine (epinephrine, norepinephrine) production is increased, which elevates the heart rate by directly stimulating the sinoatrial (SA) node and atrial and ventricular tissue. Effects of cocaine and crack can be dose related and include the following:

- Increased heart rate
- Increased force of contraction of the heart
- Increased systolic blood pressure (BP)
- Peripheral vasoconstriction, causing abdominal pain
- Atrial and ventricular dysrhythmias, including sinus tachycardia, paroxysmal supraventricular tachycardia (PSVT), atrial fibrillation and flutter, ventricular tachycardia (VT) and fibrillation, and asystole
- Increased afterload and myocardial oxygen consumption, which can lead to ischemia
- Prolongation of QT interval and QRS complex on the ECG

Coronary vasospasm, vasoconstriction, and focal endothelial damage may occur, which may increase platelet aggregation and potentiate thrombus formation. Acute myocardial infarction and cardiopulmonary arrest may occur, with or without a previous history of heart disease. Chronic, long-term cocaine abusers will develop myocarditis, pulmonary hemorrhage, and cardiomyopathy.

Alcohol

Alcohol is a central nervous system depressant that causes weakness of the heart muscle and increases cardiac failure and the risk of developing pneumonia. Cardiac changes seen with chronic abuse may include cardiomyopathy. ECG changes can be seen in the QRS complex, with the entire complex being slightly wider, upright complexes being taller, and negative complexes being more negative.

Amphetamines

Amphetamines are stimulants that enhance the release of neurotransmitters. α-adrenergic stimulation causes arterial and venous vasoconstriction. β-adrenergic stimulation produces increases in afterload, systemic vascular response, heart rate, and contractility, greatly increasing myocardial oxygen consumption. Myocardial ischemia and infarction are major concerns as vasospasm and platelet aggregation occur. Atrial and ventricular dysrhythmias also occur.

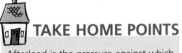

TAKE HOME POINTS

Afterload is the pressure against which the ventricle ejects blood.

Chronic amphetamine abuse can cause hypertension, congestive heart failure, cerebral and cardiac vasculitis with microaneurysms, and cardiomyopathy.

Phencyclidine

Phencyclidine (PCP) (angel dust, supergrass, ozone, wack, rocket fuel) primarily affects the central nervous system, causing agitation, rage, delusions, and irrational behavior. It can cause hypertension and, in crisis stage, it can cause hypotension, bradycardia, decreased respirations, vomiting, drooling, dizziness, memory loss, and speech difficulties. PCP can be snorted, smoked (usually mixed with mint, parsley, or oregano), or eaten.

Inhalants

Many other substances, such as crack cocaine, heroin, and methamphetamines (ice) are inhaled by abusers. Their effects are primarily seen on the central nervous and pulmonary systems (heroin exacerbates asthma, which can lead to death). These effects vary with the particular chemicals being abused. The death rate from inhalant abuse may be higher than recorded, because of direct or indirect cardiotoxicity. Patients are found in VT, leading to VF and cardiac arrest, or they are found in a state of arrest when brought to the emergency department for treatment.

Caffeine

Many people would be upset to be categorized as caffeine abusers. Caffeine has a half-life of 5 hours and is a common ingredient in products containing chocolate and in tea, soft drinks, and coffee. It is also found in some over-the-counter analgesics and herbal diuretics. Cardiac effects are dose related and can include VT and atrial fibrillation. Few people show a bradycardic response to caffeine. Caffeine also raises BP and increases serum cholesterol, unless the coffee is filtered. Thus caffeine increases risk for cardiovascular disease, particularly coronary heart disease.

Anabolic Steroids

Moderate to long-term use of anabolic steroids results in cardiac muscle and lipid metabolism changes. Anabolic steroids affect protein synthesis at the genetic level by affecting messenger RNA (mRNA) function. This alteration causes muscle cells, including cardiac cells, to hypertrophy and increase in both size and number (hyperplastic). This growth can result in cardiomegaly or left ventricular hypertrophy, resulting in decreased cardiac output. The effect of anabolic steroids on the lipid system is an increase in total choles-

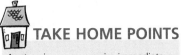

TAKE HOME POINTS

Acute crises may require immediate stabilization with cardiac drugs, depending on the dysrhythmia or situation.

People who abuse drugs are found in all ages and socioeconomic groups. It is important that you carefully evaluate patients with cardiac symptoms for drug abuse, even if they have no history of heart disease.

terol levels with a rising of low-density lipoproteins (LDLs) and a lowering of high-density lipoprotein (HDLs) levels potentiating atherosclerotic heart disease. Often results can be reversed if the steroids are discontinued.

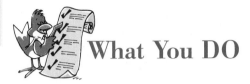

What You DO

When treating patients who could be abusing drugs, you should:

- Assess life-style and environment frequently.
- Monitor vital signs.
- Observe ECG changes.
- Support body systems.
- Treat identified dysrhythmias.
- Monitor pH of atrial blood gases (ABGs) for acidosis.
- Monitor total serum cholesterol, LDL, and HDL levels.
- Monitor for metabolic acidosis and prepare to give intravenous (IV) bicarbonate.
- Assess for changes in behavior, cognition, and level of consciousness.
- Assess for pulmonary hemorrhage (black sputum) and auscultate to detect increases in asthma symptoms

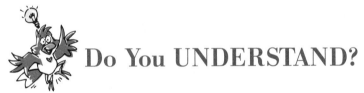

Do You UNDERSTAND?

DIRECTIONS: **Fill in the blanks.**

1. Substance abusers can have the following types of acute cardiac problems:

   _____

   _____

   _____

   _____

2. Chronic substance abusers can have the following cardiac problems:

   _____

   _____

   _____

   _____

SURGICAL THERAPY

Future challenges for effective treatment of coronary artery disease (CAD) and cardiomyopathy rests within cardiothoracic and heart transplantation surgical procedures. As a nurse, you must be able to differentiate between normal ECG changes caused by surgical approach and postoperative dysrhythmias. This section will present key points to remember in caring for patients after coronary artery bypass grafting (CABG), partial left ventriculectomy, and heart transplantation surgeries.

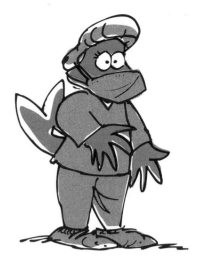

These surgical approaches to treat heart disease may directly affect the normal cardiac conduction system.

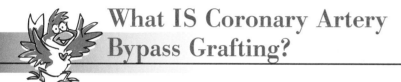

What IS Coronary Artery Bypass Grafting?

Coronary artery bypass grafting (CABG) (aortocoronary bypass grafting) is a form of surgical revascularization. This procedure bypasses coronary obstruction lesions or stenosis to restore the blood supply and flow to myocardial tissue. The procedure entails a harvested vessel or conduit (saphenous vein, internal thoracic artery, or both) being anastomosed between the aortic root (base) and a distal point to the obstruction.

CABG may be indicated for the following conditions:

- Chronic stable angina pectoris
- Significant left main coronary artery occlusion (greater than 60%)
- Unstable angina with multivessel disease
- Acute MI
- Symptoms of ischemic or impending MI
- Reocclusion after percutaneous transluminal coronary angioplasty (PTCA)
- Left ventricular failure
- Intractable ventricular irritability

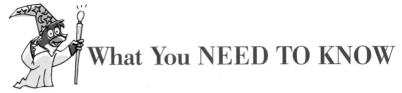

What You NEED TO KNOW

Intracellular myocardial edema, surgical manipulation, premature rewarming disruption of normal coronary perfusion, metabolic and electrolyte imbalances, atrial irritability, increased sympathetic stimulation, hypoxemia, hypotension, and other factors can cause injury to the cardiac conduction system. The cardiac dysrhythmias caused by these factors include:

- Tachydysrhythmias
- Premature ventricular contractions (PVCs)
- Bradydysrhythmias
- VT, which can occur in the immediate postoperative period

Each of these dysrhythmias must be observed and treated immediately to prevent further injury to the patient. Some dysrhythmias, such as PVCs, usually occur on the second to third postoperative day. Treatment for the dysrhythmia is aimed at preventing adverse hemodynamic effects, setting the stage for a decrease in cardiac output.

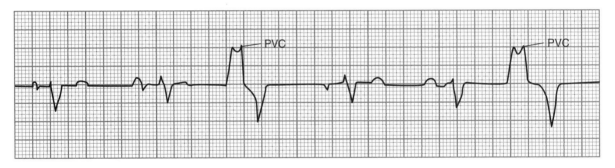

If hypoxemia and metabolic imbalances are ruled out, pharmacologic management is warranted. Depending on the dysrhythmia, drug therapy may include beta blockers, class I antidysrhythmics, and calcium channel blockers.

The most common dysrhythmia reported after CABG is atrial fibrillation and atrial flutter.

Bradydysrhythmias can be caused by injury to the conductive system during surgery. Bundle branch block (BBB) or a complete AV block may be observed. The most common treatment is the use of a temporary or dual-chamber ventricular-pacing device.

Atrial Dysrhythmias

Indications of atrial flutter:

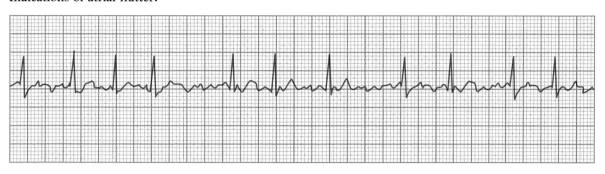

- *Rates: Atrial*—250 to 400 bpm; *ventricular*—variable, depending on degree of AV block
- *Rhythm: Atrial*—regular; *ventricular*—regular or irregular
- *P wave:* "Saw tooth" flutter waves
- *PR interval:* Not measurable
- *QRS complex:* Normal (0.04 to 0.11 seconds); unchanged conduction beyond the AV node
- *QT interval:* Not measurable

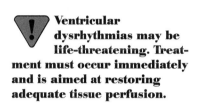

Ventricular dysrhythmias may be life-threatening. Treatment must occur immediately and is aimed at restoring adequate tissue perfusion.

Indications of atrial fibrillation:

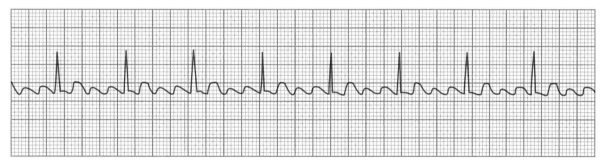

- *Rate:* Variable according to ventricular response (less than 100 bpm—*controlled atrial fibrillation*; more than 100 bpm—*uncontrolled* atrial fibrillation)
- *Rhythm:* Irregularly irregular
- *P wave:* No *true* P waves (may vary from course to fine)
- *PR interval:* Not measurable
- *QRS complex:* Usually normal; may be aberrant
- *QT interval:* Not measurable

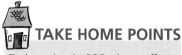

TAKE HOME POINTS

To determine the ECG adverse effects postoperatively, observe for major dysrhythmias.

Ventricular Dysrhythmias

Indications of VT:

- *Rate:* From 140 to 250 bpm
- *Rhythm:* Usually regular (may be slightly irregular)
- *P wave:* No P wave (usually buried in the wide QRS complex)
- *QRS complex:* Wide (greater than 0.11 seconds)

Indications of VF:

- *Rate:* None
- *Rhythm:* Chaotic
- *QRS complex:* No formed complexes

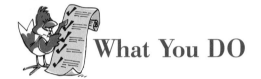

What You DO

When treating patients who have just undergone CABG, you should:

- Continuously monitor the electrocardiogram.
- Observe for the onset of dysrhythmias (especially atrial fibrillation and VT).
- Notify the health care provider as soon as you notice any dysrhythmia.
- Monitor BP, level of consciousness, and peripheral perfusion.
- Prepare for cardioversion as directed by health care provider.
- Administer prescribed medications, such as beta blockers, class I antidysrhythmics, and calcium channel blockers.
- Monitor effects of treatment.

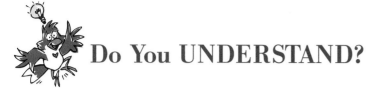

Do You UNDERSTAND?

DIRECTIONS: Fill in the blanks.

1. List five causes of potential injury to the cardiac conduction system after CABG:

   _____

   _____

   _____

   _____

   _____

2. Most common dysrhythmias reported after CABG are

   _____ and _____

   caused by increased _____.

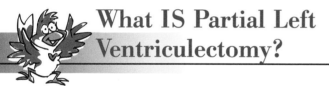

What IS Partial Left Ventriculectomy?

Partial left ventriculectomy (PLV) is a surgical procedure that is under investigation as an alternative to heart transplantation or as a treatment technique for chronic heart failure. PLV surgery removes a portion of the dilated left ventricle to create a smaller chamber to enhance the cardiac pumping mechanism. Thus PLV reduces wall tension by directly reducing the diameter of the left ventricle.

Prevention of both atrial and ventricular dysrhythmias is the goal of postoperative nursing care. Ventricular dysrhythmias are the greatest concern in the recovery phase; therefore patients are given a class III antidysrhythmic, such as amiodarone hydrochloride, (usually 400 mg daily) from the first postoperative day. The dose is reduced to 200 mg/day during long-term therapy.

Rationale for PLV is based on Laplace's law:

> Left ventricular tension (wall stress) =
> intraventricular pressure × radius of left ventricle
> ÷ ventricular wall thickness × 2

> **Because of the nature of the PLV procedure and the condition of the dilated cardiac muscle, there is an increased risk of lethal dysrhythmias.**

Answers: 1. Intracellular myocardial edema, surgical manipulation, premature rewarming, metabolic imbalances, disruption of normal coronary perfusion; 2. atrial flutter and atrial fibrillation, atrial irritability.

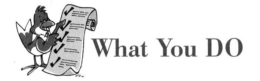

What You NEED TO KNOW

PLV is considered an investigational procedure at this time. Additional preventative measures include an ICD and temporary epicardial pacing wires to control heart rate and rhythm. Tachydysrhythmias are not tolerated postoperatively; treatment may include IV procainamide hydrochloride.

Three goals for PLV surgery have been identified:
1. Improve cardiac function
2. Eliminate mitral regurgitation
3. Reduce left ventricle size to near normal

Patients who are being considered for this procedure include those with the following:

- End-stage heart failure with idiopathic dilated cardiomyopathy
- Functional heart classification of III or IV
- Left ventricle internal diameter greater than 7 cm

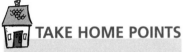

TAKE HOME POINTS

To determine ECG changes for a patient who has undergone PLV surgery, you should observe for the ventricular dysrhythmias listed in the CABG section of this chapter.

What You DO

When treating a patient who has undergone PLV surgery, you should:

- Continuously monitor the ECG for a minimum of 6 days after surgery.
- Call the health care provider if atrial or ventricular dysrhythmias appear.
- Administer amiodarone hydrochloride by mouth or IV as prescribed.
- Maintain serum potassium chloride levels at 4.5 or slightly greater and magnesium sulfate levels at 2.2 or slightly greater to prevent electrolyte disturbances
- Maintain pacemaker wires until discontinued.
- Monitor for signs and symptoms of a decrease in cardiac output.

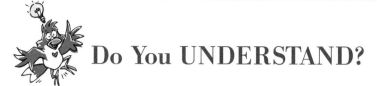

Do You UNDERSTAND?

DIRECTIONS: Read the question and fill in the short answer.

1. What are the major differences between VT and VF?

   _____

   _____

2. Removing part of the left ventricle is an experimental treatment for heart failure. What is the name of this procedure?

   _____

3. BBB can be a dysrhythmia that develops after CABG surgery. How is it treated? _____

What IS Cardiac Transplantation?

Cardiac transplantation is a surgical procedure that removes and replaces the diseased heart. The most common procedure is orthotopic transplantation, in which the posterior walls of the patient's atria remain and the rest of the diseased heart is removed. The remaining posterior atria walls are used to anchor the donor heart in place.

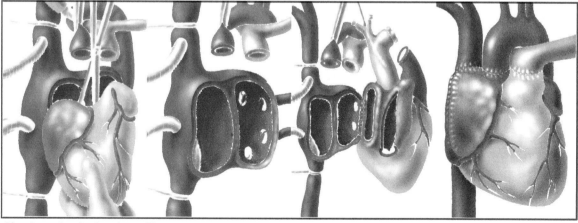

After the patient is placed on cardiopulmonary bypass, the heart is removed.

The posterior walls of the patient's left and right atria are left intact.

The left atrium of the donor heart is anastomosed to the patient's residual posterior atrial walls, and the other atrial walls, atrial septum, and great vessels are joined.

Postoperative result.

The patient cannot tolerate intense exercise or strenuous activity. Orthostatic hypotension has been observed in patients postoperatively.

The patient will exhibit ineffective responses to certain drugs (atropine or digitalis) or carotid sinus pressure.

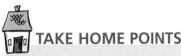 **TAKE HOME POINTS**

To determine ECG changes for patients having undergone cardiac transplantation, you should observe for the following:

- **Rate:** Resting heart rate is between 90 and 100 bpm; there is slow or no response with an increase in heart rate caused by sympathetic stimulation.
- **Rhythm:** Donor rhythm is regular; donor P waves produce a consistent PR interval.
- **P waves:** Two P waves are visible.
- **PR interval:** Donor P waves are uniform and present before each QRS complex. Recipient P waves cause an unrelated, independent atrial rate with no direct effect on cardiac contraction.
- **QRS complex:** Complexes are normal in appearance, with a width of 0.04 to 0.10 seconds unless right BBB has developed. If an immunosuppressive drug (cyclosporin) is used, the voltage of the QRS complex may be decreased.
- **QT interval:** Intervals are measurable within normal limits unless right BBB has developed.

 # What You NEED TO KNOW

The recipient's SA node remains intact. Impulses may be initiated, but they do not cross the suture line. This causes nonconducted P waves to be observed on the ECG. The SA node of the donor's heart produces the electrical impulse that results in a cardiac contraction.

In addition, a right BBB is common postoperatively, because of the disruption of normal innervation of the conduction system. Denervation (absence of autonomic innervation) effects on the transplanted heart include:

- Lack of responsiveness to vagal stimulation, causing the patient to have a resting heart rate of 90 to 110 bpm
- Slow or no response (increased heart rate, contractility, decreased cardiac output) to sympathetic stimulation (exercise or stress)
- Dependency on circulating catecholamines and an increased venous return for the management of heart rate and contractility
- Lack of anginal chest pain with recurrent CAD. Cardiac catheterization is the only diagnostic tool to evaluate recurrence of CAD.

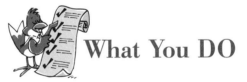 # What You DO

When treating the patient who has just undergone cardiac transplantation, you should remember to perform the following:

- Continuously monitor the ECG for atrial and ventricular dysrhythmias.
- Observe for SVT. Treatment for this dysrhythmia is limited because of denervation of the heart. Vagal maneuvers will have no effect on heart rate. Cardioversion may be required.
- Ventricular dysrhythmias may occur. Observe for the onset of premature ventricular contractions.
- Monitor vital signs and cardiac output.
- Notify health care provider of dysrhythmias.

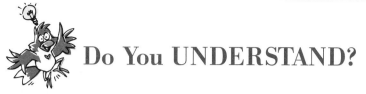

Do You UNDERSTAND?

DIRECTIONS: **Fill in the blanks.**

1. The major cause for conduction changes postcardiac transplantation is

   _____.

2. What diagnostic test is used to evaluate the recurrence of CAD?

   _____

3. Is isopruterenol (Isuprel) used to treat bradycardia or tachycardia?

   _____

> ⚠ **Because of myocardial edema, sinus bradycardia may be observed. Isoproterenol (Isuprel) may be used for treatment. Atrial dysrhythmias may been evident for up to 6 months postoperatively.**

CARDIAC TRAUMA

Are you ready to meet the challenge of cardiac trauma? Knowledge, skills, and experience with ECGs may mean the difference between life and death for your patients. Examples of cardiac trauma are cardiac contusions, penetrating wounds, and cardiac tamponade.

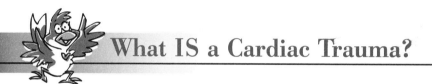

What IS a Cardiac Trauma?

Cardiac Contusion

Cardiac contusion is soft-tissue trauma caused by a blow or blunt force to the chest. Symptoms indicating cardiac contusion include:

- Ecchymosis on chest wall,
- Pericardial friction rub
- Tachycardia (see Chapter 12)
- Retrosternal angina that is unrelieved by nitroglycerin

Penetrating Wound

A penetrating wound is caused by an object piercing the heart. The heart may be penetrated either from the abdomen or back. Symptoms indicating penetrating wounds include:

- Bleeding
- Chest pain

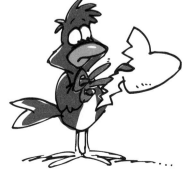

- Loss of consciousness
- Agitation
- Muffled heart sounds
- Hypotension
- Distended neck veins
- Tachycardia
- ECG readings indicating cardiac arrest (see Chapter 14)

Cardiac Tamponade

Cardiac tamponade is caused by fluid, blood, or blood clots that accumulate in the pericardial space. As fluid volume increases around the heart chambers, they are unable to completely fill with blood and cardiac output significantly decreases or stops. Tamponade occurs as the result of cardiac contusions, penetrating wounds, recent cardiac surgery, infectious pericardial neoplasm, or uremia (see Chapter 18). In addition, it may be a complication following pericardial taps, cardiac catheterization, cardiopulmonary resuscitation (CPR), or pacemaker insertion. Symptoms of cardiac tamponade include:

- Decreased cardiac output
- Pulsus paradoxus (decrease in systolic BP of greater than 15 mm Hg using cuff sphygmomanometry method during inspiration)
- Muffled heart sounds
- Jugular venous distention with clear lungs
- Hypotension
- Increased central venous pressure
- Narrowed pulse pressure

Pulse pressure is measured by subtracting the diastolic BP from the systolic BP. If the BP is 120/80, you would subtract 80 from 120 to get a pulse pressure of 40 (120 − 80 = 40). It is normally one third of the systolic BP. Pulse Pressure narrows (gets smaller) in cardiac tamponade as pressures in the heart equalize. The following ECG changes mimic myocardial injury, ischemia, or infarction:

- ST segment elevation
- T wave changes (tall T waves)
- Possibility of deep or wide Q waves
- Diminished ECG amplitude

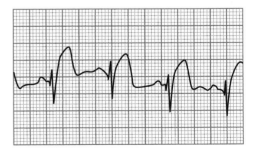

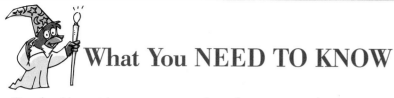

What You NEED TO KNOW

You should consider any patient with cardiac trauma to be an emergency; immediate action is required. Continuous ECG monitoring is imperative.

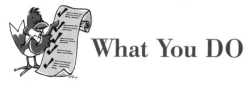

What You DO

When treating the patient in cardiac trauma, you should perform the following:

- Consider the situation an emergency and act quickly.
- Assess the ABCs.
- Notify the health care provider of any dysrhythmias.
- Continuously monitor the ECG.
- Monitor closely for shock.
- Begin IV therapy.
- Draw blood for type and cross matching.
- Get complete medical history.
- Administer oxygen.
- Assist the health care provider with insertion of chest tube or pericardiocentesis.
- Prepare for possible thoracostomy.

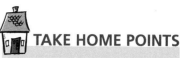

TAKE HOME POINTS

To determine ECG changes in a patient with cardiac trauma, you should observe for the following:
- **Rate:** Rapid
- **Rhythm:** Dysrhythmic
- **QRS complex:** Tall T waves; possible deep or wide Q waves
- **Rhythm:** Diminished amplitude

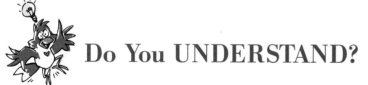

Do You UNDERSTAND?

DIRECTIONS: **Fill in the blanks.**

1. List three examples of cardiac trauma.

   _____

   _____

   _____

Answers: 1. cardiac contusion, penetrating wound, cardiac tamponade.

2. ECG changes with cardiac trauma mimic the following:

_____

_____

_____

DIRECTIONS: **Indicate in the spaces provided whether the following**
statements are *true* or *false*.

3. _____ Dysrhythmias are common in cardiac trauma.

4. _____ Cardiac tamponade is a result of a myocardial infarction.

5. _____ Suspect cardiac tamponade when ECG changes indicate a
tall T wave, diminished amplitude, and ST segment elevation.

6. _____ A flat line on the ECG indicates cardiac arrest.

References

Chapter 1

Alspach JG: *AACN core curriculum for critical care nursing,* ed 5, Philadelphia, 1998, WB Saunders.

Lamborn ML, Moseley MJ: Cardiac alterations. In Hartshorn JC, Sole ML, Lamborn ML, editors: *Introduction to critical care nursing,* ed 3, Philadelphia, 2001, WB Saunders.

McCance KL: Structure & function of the cardiovascular & lymphatic systems. In McCance KL, Huether SE, editors: *Pathophysiology: the biologic basis for disease in adults and children,* ed 3, St Louis, 1998, Mosby.

Stewart SL, Vitello-Ciccio JM: Cardiovascular clinical physiology. In Kinney et al, editors: *AACN clinical reference for critical care nursing,* ed 4, St Louis, 1998, Mosby.

Chapter 2

Boyer MJ: *Lippincott's need-to-know ECG facts,* Philadelphia, 1997, Lippincott.

Casey P: Management of patients with dysrhythmias and conduction problems. In Smeltzer S, Bare B, editors: *Bunner and Suddarth's textbook of medical-surgical nursing,* ed 9 Philadelphia, 2000, Lippincott.

Ehrat KS: *The art of EKG interpretation: a self-instructional text,* ed 4, Dubuque, IA, 1997, Kendall/Hunt.

Hartshorn JC, Sole ML, Lamborn ML: *Introduction to critical care nursing,* ed 3, Philadelphia, 2001, WB Saunders.

Huff J: *ECG workout: exercises in arrhythmia interpretation,* ed 3, Philadelphia, 1997, Lippincott.

Ignatavicius DD et al: *Medical-surgical nursing,* ed 3, Philadelphia, 1999, WB Saunders.

Lewis KM: *Sensible ECG analysis,* Albany, NY, 2000, Delmar Publishing.

Miracle VA, Sims JM: Making sense of the 12 lead ECG, *Nursing* 99(7):35, 1999.

Paul S, Hebra J: *The nurse's guide to cardiac rhythm interpretation: implications for patient care,* Philadelphia, 1998, WB Saunders.

Woods S: Dysrhythmia interpretation. In Sole LS, Lamborn ML, Hartshorn JC, editors: *Introduction to critical care nursing,* ed 3, Philadelphia, 2001, WB Saunders.

Chapter 3

Boyer MJ: *Lippincott's need-to-know ECG facts,* Philadelphia, 1997, Lippincott.

Ehrat KS: *The art of EKG interpretation: a self-instructional text,* ed 4, Dubuque, IA, 1997, Kendall/Hunt.

Lewis KM: *Sensible ECG analysis,* Albany, NY, 2000, Delmar Publishing.

Paul S, Hebra JD: *The nurse's guide to cardiac rhythm interpretation: implications for patient care,* Philadelphia, 1997, WB Saunders.

Chapter 4

Dubin D: *Rapid interpretation of EKGs,* ed 5, Tampa, 1996, Cover Publishing.

Ignatavicius DD et al: *Medical-surgical nursing,* ed 3, Philadelphia, 1999, WB Saunders.

Johns C: Arrhythmias. In Lewis SM, Heitkemper HH, Dirksen SR: *Medical-surgical nursing,* ed 5, St Louis, 2000, Mosby.

Paul S, Hebra J: *The nurse's guide to cardiac rhythm interpretation: implications for patient care*, Philadelphia, 1998, WB Saunders.

Scrima D: Foundations of arrhythmia interpretation, *Medsurg Nurs* 6:4, 1997.

Woods S: Dysrhythmia interpretation. In Sole LS, Lamborn ML, Hartshorn JC, editors: *Introduction to critical care nursing*, ed 3, Philadelphia, 2001, WB Saunders.

Chapter 5

Ignatavicius DD et al: *Medical-surgical nursing*, ed 3, Philadelphia, 1999, WB Saunders.

Paul S, Hebra J: *The nurse's guide to cardiac rhythm interpretation: implications for patient care*, Philadelphia, 1998, WB Saunders.

Woods S: Dysrhythmia interpretation. In Sole LS, Lamborn ML, Hartshorn JC, editors: *Introduction to critical care nursing*, ed 3, Philadelphia, 2001, WB Saunders.

Chapter 6

Bloomquist J, Love M: Cardiovascular assessment and diagnostic procedures. In Urden L, Stacy K, editors: *Priorities in critical care*, ed 3, St Louis, 2000, Mosby.

Huff J: *ECG workout: exercises in arrhythmia interpretation*, ed 3, Philadelphia, 1997, Lippincott.

Paul S, Hebra J: *The nurse's guide to cardiac rhythm interpretation: implications for patient care*, Philadelphia, 1998, WB Saunders.

Woods S: Dysrhythmia interpretation. In Sole LS, Lamborn ML, Hartshorn JC, editors: *Introduction to critical care nursing*, ed 3, Philadelphia, 2001, WB Saunders.

Chapter 7

Agilent Technologies: *12-lead monitoring with EASI lead system, App Note*, Palo Alto, CA, 1999, Agilent Technologies.

Boyer MJ: *Lippincott's need-to-know ECG facts*, Philadelphia, 1997, Lippincott.

Dubin D: *Rapid interpretation of EKGs*, ed 5, Tampa, FL, 1996, Cover Publishing.

Ehrat KS: *The art of EKG interpretation: a self-instructional text*, ed 4, Dubuque, IA, 1997, Kendall/Hunt.

Huff J: *ECG workout: exercises in arrhythmia interpretation*, ed 3, Philadelphia, 1997, Lippincott.

Jacobson C: Advanced ECG concepts. In Chulay M, Gizzetta C, and Dossey B, editors: *AACN handbook of critical care nursing*, Stamford, CT, 1997, Appleton & Lange.

Johns C: Nursing management of arrhythmias. In Lewis SM, Heitkemper HH, Dirksen SR, editors: *Medical-surgical nursing*, ed 5, St Louis, 2000, Mosby.

Kennedy M: Patient assessment: cardiovascular system cardiac history and physical examination. In Hudak, Gallo, Morton, editors: *Critical care nursing: a holistic approach*, Philadelphia, 1998, Lippincott.

Lewis KM: *Sensible ECG analysis*, Albany, NY, 2000, Delmar Publishing.

Lewis SM, Heitkemper HH, Dirksen SR: *Medical-surgical nursing*, ed 5, St Louis, 2000, Mosby.

Paul S, Hebra J: *The nurse's guide to cardiac rhythm interpretation: implications for patient care*, Philadelphia, 1998, WB Saunders.

Woods S: Dysrhythmia interpretation. In Sole LS, Lamborn ML, Hartshorn JC, editors: *Introduction to critical care nursing*, ed 3, Philadelphia, 2001, WB Saunders.

Chapter 8

Dubin D: *Rapid interpretation of EKG's*, ed 5, Tampa, Fla, 1996, Cover Publishing.
Huff J: *ECG workout: exercises in arrhythmia interpretation*, ed 3, Philidelphia, 1997, Lippincott.
Jacobson C: Advanced ECG concepts. In Chulay M, Gizzetta C, Dossey B, editors: *AACN handbook of critical care nursing*, Stamford, Conn, 1998, Appleton & Lange.
Kennedy M: Patient assessment: cardiovascular system cardiac history and physical examination. In Hudak, Gallo, Morton, editors: *Critical care nursing. A holistic approach*, Philidelphia, 1998, Lippincott.

Chapter 9

Dubin D: *Rapid interpretation of EKG's*, ed 5, Tampa, Fla, 1996, Cover Publishing.
Huff J: *ECG workout: exercises in arrhythmia interpretation*, ed 3, Philidelphia, 1997, Lippincott.
Jacobson C: Advanced ECG concepts. In Chulay M, Gizzetta C, Dossey B, editors: *AACN handbook of critical care nursing*, Stamford, Conn, 1998, Appleton & Lange.
Kennedy M: Patient assessment: cardiovascular system cardiac history and physical examination. In Hudak, Gallo, Morton, editors: *Critical care nursing. A holistic approach*, Philidelphia, 1998, Lippincott.

Chapter 10

Conover M: *Understanding electrocardiography*, ed 7, St Louis, 1996, Mosby.
Cummins RO, editor: *Textbook of advanced cardiac life support*, 1997, AHA.
Ehrat K: *The art of EKG interpretation: a self-instruction text*, Dubuque, 1997, Kendall/Hunt.
Hartshorn JC, Sole ML, Lamborn ML: *Introduction to critical care nursing*, ed 3, Philadelphia, 2001, WB Saunders.
Hellstedt LF: *Sorting out supraventricular tachycardias: critical care choices 98*, Springhouse, Penn, 1998, Springhouse.
Paul S, Hebra J: *The nurse's guide to cardiac rhythm interpretation: implications for patient care*, Philadelphia, 1998, WB Saunders.
Singh BN: Antiarrhythmic actions or amiodarone: a profile of a paradoxical agent, *Am J Cardiol* 78(4A):41, 1996.

Chapter 11

American Heart Association: *Advanced cardiac life support*, Dallas, 1997, The Association.
Bloomquist J, Love M: Cardiovascular assessment and diagnostic procedures. In Urden L, Stacy K, editors: *Priorities in critical care*, ed 3, St Louis, 2000, Mosby.
Boyer MJ: *Lippincott's need-to-know ECG facts*, Philadelphia, 1997, Lippincott.
Casey P: Management of patients with dysrhythmias and conduction problems. In Smeltzer S, Bare B, editors: *Brunner and Suddarth's textbook of medical-surgical nursing*, ed 9, Philadelphia, 2000, Lippincott.
Davenport J, Morton PG: Identifying nonischemic causes of life-threatening arrhythmias, *Am J Nurse* 97(11):50, 1997.

Chapter 12

Albert CT: Common supraventricular tachycardias: mechanisms and management, *AACN Clinical Issue* 12(1):100, 2001.

American Heart Association: *Advanced cardiac life support*, Dallas, 1997, The Association.

Boyer MJ: *Lippincott's need-to-know ECG facts*, Philadelphia, 1997, Lippincott.

Davenport J, Morton PG: Identifying nonischemic causes of life-threatening arrhythmias, *Am J Nurse* 97(11):50, 1997.

Hartshorn JC, Sole ML, Lamborn ML: *Introduction to critical care nursing*, ed 3, Philadelphia, 2001, WB Saunders.

Hazinski MF, Cummins RO, Field JM: *2000 handbook of emergency cardiovascular care*, Dallas, 2000, American Heart Association.

Huff J: *ECG workout: exercises in arrhythmia interpretation*, ed 3, Philadelphia, 1997, Lippincott.

Lewis KM: *Sensible ECG analysis*, Albany, NY, 2000, Delmar Publishing.

McCoy C: Nursing care of the patient with cardiac disorders. In Monahan FD, Neighbors M, editors: *Medical-surgical nursing: foundations for clinical practice*, ed 2, Philadelphia, 1998, WB Saunders.

Owen A: How to distinguish wide-complex tachycardias, www.springnet.com/criticalcare.

Paul S, Hebra J: *The nurse's guide to cardiac rhythm interpretation: implications for patient care*, Philadelphia, 1998, WB Saunders.

Chapter 13

American Heart Association: *Advanced cardiac life support*, Dallas, 1997, The Association.

Banasik J: Heart failure and dysrhythmias: common sequelae of cardiac diseases. In Copstead LC, Banasik J, editors: *Pathophysiology: biological and behavioral perspectives*, ed 2, Philadelphia, 2000, WB Saunders.

Boyer MJ: *Lippincott's need-to-know ECG facts*, Philadelphia, 1997, Lippincott.

Cohn EG, Gilroy-Doohan M: *Flip and see ECG*, Philadelphia, 1995, WB Saunders.

Davenport J, Morton, PG: Identifying nonischemic causes of life-threatening arrhythmia's, *Am J Nurs* 97(11):50, 1997.

Hartshorn JC, Sole ML, Lamborn ML: *Introduction to critical care nursing*, ed 3, Philadelphia, 2001, WB Saunders.

Huff J: *ECG workout: exercises in arrhythmia interpretation*, ed 3, Philadelphia, 1997, Lippincott.

Lewis KM: *Sensible ECG analysis*, Albany, NY, 2000, Delmar Publishing.

McCoy C: Nursing care of the patient with cardiac disorders. In Monahan FD, Neighbors M, editors: *Medical-surgical nursing: foundations for clinical practice*, ed 2, Philadelphia, 1998, WB Saunders.

Owen A: *How to distinguish wide-complex tachycardias*, www.springnet.com/criticalcare.

Paul S, Hebra J: *The nurse's guide to cardiac rhythm interpretation: implications for patient care*, Philadelphia, 1998, WB Saunders.

Chapter 14

American Heart Association: *Advanced cardiac life support*, Dallas, 1997, The Association.

Boyer MJ: *Lippincott's need-to-know ECG facts*, Philadelphia, 1997, Lippincott.

Clochesy JM, Breu C, Cardin S, Whittaker AA, Rudy E: *Critical care nursing, ed 2*, Philadelphia: 1996, WB Saunders.

Davenport J, Morton, PG: Identifying nonischemic causes of life-threatening arrhythmia's, *Am J Nurs* 97(11):50, 1997.

Earl W: *Procedures checklists: fundamentals of nursing—concepts, process, and practice*, Aspen, CO, 2000, Saddle Ruin: Prentice Hall Health.

Hartshorn JC, Sole ML, Lamborn ML: *Introduction to critical care nursing, ed 3*, Philadelphia, 2001, WB Saunders.

Huff J: *ECG workout: exercises in arrhythmia interpretation, ed 3*, Philadelphia, 1997, Lippincott.

Ignatavicius DD, Workman ML, Mishler MA: *Medical-surgical nursing across the health care continuum*, Philadelphia, 1999, WB Saunders.

Lewis KM: *Sensible ECG analysis*, Albany, NY, 2000, Delmar Publishing.

McCoy C: Nursing care of the patient with cardiac disorders. In Monahan FD, Neighbors M, editors: *Medical-surgical nursing: foundations for clinical practice, ed 2*, Philadelphia, 1998, WB Saunders.

Owen A: *How to distinguish wide-complex tachycardias*, www.springnet.com/criticalcare.

Paul S, Hebra J: *The nurse's guide to cardiac rhythm interpretation: implications for patient care*, Philadelphia, 1998, WB Saunders.

Chapter 15

Boyer MJ: *Lippincott's need-to-know ECG facts*, Philadelphia, 1997, Lippincott.

Copstead LE, Banasik J: Pathophysiology: biological and behavioral perspectives, ed 2, Philadelphia, 2000, WB Saunders.

Huff J: ECG workout: exercises in arrhythmia interpretation, ed 3, Philadelphia, 1997, Lippincott.

Lewis KM: *Sensible ECG analysis*, Albany, NY, 2000, Delmar Publishing.

Springhouse Corporation: *ECG interpretation made incredibly easy*, Springhouse, PA, 1997, Springhouse Corporation.

Chapter 16

Adams SL et al: Ambulatory blood pressure and Holter monitor of emergency physicians before, during, and after a night shift, *Acad Emerg Med* 5(9):871, 1998.

Carlson MD, Thames MD: Approach to the patient with syncope. In WN Kelley: *Textbook of internal medicine*, Philadelphia, 1997, Lippincott-Raven.

Chernecky C, Berger B: *Laboratory tests and diagnostic procedures, ed 3*, Philadelphia, 2001, Saunders.

Elhendy A et al: Safety and feasibility of dobutamine-atropine stress echocardiography for the diagnosis of coronary artery disease in diabetic patients unable to perform an exercise stress test, *Diabetes Care* 21(11):1797, 1998.

Futterman LG, Lemberg L: The ECG in cardiac stress testing: a valuable, but unappreciated source of clues, *Am J Crit Care* 7(4):320, 1998.

Hill JM, Newton JL: Contrast echo: your role at the bedside, *RN* 61(10):32, 1998.

Kinney M et al: *AACN clinical reference for critical care nursing, ed 4*, St Louis, 1998, Mosby.

Koca V et al: Left ventricular thrombi detection with multiplane transesophageal echocardiography: an echocardiographic study with surgical verification, *J Heart Valve Dis* 8(1):63, 1999.

Quittan M, Cristal N, Ernst E: Exercise testing in coronary artery disease—procedures and clinical implications, *Eur J Phys Med Rehabil* 7(5):142, 1997.

Roelandt JR: Three-dimensional echocardiography: the future today, *Acta Cardiol* 53(6):323, 1998.

Sergeant LL: Tracking your outpatient's EKG with a Holter monitor, *Nursing* 16(10):47, 1986.

Yamada T et al: An approach to the detection of autonomic neuropathy by use of signal-averaged electrocardiography, *Pacing Clin Electrophysiol* 20(2):261, 1999.

Yamada T et al: Dispersion of signal-averaged P wave duration on precordial body surface in patients with paroxysmal atrial fibrillation, *Eur Heart J* 20(3):171, 1999.

Zitkus BS: Diagnostic tests. Transesophageal echocardiography, *Am J Nurse* 97(9):17, 1997.

Chapter 17

Bucher L: Acute myocardial infarction. In Bucher L, Melander S: *Critical care nursing*, Philadelphia, 1999, WB Saunders.

Ehrat K: *The art of EKG interpretation*, ed 4, Dubuque, IA, 1997, Kendall-Hunt.

Halm M, Penque S: Heart disease in women, *Am J Nurs* 99(4):26, 1999.

Miracle V, Sims J: Making sense of the 12-lead ECG, *Nursing* 29(7):34, 1999.

O'Donnell M, Dirks J: Cardiovascular disorders. In Urden L, Stacy K: *Priorities in critical care nursing*, ed 3, St Louis, 2000, Mosby.

Perrin KQ: Interventions for critically ill patients with coronary artery disease. In Ignatavicius DD, Workman M, Mishler M: *Medical-surgical nursing across the health care continuum*, vol 1, ed 3, Philadelphia, 1999, WB Saunders.

Chapter 18

Anderson K: *Mosby's medical, nursing, and allied health dictionary*, ed 5, St Louis, 1998, Mosby.

Copstead LEC, Banasik JC: *Pathophysiology: biological and behavioral perspectives*, ed 2, Philadelphia, 2000, WB Saunders.

Davenport J, Morton PG: Identifying nonischemic causes of life-threatening arrhythmias, *Am J Nurs* 97(11):50, 1997.

Dugan K: Caring for patients with pericarditis, *Nursing* 28(3):50, 1998.

Ehrat K: *The art of EKG interpretation: a self-instructional text*, ed 4, Dubuque, IA, 1997, Kendal Hunt.

Grauer K: *A practical guide to ECG interpretation*, St Louis, 1992, Mosby.

Huszar R: *Basic dysrhythmias: interpretation and management*, ed 2, St Louis, 1994, Mosby.

Kotecki CN: Infectious cardiac disorders. In Bucher L, Melander S: *Critical care nursing*, Philadelphia, 1999, WB Saunders.

Kupper NS, Duke ES: Inflammatory and valvular heart disease. In Lewis SM, Heitkemper MM, Dirksen SR: *Medical surgical nursing: assessment and management of clinical problems*, ed 5, St Louis, 2000, Mosby.

Lamborn ML, Moseley MJ: Cardiac alterations. In Hartshorn JC, Sole ML, Lamborn ML, editors: *Introduction to critical care nursing*, ed 3, Philadelphia, 2001, WB Saunders.

Lazzara D, Sellergren C: Chest pain: making the right call when the pressure is on, *Nursing 96* 26(11):42, 1996.

Makrevis C: Understanding non-Q wave MI, *Nursing 94* 24(8):32CC, 1994.

McCoy C, Livingston N: Cardiovascular laboratory and diagnostic tests. In Bucher L, Melander S: *Critical care nursing,* Philadelphia, 1999, WB Saunders.

Pierce CO: Acute post-MI pericarditis, *J Cardiovasc Nurs* 6(4):46, 1992.

Sims JM, Miracle V: Using the ECG to detect myocardial infarction, *Nursing* 29(8):41, 1999.

Skidmore L: *Mosby's drug guide for nurses,* St Louis, 2001, Mosby.

Thelan LA, Urden LD, Lough ME, Stacy KM: *Critical care nursing: diagnosis and management,* ed 3, St Louis, 1998, Mosby.

Wharton JM, Goldschlager N: *Guide to interpreting 12-lead ECGs,* Oradell, NJ, 1984, Medical Economics Books.

Chapter 19

Anderson K, editor: *Mosby's medical, nursing and allied health dictionary,* ed 5, St Louis, 1998, Mosby.

Chemecky C, Berger B: *Laboratory tests and diagnostic procedures,* ed 3, Philadelphia, 2001, WB Saunders.

Copstead LEC, Banasik JC: *Pathophysiology: biological and behavioral perspectives,* ed 2, Philadelphia, 2000, WB Saunders.

Davenport J, Morton PG: Identifying nonischemic causes of life-threatening arrhythmias, *Am J Nurs* 97(11):50, 1997.

Ehrat K: *The art of EKG interpretation: a self-instructional text,* ed 4, Dubque, IA, 1997, Kendal Hunt.

Lamborn ML, Moseley MJ: Cardiac alterations. In Hartshorn JC, Sole ML, Lamborn ML, editors: *Introduction to critical care nursing,* ed 3, Philadelphia, 2001, WB Saunders.

McCoy C, Livingston N: Cardiovascular laboratory and diagnostic tests. In Bucher L, Melander S: *Critical care nursing,* Philadelphia, 1999, WB Saunders.

Skidmore L: *Mosby's drug guide for nurses,* St Louis, 2001, Mosby.

Thelan LA, Urden LD, Lough ME, Stacy KM: *Critical care nursing: diagnosis and management,* ed 3, St Louis, 1998, Mosby.

Chapter 20

Anderson K: *Mosby's medical, nursing, and allied health dictionary,* ed 5, St Louis, 1998, Mosby.

Conover MB: Understanding electrocardiography, ed 5, St Louis, 1988, Mosby.

Copstead LEC, Banasik JC: *Pathophysiology: biological and behavioral perspectives,* ed 2, Philadelphia, 2000, WB Saunders.

Cummins RO: Advanced cardiac life support, Dallas, 1997, American Heart Association.

Davenport J, Morton PG: Identifying nonischemic causes of life-threatening arrhythmias, *Am J Nurs* 97(11):50, 1997.

Dugan K: Caring for patients with pericarditis, *Nursing* 28(3):50, 1998.

Ehrat K: *The art of EKG interpretation: a self-instructional text,* ed 4, Dubuque, IA, 1997, Kendal Hunt.

Grauer K: *A practical guide to ECG interpretation,* St Louis, 1992, Mosby.

Huszar R: *Basic dysrhythmias: interpretation and management,* ed 2, St Louis, 1994, Mosby.

Kotecki CN: Infectious cardiac disorders. In Bucher L, Melander S: *Critical care nursing,* Philadelphia, 1999, WB Saunders.

Kupper NS, Duke ES: Inflammatory and valvular heart disease. In Lewis SM, Heitkemper MM, Dirksen SR: *Medical surgical nursing: assessment and management of clinical problems,* ed 5, St Louis, 2000, Mosby.

Lamborn ML, Moseley MJ: Cardiac alterations. In Hartshorn JC, Sole ML, Lamborn ML, editors: *Introduction to critical care nursing,* ed 3, Philadelphia, 2001, WB Saunders.

Lazzara D, Sellergren C: Chest pain: making the right call when the pressure is on, *Nursing 96* 26(11):42, 1996.

Makrevis C: Understanding non-Q wave MI, *Nursing 94* 24(8):32CC, 1994.

McCoy C, Livingston N: Cardiovascular laboratory and diagnostic tests. In Bucher L, Melander S: *Critical care nursing,* Philadelphia, 1999, WB Saunders.

Pierce CO: Acute post-MI pericarditis, *J Cardiovasc Nurs* 6(4):46, 1992.

Sims JM, Miracle V: Using the ECG to detect myocardial infarction, *Nursing* 29(8):41, 1999.

Skidmore L: *Mosby's drug guide for nurses,* St Louis, 2001, Mosby.

Thelan LA, Urden LD, Lough ME, Stacy KM: *Critical care nursing: diagnosis and management,* ed 3, St Louis, 1998, Mosby.

Wharton JM, Goldschlager N: *Guide to interpreting 12-lead ECGs,* Oradell, NJ, 1984, Medical Economics Books.

Chapter 21

Donnerstein RL et al: Acute effects of caffeine ingestion on signal-averaged electrocardiograms, *Am Heart J* 136(4):643, 1998.

James JE: Is habitual caffeine use a preventable cardiovascular risk factor? *Lancet* 349(9047):279, 1997.

Mason MG: The "crackbelly": newly recognized bowel sequelae after crack cocaine intoxication, *J Emerg Nurs* 25(5):373, 1999.

Occhetta E et al: Implantable cardioverter defibrillators and cellular telephones: is there any interference? *Pacing Clin Electrophysiol* 22(17):983, 1999.

Perera R, Kraebber A, Schwartz MJ: Prolonged QT interval and cocaine use, *J Electrophysiol* 30(4):337, 1997.

Perrin KO: Assessment of the cardiovascular system. In Ignatavicius DD, Workman ML, Mishler MA: *Medical surgical nursing across the health care continuum,* ed 3, Philadelphia, 1999, WB Saunders.

Petrin CJ: Interventions for patients with dysrhythmias. In Ignatavicius DD, Workman ML, Mishler MA: *Medical surgical nursing across the health care continuum,* ed 3, Philadelphia, 1999, WB Saunders.

Philbin DM et al: Inappropriate shocks delivered by an ICD as a result of sensed potentials form a TENS unit, *Pacing Clin Electrophysiol* 21(10):2010, 1998.

Poterfield LM, Morton PG, Butze E: The evolution of internal defibrillators, *Crit Care Nurs Clin North Am* 11(3):303, 1999.

Santucci PA et al: Interference with an implantable defibrillator by an electronic antitheft surveillance device, *N Engl J Med* 339(19):1371, 1998.

Tse HF et al: Effect of implantable arterial defibrillator on the natural history of atrial fibrillation, *J Cardiovasc Electrophysiol* 10(9):1200, 1999.

Wang RY: pH-dependent cocaine-induced cardiotoxicity, *Am J Emerg Med* 17(4):364, 1999.

Color Insert (Atrial Fibrillation/Atrial Flutter Algorithm)

Chapman MJ et al: Management of atrial tachyarrhythmias in the critically ill: a comparison of intravenous procainamide and amiodarone, *Intensive Care Med* 19:48, 1993.

Clemo HF et al: Intravenous amiodarone for acute heart rate control in the critically ill patient with atrial tachyarrhythmias, *Am J Cardiol* 81:594, 1998.

Cotter G et al: Conversion of recent onset paroxysmal atrial fibrillation to normal sinus rhythm: the effect of no treatment and high-dose amiodarone: a randomized, placebo-controlled study, *Eur Heart J* 20:1833, 1999.

Ellenbogen KA et al: A placebo-controlled trial of continuous intravenous diltiazem infusion for 24-hour heart rate control during atrial fibrillation and atrial flutter: a multicenter study, *J Am Coll Cardiol* 18:891, 1991.

Salerno DM et al: Efficacy and safety of intravenous diltiazem for treatment of atrial fibrillation and atrial flutter, *Am J Cardiol* 63:1046, 1989.

Illustration Credits

Text

Page 2 (*top*): Redrawn from Guyton, Hall: *Textbook of medical physiology*, ed 7, Philadelphia, 1986, WB Saunders, as presented in Sole, Hartshorn, Lamborn: *Introduction to critical care nursing*, ed 3, Philadelphia, 2001, WB Saunders, p. 235.

Page 4: Redrawn from Thibodeau, Patton: *Anatomy & physiology*, ed 1, St Louis, 1987, Mosby, as presented in McCance, Huether: *Pathophysiology: the biological basis for disease in adults & children*, ed 3, St Louis, 1998, Mosby, p. 971.

Page 5 (*top*): Redrawn from Thibodeau, Patton: *Anatomy & physiology*, ed 1, St Louis, 1987, Mosby, as presented in McCance, Huether: *Pathophysiology: the biological basis for disease in adults & children*, ed 3, St Louis, 1998, Mosby, p. 974.

Page 7: Redrawn from Thibodeau, Patton: *Anatomy & physiology*, ed 1, St Louis, 1987, Mosby, as presented in McCance, Huether: *Pathophysiology: the biological basis for disease in adults & children*, ed 3, St Louis, 1998, Mosby, p. 977.

Page 18: Redrawn from Phipps, Sands, Marek: *Medical-surgical nursing: concepts and clinical practice*, ed 6, St Louis, 1999, Mosby, p. 675.

Page 25: Redrawn from Sole, Hartshorn, Lamborn: *Introduction to critical care nursing*, ed 3, Philadelphia, 2001, WB Saunders, p. 52.

Page 26 (*bottom*): Redrawn from Sole, Hartshorn, Lamborn: *Introduction to critical care nursing*, ed 3, Philadelphia, 2001, WB Saunders, p. 52.

Page 62: From Hudak, Gallo, Morton, editors: *Critical care nursing: a holistic approach*, ed 6, Philadelphia, 1998, Lippincott, p. 204.

Page 67: Modified from Huff: *ECG workout: exercises in arrhythmia interpretation*, ed 3, Philadelphia, 1997, Lippincott, p. 3.

Page 68: From Hudak, Gallo, Morton, editors: *Critical care nursing: a holistic approach*, ed 6, Philadelphia, 1998, Lippincott, p. 189.

Page 82: From Hudak, Gallo, Morton, editors: *Critical care nursing: a holistic approach*, ed 6, Philadelphia, 1998, Lippincott, p. 203.

Page 87: Redrawn from Franks: *3D view of the heart; application note, 12-Lead monitoring with EASI lead system*, October 1999, Agilent Technologies.

Page 88 (*top*): Redrawn from Franks: *3D view of the heart; application note, 12-Lead monitoring with EASI lead system*, United States, October 1999, Agilent Technologies.

Page 88 (*bottom*): Redrawn from Franks: *3D view of the heart; application note, 12-Lead monitoring with EASI lead system*, United States, October 1999, Agilent Technologies.

Page 93: Redrawn from Cohn, Gilroy-Doohan: *Flip and see ECG*, Philadelphia, 1996, WB Saunders, p. 77.

Page 95: Redrawn from Cohn, Gilroy-Doohan: *Flip and see ECG*,Philadelphia, 1996, WB Saunders, p. 77.

Page 96: Redrawn from Cohn, Gilroy-Doohan: *Flip and see ECG*, Philadelphia, 1996, WB Saunders, p. 75.

Page 98: Redrawn from Cohn, Gilroy-Doohan: *Flip and see ECG*, Philadelphia, 1996, WB Saunders, p. 75.

Page 99: Redrawn from Cohn, Gilroy-Doohan: *Flip and see ECG*, Philadelphia, 1996, WB Saunders, p. 73.

Page 101: Redrawn from Cohn, Gilroy-Doohan: *Flip and see ECG*, Philadelphia, 1996, WB Saunders, p. 75.

Page 101: Redrawn from Cohn, Gilroy-Doohan: *Flip and see ECG*, Philadelphia, 1996, WB Saunders, p. 73.

Page 102: Redrawn from Cohn, Gilroy-Doohan: *Flip and see ECG*, Philadelphia, 1996, WB Saunders, p. 77.

Page 103: Redrawn from Paul, Hebra: *The nurse's guide to cardiac rhythm interpretation*, Philadelphia, 1998, WB Saunders, p. 67.

Page 108 *(bottom)*: Redrawn from Cohn, Gilroy-Doohan: *Flip and see ECG*, Philadelphia, 1996, WB Saunders, p. 79.

Page 109: Redrawn from Alpert: *Cardiac arrhythmias*, St Louis, 1980, Mosby, p. 34.

Page 110 *(top)*: Redrawn from Alpert: *Cardiac arrhythmias*, St Louis, 1980, Mosby, p. 41.

Page 110 *(middle)*: Redrawn from Alpert: *Cardiac arrhythmias*, St Louis, 1980, Mosby, p. 36.

Page 110 *(bottom)*: Redrawn from Alpert: Cardiac arrhythmias, St Louis, 1980, Mosby, p. 39.

Page 112: Redrawn from Cohn, Gilroy-Doohan: *Flip and see ECG*, Philadelphia, 1996, WB Saunders, p. 79.

Page 113 *(top)*: Redrawn from Phipps, Sands, Marek: *Medical-surgical nursing: concepts and clinical practice*, ed 6, St Louis, 1999, Mosby, p. 670.

Page 114: Redrawn from Paul, Hebra: *The nurse's guide to cardiac rhythm interpretation*, Philadelphia, 1998, WB Saunders, p. 89.

Page 115: Redrawn from Alpert: *Cardiac arrhythmias*, St Louis, 1980, Mosby, p. 53.

Page 116: Redrawn from Alpert: *Cardiac arrhythmias*, St Louis, 1980, Mosby, p. 57.

Page 118 *(bottom)*: Redrawn from Cohn, Gilroy-Doohan: *Flip and see ECG*, Philadelphia, 1996, WB Saunders, p. 83.

Page 120 *(top)*: Redrawn from Paul, Hebra: The nurse's guide to cardiac rhythm interpretation, Philadelphia, 1998, WB Saunders, p. 100.

Page 120 *(bottom)*: Redrawn from Paul, Hebra: *The nurse's guide to cardiac rhythm interpretation*, Philadelphia, 1998, WB Saunders, p. 85.

Page 121: Redrawn from Alpert: *Cardiac arrhythmias*, St Louis, 1980, Mosby, p. 68.

Page 122 *(top)*: Redrawn from Alpert: *Cardiac arrhythmias*, St Louis, 1980, Mosby, p. 68.

Page 126: Redrawn from Paul, Hebra: *The nurse's guide to cardiac rhythm interpretation*, Philadelphia, 1998, WB Saunders, p. 111.

Page 128: Redrawn from Paul, Hebra: *The nurse's guide to cardiac rhythm interpretation*, Philadelphia, 1998, WB Saunders, p. 108.

Page 130: Redrawn from Paul, Hebra: *The nurse's guide to cardiac rhythm interpretation*, Philadelphia, 1998, WB Saunders, p. 83.

Page 133 *(top)*: Redrawn from Paul, Hebra: *The nurse's guide to cardiac rhythm interpretation*, Philadelphia, 1998, WB Saunders, p. 61.

Page 133 *(bottom)*: Redrawn from Paul, Hebra: *The nurse's guide to cardiac rhythm interpretation*, Philadelphia, 1998, WB Saunders, p. 102.

Page 136: Redrawn from Paul, Hebra: *The nurse's guide to cardiac rhythm interpretation*, Philadelphia, 1998, WB Saunders, p. 113.

Page 140: Redrawn from Phipps, Sands, Marek: *Medical-surgical nursing: concepts and clinical practice*, ed 6, St Louis, 1999, Mosby, p. 673.

Page 140: Redrawn from Phipps, Sands, Marek: *Medical-surgical nursing: concepts and clinical practice*, ed 6, St Louis, 1999, Mosby, p. 673.

Page 141 *(top)*: Redrawn from Paul, Hebra: *The nurse's guide to cardiac rhythm interpretation*, Philadelphia, 1998, WB Saunders, p. 131.

Page 142: Redrawn from Ignatavicius, Workman, Mishler: *Medical-surgical nursing across the health care continuum*, ed 2, Philadelphia, 1995, WB Saunders, p. 852.

Page 145: Redrawn from Cohn, Gilroy-Doohan: *Flip and see ECG*, Philadelphia, 1996, WB Saunders, p. 89.

Page 150: Redrawn from Paul, Hebra: *The nurse's guide to cardiac rhythm interpretation*, Philadelphia, 1998, WB Saunders, p. 163.

Page 155: Redrawn from Cohn, Gilroy-Doohan: *Flip and see ECG*, Philadelphia, 1996, WB Saunders, p. 91.

Page 161: Redrawn from Ignatavicius, Workman, Mishler: *Medical-surgical nursing across the health care continuum*, ed 2, Philadelphia, 1995, WB Saunders, p. 852.

Page 162: Redrawn from Ignatavicius, Workman, Mishler: *Medical-surgical nursing across the health care continuum*, ed 2, Philadelphia, 1995, WB Saunders, p. 854.

Page 167: Redrawn from Cohn, Gilroy-Doohan: *Flip and see ECG*, Philadelphia, 1996, WB Saunders, p. 97.

Page 170: Redrawn from Ignatavicius, Workman, Mishler: *Medical-surgical nursing across the health care continuum*, ed 2, Philadelphia, 1995, WB Saunders, p. 852.

Page 171: Redrawn from Ignatavicius, Workman, Mishler: *Medical-surgical nursing across the health care continuum*, ed 2, Philadelphia, 1995, WB Saunders, p. 854.

Page 173: Redrawn from Cohn, Gilroy-Doohan: *Flip and see ECG*, Philadelphia, 1996, WB Saunders, p. 103.

Page 188 *(top)*: Redrawn from Copstead, Banasik: *Pathophysiology*, ed 2, Philadelphia, 2000, WB Saunders, p. 420.

Page 188 *(bottom)*: Redrawn from Guyton, Hall: *Textbook of medical physiology*, ed 7, Philadelphia, 1986, WB Saunders, p. 133.

Page 189 *(top)*: Redrawn from Guyton, Hall: *Textbook of medical physiology*, ed 7, Philadelphia, 1986, WB Saunders, p. 133.

Page 189 *(bottom)*: Redrawn from Guyton, Hall: *Textbook of medical physiology*, ed 7, Philadelphia, 1986, WB Saunders, p. 133.

Page 190: Redrawn from Copstead, Banasik: *Pathophysiology*, ed 2, Philadelphia, 2000, WB Saunders, p. 421.

Page 191: Redrawn from Copstead, Banasik: *Pathophysiology*, ed 2, Philadelphia, 2000, WB Saunders, p. 421.

Page 192: Redrawn from Copstead, Banasik: *Pathophysiology*, ed 2, Philadelphia, 2000, WB Saunders, p. 421.

Page 194 *(top)*: Redrawn from Bucher, Melander: *Critical care nursing*, Philadelphia, 1999, WB Saunders, p. 189.

Page 194 *(bottom)*: Redrawn from Bucher, Melander: *Critical care nursing*, Philadelphia, 1999, WB Saunders, p. 189.

Page 195: Redrawn from Bucher, Melander: *Critical care nursing*, Philadelphia, 1999, WB Saunders, p. 189.

Page 198: Redrawn from Huszar: *Pocket guide to basic dysrhythmias*, ed 2, St Louis, 1995, Mosby, p. 80.

Page 199: Redrawn from Bucher, Melander: *Critical care nursing*, Philadelphia, 1999, WB Saunders, p. 191.

Page 201: Redrawn from Huszar: *Pocket guide to basic dysrhythmias*, ed 2, St Louis, 1995, Mosby, p. 84.

Page 204: Redrawn from Bucher, Melander: *Critical care nursing*, Philadelphia, 1999, WB Saunders, p. 295.

Page 209: Redrawn from Lipman, Lipman: *ECG pocket guide*, St Louis, 1987, Mosby, p. 120.

Page 212: Redrawn from Bucher, Melander: *Critical care nursing*, Philadelphia, 1999, WB Saunders, p. 185.

Page 218 *(left)*: Redrawn from Chernecky, Macklin, Murphy-Ende: *Real-world nursing survival guide: fluids & electrolytes*, Philadelphia, 2001, WB Saunders.

Page 221 *(left)*: Redrawn from Chernecky, Macklin, Murphy-Ende: *Real-world nursing survival guide: fluids & electrolytes*, Philadelphia, 2001, WB Saunders.

Page 231: Redrawn from Paul, Hebra: *The nurse's guide to cardiac rhythm interpretation*, Philadelphia, 1998, WB Saunders, p. 252.

Page 232: Redrawn from Paul, Hebra: *The nurse's guide to cardiac rhythm interpretation*, Philadelphia, 1998, WB Saunders, p. 244.

Page 233: Redrawn from Paul, Hebra: *The nurse's guide to cardiac rhythm interpretation*, Philadelphia, 1998, WB Saunders, p. 244.

Page 239: Redrawn from Ignatavicius, Workman, Mishler: *Medical-surgical nursing across the health care continuum*, ed 2, Philadelphia, 1995, WB Saunders, p. 781.

Page 240: Redrawn from Cohn, Gilroy-Doohan: *Flip and see ECG*, Philadelphia, 1996, WB Saunders, p. 91.

Page 242: Redrawn from Ignatavicius, Workman, Mishler: *Medical-surgical nursing across the health care continuum*, ed 2, Philadelphia, 1995, WB Saunders, p. 792.

Page 244 *(top)*: Redrawn from Ignatavicius, Workman, Mishler: *Medical-surgical nursing across the health care continuum*, ed 2, Philadelphia, 1995, WB Saunders, p. 795.

Page 244 *(bottom)*: Redrawn from Ignatavicius, Workman, Mishler: *Medical-surgical nursing across the health care continuum*, ed 2, Philadelphia, 1995, WB Saunders, p. 795.

Page 253 *(top)*: Redrawn from Cohn, Gilroy-Doohan: *Flip and see ECG*, Philadelphia, 1996, WB Saunders, p. 85.

Page 253 *(bottom)*: Redrawn from Cohn, Gilroy-Doohan: *Flip and see ECG*, Philadelphia, 1996, WB Saunders, p. 83.

Page 260: Redrawn from Ignatavicius, Workman, Mishler: *Medical-surgical nursing across the health care continuum*, ed 2, Philadelphia, 1995, WB Saunders, p. 835.

Color insert

Page 1: From Thibodeau, Patton: *The human body in health and disease*, ed 3, St Louis, 2001, Mosby.

Page 2: From Thibodeau, Patton: *The human body in health and disease*, ed 3, St Louis, 2001, Mosby.

Page 3: From Thibodeau, Patton: *The human body in health and disease*, ed 3, St Louis, 2001, Mosby.

Page 4: From Aehlert: *ACLS quick review study guide*, St Louis, 2002, Mosby.

NCLEX Section

CHAPTER *1*

1. What chamber of the heart pumps oxygenated blood back into the circulatory system?
   1 Right atrium
   2 Right ventricle
   3 Mitral valve
   4 Left ventricle

2. Another name for ventricular contraction is:
   1 Systole
   2 Diastole
   3 Cyanosis
   4 Sternum

3. The electrical power source of the heart is the SA node. It is located in the:
   1 Right ventricle
   2 Right atrium
   3 Aorta
   4 Left atrium

4. Which of the following medications do not have a positive inotropic effect on the myocardium?
   1 Dobutamine
   2 Digitalis
   3 Propranolol
   4 Epinephrine

2. The student you are tutoring is studying a rhythm strip. You know there is understanding when the student states:
   1 "There should be an isoelectric line after the PR interval."
   2 "P waves should be upright in lead II."
   3 "Q waves are always present in a QRS complex."
   4 "T waves are notched at their peak."

3. When the flow of electrical energy moves toward the positive electrode and then turns toward the negative, what waveform is recorded?
   1 Positive
   2 Negative
   3 Biphasic
   4 Isoelectric

CHAPTER *2*

1. The part of the rhythm that indicates the time it takes for the SA node to fire and the atria to depolarize is known as the:
   1 P wave
   2 R wave
   3 S wave
   4 T wave

Notes

NCLEX CHAPTER *1* Answers

1.4 The left ventricle pumps blood into the systemic circulation. The right atrium pumps blood to the right ventricle. The mitral valve is not a heart chamber. The right ventricle pumps blood to the lungs.

2.1 Systole is ventricular contraction. Diastole is ventricular filling. Cyanosis is a bluish tint to the skin and oral mucosa because of a lack of oxygen. The sternum is the breast bone.

3.2 The sinoatrial node is located in the right atrium. The right ventricle leads to the pulmonary artery. The aorta is the main blood vessel leading to the body. The left atrium is the heart chamber that receives oxygenated blood from the lungs.

4.3 Propranolol has a negative inotropic effect on the myocardium (decreasing cardiac contractility). Dobutamine, digitalis, and epinephrine are positive inotropic drugs.

NCLEX CHAPTER *2* Answers

1.1 P waves indicate atrial depolarization. R and S waves indicate ventricular depolarization. T waves indicate ventricular repolarization.

2.2 P waves are positive in lead II because the positive electrode in lead II is below the heart and sees the normal atrial depolarization waves coming toward it. The PR interval is an isoelectric line. The QRS complex is after the PR interval. Q waves are not always present in the QRS complex. T waves are normally rounded. Notching may indicate a P wave sitting on top of a T wave.

3.3 A biphasic or two-phased waveform is caused when the wave of stimulation goes toward the positive and then the negative electrode. A positive waveform is caused when the electrical current flows toward a positive electrode. A negative waveform is caused by the wave of depolarization flowing toward the negative electrode. An isoelectric waveform is caused when the electrical flow is perpendicular or between a positive and negative electrode.

CHAPTER *2*—cont'd

4. The relative refractory period of the heart is:
   1 During the P wave
   2 In the middle of the R wave
   3 The first part of the S wave
   4 In the middle of the T wave

CHAPTER *3*

1. You are preparing a presentation on the basics of analyzing ECGs for a group of graduate nurses. Which of the following areas is most important to cover in your discussion?
   1 Voltage measurements
   2 Time measurements
   3 Use of calipers
   4 Heart size

2. A student nurse has measured Mr. O'Brien's QRS complex to be seven small boxes wide. What time interval would this indicate?
   1 0.04 seconds
   2 0.20 seconds
   3 0.28 seconds
   4 1.4 seconds

3. While discussing changes on Ms. Laticia's ECG, you identify a waveform that measures five small boxes vertically on the ECG paper. This indicates:
   1 1 mm
   2 0.12 mm
   3 5 mm
   4 10 mm

4. Documentation on a rhythm strip should include all of the following except:
   1 Date and time
   2 Full name and title
   3 Signature of the reviewing physician
   4 Rhythm analysis

5. While reviewing Mr. Jackson's ECG, you find that his waveforms have increased in height. This may be an indication of which of the following conditions?
   1 Cardiac hypertrophy
   2 Cardiac tamponade
   3 Cardiac standstill
   4 Rheumatoid arthritis of the neck

CHAPTER *4*

1. When determining heart rate in a normal heart, you should remember that the atrial rate is:
   1 Always slower than the ventricular rate
   2 The preferred rate to measure
   3 Always faster than the ventricular rate
   4 Always equal to the ventricular rate

Notes

NCLEX CHAPTER 2 Answers—cont'd

4.4 The relative refractory period is the middle of the T wave. The T wave is ventricular repolarization and the middle of the T wave is where the cardiac cells try to regain their negativity. If stimulated here, the heart can go into electrical chaos. The P wave indicates atrial depolarization. The R and S waves indicate ventricular depolarization.

NCLEX CHAPTER 3 Answers

1.2 It is most important for the nurse to be able to accurately determine heart rate and regularity, which are time measurements. The other areas (voltage measurement, use of calipers, and heart size) are necessary to the discussion, but time measurements are the priority.

2.3 0.28 seconds. Seven small boxes × 0.04 seconds (time allotted for each box) = 0.28 seconds.

3.3 Vertical small blocks indicate 1 mm. Therefore 1 mm times five little vertical blocks equals 5 mm.

4.3 The physician or advanced practice nurse need not sign that he or she has reviewed the rhythm. Date, time, full name, title, and rhythm analysis are written either on the strip or in the health care provider's notes (or wherever hospital protocol dictates).

5.1 Enlarged heart muscle (cardiac hypertrophy) causes an increase in numbers of vertical boxes and voltage on the ECG. Cardiac tamponade would decrease voltage, and cardiac standstill has no voltage. Rheumatoid arthritis would not affect the ECG.

NCLEX CHAPTER 4 Answers

1.4 In the normal heart, the atrial and ventricular rates should be equal. An atrial rate slower than the ventricular rate would indicate bradycardia. Ventricular rates, not atrial rates, are the preferred rate to measure because they are more easily identified. An atrial rate faster than the ventricular rate would indicate tachycardia.

CHAPTER *4*—cont'd

2. While discussing the estimated methods of heart-rate calculation with a group of students, which of the following methods would you identify as most accurate?
   1 Six-second method
   2 Rule of 1500s
   3 Rule of 300s
   4 Rule of 5s

3. The 6-second method is the only one that can be used for:
   1 Measuring regular and irregular heart rates
   2 Measuring R-to-R time intervals
   3 Measuring P-to-P time intervals
   4 Measuring small boxes

4. Mr. Sylvester's heart rate is 120 beats per minute. You would be correct in describing this rate as a:
   1 Bradycardia
   2 Normal rate
   3 Tachycardia
   4 Heart block

5. Using the 6-second method or the rule of 10s, which of the following is the atrial rate if the number of P waves on a 6-second strip is 5.
   1 300
   2 30
   3 50
   4 25

CHAPTER *5*

1. When using the eight-step method, you should look at configuration and location of which of the following?
   1 P waves
   2 PRI
   3 ST segments
   4 Absolute refractory period

2. Conduction times in ECG analysis refers to:
   1 P waves
   2 PRI
   3 ST segments
   4 P-to-P interval

Notes

2.2 The rule of 1500s gives a precise heart rate. The 6-second method is for a quick estimation of rates and can be used for both regular and irregular rhythms. The rule of 300s can be performed without a calculator and is used to calculate approximate rates for regular rhythms only. There is no rule of 5s.

3.1 The 6-second method looks at number of beats and therefore can be used to determine rates for regular and irregular rhythms. Measuring R-to-R intervals and P-to-P intervals and counting only small boxes can be done with the rule of 1500s or the rule of 300s.

4.3 Rates greater than 100 are described as tachycardia. A bradycardia is a heart rate below 60. A normal rate is between 60 and 100. A heart block involves looking at the PR interval and its relationship to the QRS.

5.3 10×5 (number of P waves) $= 50$.

NCLEX CHAPTER *5* **Answers**

1.1 The configuration and location of P waves that look the same indicate the rhythm is coming from the SA node. P waves that are inverted or notched are usually from an ectopic focus. The PRI is a measure of conduction. The ST segment is not viewed solely from a rhythm strip; a 12-lead ECG must be examined. The absolute refractory period is located in the middle of the T wave; this is examined in relationship to an R wave.

2.2 The PRI is indicative of conduction above the ventricle conduction. The P waves are not measured in length alone. They are, however, part of the PRI, which is a measurement of conduction. The ST segments are not measured for time; they are measured up and down in a 12-lead ECG. The P-to-P interval is measured to determine atrial regularity.

CHAPTER **5**—cont'd

3. A health care provider you are tutoring shows you a rhythm strip that has been run on a new patient with unstable angina. To help analyze this strip, the best thing to tell the provider is:
   1 "Don't worry. Just put it on the chart and call it to the physician's attention during rounds this morning."
   2 "Try to describe the rhythm using as much descriptive language as possible."
   3 "Give it to me, and I will do the analysis."
   4 "The ECG technician will help you with it in a minute."

4. A cause of 60-cycle interference is:
   1 Jumping up and down
   2 An ungrounded electrical shaver
   3 A straight razor
   4 A battery-operated radio

Notes _____

CHAPTER **6**

1. When a patient's ECG alarm goes off because of a suggested artifact, your first action should be to:
   1 Ignore the warning.
   2 Call the prescribing professional in charge of the patient and ask for an interpretation of the rhythm strip.
   3 Assess the patient to ensure his or her safety.
   4 Ask a more experienced provider for direction.

2. A wandering baseline is caused by:
   1 Improperly grounded electrical equipment
   2 A monitor that does not count each QRS
   3 Chest movement during respiration
   4 Shivering from a high fever

3. Which of the following is not a cause of artifact?
   1 Hiccup
   2 Convulsions
   3 Shivering
   4 Tachycardia

NCLEX CHAPTER **5** **Answers**—cont'd

3.2 Even if the health care provider does not know exactly what the rhythm is, he or she needs to go through the steps to tell what characteristics the rhythm has so that he or she can more fully describe the rhythm to other health care practitioners. Telling a provider "not to worry" is belittling; rather, he or she should be given every opportunity to learn the correct way to determine rhythm strips. Doing it for the provider will not help the learning process. He or she needs to practice under direct supervision. The ECG technician, although a good resource person, is not the legal professional in charge of the patient's care.

NCLEX CHAPTER **6** **Answers**

1.3 A health care provider should always check the patient first if the monitor alarm goes off. Alarms should never be ignored. The physician or advanced practice nurse only needs to be called if the patient requires medical treatment for a change in rhythm. The advice of a more experienced provider is not needed until the situation is assessed and found to be beyond your ability to understand.

2.3 Chest movements up and down during respiration will cause the rhythm strip to move up and down in a regular cyclic pattern. Improperly grounded electrical equipment causes 60-cycle interference (electrical). Weak signals may cause the monitor to miss QRS complexes and therefore record a falsely low heart rate. High fevers can cause artifact or picking up of muscular tremors.

3.4 Tachycardia is a fast heart rate and not artifact. Hiccup, convulsions, and shivering can cause artifact because they cause strong muscular movements.

4.2 An ungrounded electrical device (in this case, a shaver) can cause leakage of electrical current and therefore electrical interference. Jumping up and down will cause muscular interference. A straight razor and a battery-operated radio do not run on electrical current and therefore are acceptable for patient use.

CHAPTER 7

1. Provider Jones has worked in the coronary care unit for 6 years and is overseeing the training of Ms. Confer, GN. Provider Jones knows Ms. Confer understands the rationale for a ground electrode when she states:
   1 "The ground electrode magnifies the lead of the heart so that the nurse can see it."
   2 "The ground electrode changes the lead of the heart."
   3 "The ground electrode prevents electrical shock to the patient."
   4 "The ground electrode records the current of electricity, from positive to negative."

2. Which of the following best describes lead II?
   1 Negative on the right arm, positive on the left arm
   2 Negative on the left arm, positive on the right arm
   3 Negative on the right arm, positive on the left lower chest
   4 Negative on the left arm, positive on the right lower chest

3. A 12-lead ECG is being recorded by an unlicensed assistive person. The waveform looks unusual in aVR. The health care provider checks the lead on the patient's chest and knows that aVF is recorded as:
   1 Left arm positive, heart negative
   2 Right arm positive, heart negative
   3 Right leg positive, heart negative
   4 Right arm negative, left leg positive

4. The health care provider is performing a 12-lead ECG on a patient. The patient asks the provider to explain why so many electrodes are needed across the chest. Which of the following is the best explanation for this patient?
   1 Electrode placement across the chest ensures accuracy of heart conduction.
   2 The six sticky tabs across your chest look at the heart from top to bottom.
   3 These electrodes are needed to look at your heart in the frontal plane.
   4 These electrodes will tell me about your heart, from right to left.

CHAPTER 8

1. When reviewing the characteristics of normal sinus rhythm, the health care provider knows that if the sinoatrial node is the dominant pacemaker in a rhythm strip being evaluated, the strip will show:
   1 R-to-R intervals equal to the PR intervals
   2 A regular rhythm
   3 P waves, consistently rounded and uniform in shape, preceding all QRS complexes
   4 That the dominant pacemaker cannot be determined from a rhythm strip

2. In analyzing an ECG strip, the health care practitioner suspects that the atrial tissue is ischemic (lacks oxygen) and not capable of conducting the sinoatrial node–initiated heart beat. Which observation did the health care practitioner consider initially when determining atrial ischemia?

1 The heart rate is 110 bpm.

2 The P waves are irregular in their shape and location.

3 Every fourth beat is blocked at the atrioventricular junction.

4 Some contractions are occurring prematurely in the cardiac cycle.

Notes

NCLEX CHAPTER *7* Answers

1. 3 A ground wire prevents leakage of current and electrical shock. The augmented leads magnify the view of the heart. The placement of the positive and negative electrodes changes the lead. The axis of the lead describes where the flow of energy goes.

2. 4 In lead II, the negative electrode is on the left shoulder and the positive electrode is on the right lower chest area. "Left arm positive, heart is negative" does not describe any lead. "Negative on the left arm, positive on the right arm" describes lead I. "Right leg positive, heart is negative" describes lead III.

3. 2 In aVR, the right arm is positive and the heart is negative. In the augmented leads, the positive electrode is on the appendage of the last letter in its abbreviation. "Right leg positive, heart negative" best describes aVF. "Right arm negative, left leg positive" does not describe any lead of the 12-lead ECG.

4. 4 The electrode placement in the V leads looks at the heart from right ventricle (V1) to left ventricle (V6). Electrode placement across the chest ensures accuracy of heart conduction and describes the V leads, but it does not state why or answer the patient's questions. The leads do not look at the heart from top to bottom; they look at it from right to left. The V leads look at the heart in the horizontal plane.

NCLEX CHAPTER *8* Answers

1. 3 A P wave denotes the conduction of the sinoatrial node stimulus through the atria. The R-to-R intervals are not equal to PR intervals. Equal R-to-R intervals define a regular rhythm, but this can be true in nonsinoatrial node–initiated situations such as nodal tachycardia or ventricular tachycardia. The purpose of evaluating the rhythm strip is to determine information about all aspects of the conduction system, including the dominant pacemaker.

2. 2 The presence of P waves will show that the stimulus has resulted in contraction of the atria, but their lack of uniformity suggests an irritable transmission through the atria. The heart rate itself is not the determinant of oxygen availability; however, more oxygen is consumed with the higher rate and the health care practitioner should be aware of this factor. Blocked beats and premature contractions do not give direct information about ischemia.

CHAPTER *8*—cont'd

3. Mr. Peters arrives in the emergency department complaining of palpitations, shortness of breath, and dizziness. His ECG reveals sinus tachycardia. What is the probable cause of his dizziness?
   1   An overstimulation of the parasympathetic nervous system
   2   An increase in cardiac output
   3   A decrease in ventricular filling time
   4   An increase in blood pressure

4. Ms. Houser is a patient with cardiac disease who is now experiencing sinus tachycardia. The health care practitioner is aware that this dysrhythmia could trigger congestive heart failure because:
   1   The cardiac muscle may be unable to sustain the heart rate.
   2   It is well known that this condition occurs with sinus node abnormalities.
   3   The slow heart rate is insufficient to deliver blood to the heart muscle.
   4   Cardiac medications eventually become ineffective, and any dysrhythmia results in heart failure.

5. The heart monitor alarm frequently rings because the patient's usual heart rate of 58 is lower than the preset 60 as lower limit rate. What action should the health care provider take?
   1   Turn off the alarm but look more frequently at the remote ECG screen in the provider's station.
   2   Check the hospital's policy and reset the lower limit to a lower value accordingly.
   3   Turn down the alarm and turn off the graphing device that triggers when the alarm sounds, because monitors are permanently set with their upper and lower limits.
   4   Lower the limit on the monitor as necessary because this would be considered an independent provider judgment.

Notes

3.3   Because of the fast heart rate, there is less time for the ventricles to receive full stroke volume. This results in smaller blood volumes with each heartbeat and therefore insufficient oxygenation to the brain, resulting in dizziness. Overstimulation of the parasympathetic nervous system would be responsible for an increased heart rate. Although a decrease in cardiac output could account for decreased cerebral perfusion and thus dizziness, this is not true of an increase. A decrease rather than an increase in blood pressure might result in insufficient oxygenation to the brain in this particular situation.

4.1   The increased workload of the heart muscle based on the rapid heart rate can result in decompensation of the muscle, resulting in heart failure. Sinus node abnormalities are not directly known to result in heart failure. Congestive heart failure can occur with any long-term disease related to heart muscle, valvular problems, or high blood pressure. Sinus tachycardia is a rapid heart rate (>100 bpm), whereas sinus bradycardia is a slow heart rate (< 60 bpm). There is no direct relationship between long-term use of medications and heart failure.

5.2   Although monitors are typically preset for bradycardia and tachycardia values (< 60 bpm and >100 bpm), patients are often monitored for these types of dysrhythmias as their underlying cardiac problems. The hospital policy will identify the health care provider's action. The alarm must remain on at all times. Even the most astute provider cannot be expected to observe multiple heart monitors for potentially lethal dysrhythmias. Limits may be changed in accordance with the hospital's policy; other interventions to control the sound or graphing would be inappropriate. The appropriate judgment for the health care provider is that the policy needs to be checked because a constantly sounding alarm defeats the purpose for which it was intended; however, changing it without this review or determination could result in harm to the patient.

CHAPTER 9

1. Mr. Willow's ECG shows five premature atrial contractions in a 1-minute strip. What action should the health care practitioner take?
   1. Notify the physician immediately because these ectopic beats may quickly lead to life-threatening dysrhythmias.
   2. Disregard these beats but take the patient's blood pressure more often to access cardiac output.
   3. Change the patient's dietary order to include only decaffeinated beverages.
   4. Monitor Mr. Willow's ECG and notify the physician if six or more premature atrial contractions occur in a 1-minute strip.

2. The health care provider is assessing the patient's apical rate, which is very irregular at a varying rate of 60 to 150 bpm. What might the provider conclude from this assessment?
   1. The patient is in atrial flutter with a varying degree of block.
   2. The patient is in atrial fibrillation because this would be heard as an irregular heart beat.
   3. The patient's ECG needs to be observed to determine the nature of the dysrhythmia.
   4. The patient is in an accelerated junctional tachycardia because a varying rate is a hallmark feature of this dysrhythmia.

3. Ms. Belfry has been diagnosed with atrial flutter and is scheduled for a cardioversion. When assisting with this procedure, the health care practitioner anticipates that the shock will be given at what point on the ECG waveform?
   1. On the P wave
   2. On the R wave
   3. On the T wave
   4. During the PR interval

4. The health care provider suspects that a patient with a paroxysmal supraventricular tachycardia may be experiencing a decrease in cardiac output. Which of the following assessment findings supports this concern?
   1. Flushed face and warm extremities
   2. Capillary refill less than 3 seconds
   3. A complaint of chest pain, subsiding as output lowers and oxygen demands decrease
   4. Dizziness when the patient sits in a chair

Notes

NCLEX CHAPTER *9* Answers

1. 4 The new development of six or more premature atrial contractions in 1 minute would be cause for notifying the physician, because their presence suggests a possible new irritability that should be investigated further. Fewer than six premature atrial contractions per minute are not considered life threatening. In general, the health care provider should be aware of new developments in rhythms. Therefore if Mr. Willow developed premature atrial contractions when none were evident before, it would be good to alert the physician on the next regular contact; however, this is not an emergency. Provided there is not a significant change in the ventricular rate of this patient, cardiac output should not be changed. Caffeinated beverages can contribute to premature atrial contractions, but the practitioner would not be the one initiating a dietary change.

2. 3 Although it is possible to use the generic labels of bradycardia or tachycardia for slow and rapid heart rates, respectively, precise dysrhythmias can only be documented with an ECG. It is not possible to identify atrial flutter, atrial fibrillation, or accelerated junctional tachycardia through auscultation.

3. 2 This type of cardioversion is called synchronous; a shock at this time directs conduction and systole to occur simultaneously, reestablishing the normal conduction pathway. Once the P wave is initiated, the QRS would follow and the conduction system would not be reset. The T wave is the time for ventricular repolarization or diastole; a shock at this time would be dangerous because the ventricle should not be contracting and life-threatening dysrhythmias can result (ventricular fibrillation).

4. 4 Dizziness occurs because of the reduced stroke volume (a result of shortened ventricular filling time) with the rapid rate and the small subsequent quantities of blood perfusing the cerebral tissue. Warm face and extremities would suggest that cardiac output is adequate. Capillary refill should be less than 3 seconds if there is sufficient cardiac output. Lower oxygen demands on the myocardium decrease chest pain, but this occurs when cardiac output is sufficient and not lowered.

CHAPTER **9**—cont'd

5. The heart conduction system includes inherent pacemakers at varying locations. Which of the following ECG tracing descriptions might the health care provider observe if the atrioventricular node were the primary pacemaker?
   1 Absence of P waves and a ventricular rate less than 40 bpm
   2 Abnormally-shaped QRS complexes
   3 Abnormal or inverted P waves and a ventricular rate between 40 and 60 bpm
   4 Depressed ST segments

6. A patient's heart rate has decreased over several days from 70 to 54 bpm. Which of the following drugs may be responsible for the change?
   1 Adenosine (Adenocard)
   2 Furosemide (Lasix)
   3 Digoxin (Lanoxin)
   4 Atropine (Atropine Sulfate, Isopto-Atropine)

7. Mr. Carson develops paroxysmal supraventricular tachycardia during a time of high stress in his life. Despite efforts to reduce his stress, his condition continues. What initial therapy might be attempted to end paroxysmal supraventricular tachycardia?
   1 Vagal stimulation
   2 Cardioversion
   3 Intravenous adenosine (Adenocard)
   4 Intravenous epinephrine (Adrenaline)

CHAPTER **10**

1. Mrs. Anthony was admitted with an accelerated junctional tachycardia. In obtaining Mrs. Anthony's drug history, which medication should alert the health care provider as to a possible cause for this dysrhythmia?
   1 Stool softener
   2 Sedative
   3 Antihypertensive
   4 Digitalis glycoside

Notes

NCLEX CHAPTER **9** Answers—cont'd

5.3 Abnormal or inverted P waves and a ventricular rate between 40 and 60 bpm suggests that the atrioventricular node is the primary pacemaker because atrial contraction is seen in retrograde fashion as inverted P waves. The absence of P waves and a ventricular rate less than 40 bpm suggests that the ventricular tissue is the primary pacemaker. Abnormally shaped QRS complexes suggest abnormal conduction in the bundle of His or may refer to QRS complexes seen in premature ventricular contractions. Depressed ST segments suggest myocardial injury. Elevated ST segments suggest myocardial ischemia or oxygen deficiency.

6.3 Digoxin, as a chronotropic drug, promotes a decrease in rate because it prolongs the refractory (resting) time of the atrioventricular node. Fewer sinoatrial or atrial stimuli are thus conducted to the ventricle and the heart rate decreases. Adenosine is used to suppress paroxysmal supraventricular tachycardia. Furosemide is a loop diuretic; it promotes water elimination and thus can assist in the reduction of blood pressure, but it does not directly lower heart rate. Atropine is given to increase heart rate and is used in the treatment of bradycardia.

7.1 Stimulation of the vagus nerve through carotid massage, eyeball pressure, or initiation of the Valsalva maneuver (bearing down, as in defecation) may be successful in reducing the heart rate and is the initial approach to paroxysmal supraventricular tachycardia in most patients. Cardioversion may be tried when vagal stimulation and drug therapy fail. Adenosine is the drug of choice and is usually given if vagal stimulation is unsuccessful. Epinephrine would increase the heart rate and is not used in paroxysmal supraventricular tachycardia.

NCLEX CHAPTER **10** Answers

1.4 Digoxin, a digitalis glycoside, is often the culprit in initiating junctional tachycardia. Additional doses of digoxin could be lethal in this situation. A stool softener is given to decrease a vagal response that could cause sinus bradycardia or heart block. A sedative usually slows the heart rate rather than increases it. An antihypertensive drug, which is a centrally acting sympatholytically, reduces cerebral sympatholytic outflow, thereby decreasing sympathetic responses (decreasing heart rate) and peripheral resistance.

CHAPTER *10*—cont'd

2. The conduction system of the heart includes inherent pacemakers at varying locations. Which of the following ECG tracing descriptions might the health care practitioner observe if the atrioventricular node is the primary pacemaker?
    1   Absence of P waves and a ventricular rate less than 40 bpm
    2   Abnormally shaped QRS complexes
    3   Abnormal or inverted P waves and a ventricular rate between 40 and 60 bpm
    4   Depressed ST segments

3. Mr. Collins develops paroxysmal supraventricular tachycardia. What initial therapy might be attempted?
    1   Cardioversion
    2   Intravenous atropine
    3   Intravenous epinephrine
    4   Vagal stimulation

4. All the following are indicators of junctional beats *except*:
    1   PR interval less than 0.12 seconds
    2   No P wave
    3   PR interval greater than 0.20 seconds
    4   Retrograde or inverted P wave in lead II

5. In paroxysmal supraventricular tachycardia, cardiac output is reduced because of:
    1   Wide QRS complexes
    2   Shortened diastolic filling time
    3   Increased stroke volume
    4   Slowed heart rate

6. A junctional rhythm with a ventricular rate exceeding 60 bpm but less than 100 bpm is referred to as:
    1   Ventricular escape rhythm
    2   Junctional tachycardia
    3   Bradycardia
    4   Accelerated junctional rhythm

7. Supraventricular tachycardias may occur in what group(s) of people because of immature sympathetic nervous system development?
    1   Teenagers and young adults
    2   Neonates and children
    3   Mature adults
    4   Infants and teenagers

Notes

Notes

2.3 A junctional rhythm may have abnormal or inverted P waves. The inherent rate for the atrioventricular node is 40 to 60 bpm. Absence of P waves with a ventricular rate of less than 40 is slower than a typical junctional rhythm. In a junctional rhythm the QRS complexes should be less than 0.12 seconds wide and shaped normally. In a junctional rhythm the ST segments are normally isoelectric, unless there is some ischemia.

3.4 Vagal maneuvers are used initially to slow the heart rate and allow the sinus node to resume pacemaker activities; however, if this is not successful, cardioversion is used. Cardioversion may be used if the patient is unstable or the rate is greater than 150 bpm. Intravenous atropine is administered to increase heart rate. Intravenous epinephrine is a sympathomemetic medication and will increase heart rate.

4.3 A PR interval greater than 0.2 seconds indicates a first-degree atrioventricular block. Junctional beats may have P waves and short PR intervals (less than 0.12 seconds). Junctional beats may have no P waves. A junctional rhythm may have inverted P waves in lead II.

5.2 Cardiac output is a result of stroke volume times heart rate. In tachycardias, the increased heart rate shortens diastolic filling time, thus decreasing stroke volume and cardiac output. Wide QRS complexes indicate slowed conduction through the ventricles. Increased stroke volume would occur when there is adequate diastolic filling time, normal afterload, and appropriate contractility. Heart rate is one of the components in the cardiac output formula. Slowed rates decrease cardiac output if the stroke volume does not increase.

6.4 The definition of an accelerated rhythm is a rhythm that is faster than the inherent rate but not fast enough to be a tachycardia. An accelerated junctional rhythm has a rate between 60 and 100 bpm. A ventricular escape rhythm has a rate between 20 and 40 bpm. A junctional tachycardia has a rate greater than 100 bpm. A bradycardia has a rate less than 60 bpm.

7.2 Neonates and children have not developed a mature sympathetic nervous system and therefore may experience supraventricular tachycardias. Teenagers, young adults, and mature adults should have a mature sympathetic nervous system.

CHAPTER *10*—cont'd

8. The health care provider is assessing a rhythm strip and having difficulty identifying P waves. The QRS complexes are less than 0.12 seconds wide. The ventricular rate is 122. The rhythm strip most probably should be identified as:
   1 Ventricular tachycardia
   2 A junctional rhythm
   3 Sinus tachycardia
   4 Supraventricular tachycardia

9. A junctional rhythm with retrograde atrial conduction would be indicated by which of the following?
   1 PR interval greater than 0.28 seconds
   2 PR interval less than 0.12 seconds
   3 P waves upright in lead II
   4 P waves negative in lead II

10. All of the following therapies might be used to treat supraventricular tachycardia °
    1 Atropine
    2 Adenosine
    3 Cardioversion
    4 Vagal maneuvers

CHAPTER *11*

1. Why would a patient have premature ventricular contractions during endotracheal suctioning?

2. You are counseling Ms. Frost after she visits your clinic complaining of palpitations. Her ECG is normal but her Holter monitor shows premature ventricular contractions during her waking hours. Which of the following could you counsel Ms. Frost to avoid to reduce her symptoms?
   1 Cheese
   2 Milk products
   3 Nicotine
   4 Red wine

3. Mr. Landry is admitted to your telemetry unit for congestive heart failure. His laboratory results reveal the following: sodium of 140 mEq/L , potassium of 3.2 mEq/L, calcium of 10 mg/dL, and magnesium of 1.5 mEq/L. Which of these levels could be responsible for the premature ventricular contractions he is having with increasing frequency?
   1 Sodium
   2 Potassium
   3 Calcium
   4 Magnesium

Notes

8. 4 A supraventricular tachycardia has a rate greater than 100 with difficulty identifying P waves and the QRS complexes are normal (< 0.12 seconds wide). A ventricular tachycardia will have a rate greater than 100 with no apparent P waves; however, the QRS complexes will be wide (> 0.12 seconds). A junctional rhythm will have a rate between 40 and 60 bpm. A sinus tachycardia will have a rate greater than 100 with a normal-width QRS; however, in a sinus tachycardia P waves should be identifiable.

9. 4 Negative P waves in lead II indicate retrograde conduction and are indicative of a junctional rhythm. A PR interval greater than 0.28 seconds would be indicative of a first-degree atrioventricular block. A junctional rhythm may have a PR interval less than 0.12 seconds; however, if retrograde conduction occurs, the P wave will be inverted in lead II. In a junctional rhythm with retrograde conduction the P wave is inverted, not upright, in lead II.

10. 1 Atropine is used to treat symptomatic bradycardias. Adenosine may be used to treat narrow complex tachycardias. Cardioversion is used in supraventricular tachycardias when the patient is symptomatic or rates exceed 150 bpm, usually after vagal maneuvers are used. Vagal maneuvers are initially used to slow a supraventricular tachycardia in an attempt to allow the sinus node to regain control.

NCLEX CHAPTER *11* Answers

1. Suctioning removes oxygen along with secretions. Hypoxemia causes premature ventricular contractions.

2. 3 Nicotine stimulates the sympathetic nervous system to increase the heart rate and can cause premature ventricular contractions in a normal person. Milk, cheese, and red wine do not stimulate the sympathetic nervous system.

3. 2 Hypokalemia related to potassium is a frequent and notorious cause of premature ventricular contractions. All of Mr. Landry's other laboratory levels (sodium, magnesium, calcium) are within normal limits.

CHAPTER *11*—cont'd

4. Mr. Yodlowski is experiencing ventricular bigeminy and low blood pressure. Why?

5. According to the American Heart Association, should lidocaine be given prophylactically to patients with acute myocardial infarction to prevent the onset of ventricular tachycardia?

CHAPTER *12*

1. Ventricular tachycardia is defined as:
   1   Atrial rate above 100 bpm
   2   Atrial rate between 90 and 160 bpm
   3   Ventricular rhythm between 100 and 220 bpm
   4   Sinus tachycardia with a ventricular rate greater than 150 bpm

2. According to Advanced Cardiac Life Support protocols, the first line drug for stable ventricular tachycardias is:
   1   Adenosine
   2   Lidocaine
   3   Atropine
   4   Pronestyl

3. According to Advanced Cardiac Life Support, how is the proper treatment for ventricular tachycardia determined?

4. Mrs. Murphy is in ventricular tachycardia at 180 bpm. She is complaining of lightheadedness and shortness of breath. Her blood pressure is 80/60. What action needs to be taken?
   1   Immediately defibrillate at 200 joules.
   2   Administer verapamil 15 mg IV push.
   3   Immediately cardiovert at 100 joules after considering sedation.
   4   Obtain a 12-lead ECG to differentiate ventricular tachycardia from supraventricular tachycardia.

5. First-line treatment for ventricular tachycardia with no pulse is
   1   Defibrillation at 200 joules
   2   Synchronized cardioversion at 50 joules
   3   Lidocaine 1 mg/kg IV push
   4   Bretylium 5 mg/kg IV push

NCLEX CHAPTER *11* **Answers—cont'd**

4. Cardiac output is decreased because every other beat in the premature ventricular contraction represents incomplete ventricular filling; thus blood pressure is decreased.

5. Advanced Cardiac Life Support protocols state that lidocaine should not be used to prevent ventricular dysrhythmias—only to TREAT ventricular dysrhythmias. Lidocaine can cause decreased contractility, seizures, hypotension, and asystole.

NCLEX CHAPTER *12* **Answers**

1. 3 Ventricular tachycardia originates in the ventricles and is therefore a ventricular rhythm. The atrial rate is not significant. Sinus tachycardia is not the same as ventricular tachycardia.

2. 2 Lidocaine is the drug of choice to control irritable foci in the ventricle. Adenosine is indicated in supraventricular, not ventricular, rhythms. Atropine is administered to increase the heart rate in bradycardias. Pronestyl would be given next if lidocaine is ineffective.

3. Advanced Cardiac Life Support protocols recommends assessing the clinical effects of the tachycardia on the patient and then using the appropriate algorithm for either stable ventricular tachycardia, unstable ventricular tachycardia, or pulseless ventricular tachycardia.

4. 3 If the patient is exhibiting chest pain, hypotension, decreased level of consciousness, shortness of breath, or pulmonary edema, the ventricular tachycardia is considered unstable. This patient is in unstable ventricular tachycardia, which requires immediate synchronized cardioversion. Defibrillation is not indicated because she has a pulse and is awake. Verapamil is not indicated; it is used for supraventricular tachycardia and can lower the blood pressure. Since the patient is unstable, time should not be wasted to differentiate the source of the tachycardia by doing a 12-lead ECG.

5. 1 Defibrillation is the treatment of choice for ventricular tachycardia with no pulse. In pulseless ventricular tachycardia, it would not be effective to give lidocaine or bretylium or to perform synchronized cardioversion.

CHAPTER *13*

1. Jamie Funk is a student working in your telemetry unit and taking care of Mr. Johns, who has been known to go into ventricular fibrillation. Jamie wants to be prepared to help with Mr. Johns. You know she understands the concept of defibrillation when she states:
   1 "We will be using a small amount of energy to shock his heart."
   2 "We must set the machine up to avoid the R wave and fire on the T."
   3 "We will give Mr. Johns sedation before shocking him."
   4 "Up to three consecutive shocks (at energy settings of 200, 300 and 360) may need to be delivered."

2. Which of the following describes ventricular fibrillation:
   1 Countable
   2 Regular
   3 Synchronous
   4 Chaotic

3. Ventricular fibrillation may be caused by:
   1 Ventricular tachycardia
   2 Pericarditis
   3 Tuberculosis
   4 Complete heart block

4. Mr. Maiorino has been brought into the emergency department with hypoxia, acidosis, and severe electrolyte imbalances. His cardiac status is of utmost concern to you because:
   1 These are causes of ventricular fibrillation, which can lead to cardiac arrest.
   2 Hypoxia can lead to further lung failure.
   3 Acidosis causes cardiac necrosis.
   4 Electrolyte imbalances cause pericarditis, which can lead to cardiac dysrhythmias.

5. Lidocaine, Atropine, Narcan, and Epinephrine (LANE) are often given by what route to a ventilated patient in ventricular fibrillation?
   1 Intravenous
   2 Down the endotracheal tube
   3 Subcutaneous
   4 Intrathecally into the spinal cord

CHAPTER *14*

1. Which of the following treatments is used for asystole?
   1 Defibrillation
   2 Cardioversion
   3 Pacemaker insertion
   4 Lidocaine

2. The initial treatment for ventricular standstill is:
   1 Cardiopulmonary resuscitation
   2 Defibrillation
   3 Cardioversion
   4 Pacemaker insertion

Notes

NCLEX CHAPTER *13* Answers

1.4 In defibrillation, a 200-joule charge is initially delivered to the precordial surface. If this does not convert the ventricular fibrillation rhythm, the charge is increased to 300 joules. If this still does not convert the rhythm, the charge is increased to the maximal power of 360 joules. Defibrillation delivers a strong electrical charge to the heart, firing all cardiac cells at once. Setting up the machine to fire on the T wave refers to cardioversion. The patient will be unconscious and therefore not need sedation before defibrillation.

2.4 There is no regular pattern or synchrony to the ventricular fibrillation rhythm, which therefore is chaotic. Ventricular fibrillation is not countable as there are no P waves or QRS complexes. Ventricular fibrillation is irregular because of the ventricles quivering.

3.1 An untreated ventricular tachycardia may cause ventricular fibrillation. Pericarditis is an inflammation of the pericardium, which is usually not life threatening unless it develops into cardiac tamponade. Tuberculosis may lead to hemorrhage but not to ventricular fibrillation in and of itself. Complete heart block may lead to asystole but not ventricular fibrillation.

4.1 Ventricular fibrillation has electrolyte disturbances, hypoxia, and acidosis as risk factors and can lead to cardiac arrest.

5.2 Lidocaine, Atropine, Narcan, and Epinephrine medications are administered down the endotracheal tube so they can reach the alveoli blood supply quickly.

NCLEX CHAPTER *14* Answers

1.3 Pacemakers try to stimulate the heart when there is no stimulus from the heart itself. Defibrillation treats ventricular fibrillation. Cardioversion treats tachycardia. Lidocaine is used to treat ventricular dysrhythmias.

2.1 Cardiopulmonary resuscitation is performed because the body has no perfusion to the brain and vital organs. Defibrillation is the treatment for ventricular fibrillation. Cardioversion is the treatment for ventricular tachycardia. Pacemaker insertion comes after cardiopulmonary resuscitation because it is not as immediately available.

CHAPTER *14*—cont'd

3. All of the following rhythms may cause a patient to be pulseless except:
   1 Ventricular tachycardia
   2 Ventricular fibrillation
   3 Asystole
   4 Premature ventricular contractions

4. In a person experiencing cardiac standstill, how will the pupils look?

5. The first drug administered in cardiac standstill is:
   1 Intravenous epinephrine
   2 Intravenous digoxin
   3 Intravenous potassium
   4 Intravenous lidocaine

3. What is the treatment for first-degree heart block?

4. All of the following symptoms may be associated with heart block except
   1 Hypertension
   2 Syncope
   3 Decreased urinary output
   4 Confusion

Notes _____

CHAPTER *15*

1. Which of the following best describes a complete heart block?
   1 Prolonged PR interval
   2 Progressive prolongation of the PR with occasional dropped QRSs
   3 Every other P wave dropped
   4 Ps and QRSs each in a regular pattern but beating independently of each other

2. Mr. Brown is admitted to the progressive telemetry unit with a suspected MI. His rhythm strip indicates the development of second-degree heart block, or Mobitz II. Which of the following medications would you hold until making his primary health care provider aware of the situation?
   1 Digoxin
   2 Atropine
   3 Sublingual nitroglycerin
   4 Dopamine (Intropin)

Notes

3. 4 Premature ventricular contractions produce a weak but palpable pulse. The other rhythms (ventricular tachycardia, ventricular fibrillation, and asystole) usually do not have an obtainable pulse because of a quick drop in blood pressure.

4. Cardiac standstill creates pupils that are dilated and fixed due to absence of blood supply to the brain.

5. 1 Epinephrine is administered to try to quickly and efficiently restart the heart. Digoxin, as a chronotropic drug, promotes a decrease in rate because it prolongs the refractory or resting time of the atrioventricular node. Potassium is administered to correct fluid and electrolyte balance. Lidocaine is used to treat ventricular dysrhythmia.

NCLEX CHAPTER *15* Answers

1. 4 Complete heart block is described as Ps and QRSs in a regular pattern but beating independently of each other. Prolonged PR interval describes first-degree heart block. Progressive prolongation of the PR with occasional dropped QRSs is second-degree heart block, or Wenckebach. "Every other P wave dropped" is the definition for second-degree heart block or Mobitz II.

2. 1 Digoxin, as a chronotropic drug, promotes a decrease in rate because it prolongs the refractory, or resting, time of the atrioventricular node. Atropine is given for symptomatic second-degree heart block. Nitroglycerin is given for chest pain and is contraindicated in hypotension. Dopamine is given in larger intravenous doses for hypotension, which could result from second-degree heart block.

3. First-degree heart block is relatively benign, and there is no specific treatment unless the heart rate drops too low; in this case, the treatment would be of the bradycardia, not the first-degree heart block itself. The first-degree block should be closely observed to ensure that it does not advance to a higher level.

4. 1 Hypotension, but not hypertension, can be a result of heart block. Syncope, decreased urinary output, and confusion are symptoms that can be caused by heart block as a result of lack of oxygen to the brain and kidneys.

CHAPTER *15*—cont'd

5. Ventricular escape beats are treated with
   1 Nothing
   2 Procainamide
   3 Cardioversion
   4 Lidocaine

CHAPTER *16*

1. An acoustic image that looks at the size and shape of the heart and heart valves in called an:
   1 Electrocardiogram
   2 Electroencephalogram
   3 Endoscopic vesselogram
   4 Echocardiogram

2. To evaluate prosthetic heart valves in an obese person, the best cardiac diagnostic test to perform would be a(n):
   1 ECG
   2 Holter monitor
   3 Transesophageal echocardiogram
   4 Sinoatrial ECG

3. Mrs. Eckroid's Holter monitor indicates pacemaker failure. What two symptoms are usually associated with this?
   1 Dizziness and syncope
   2 Diarrhea and fever
   3 Shortness of breath and leg cramps
   4 Headache and vomiting

4. A Holter monitor is commonly used to evaluate what type of drug therapy?
   1 Antihypertensive
   2 Antidiarrheal
   3 Antispasmodic
   4 Antidysrhythmic

5. The patient's apical pulse is tachycardic, and he is complaining of angina, shortness of breath, and syncope. He has a history of dizziness for the past 3 days. Based on this information, what might the patient's diagnosis be?
   1 Renal failure
   2 Cardiac dysrhythmia
   3 Brain tumor
   4 Hypertension

6. Which of the following will create artifact on the sinoatrial ECG? The patient:
   1 Is lying still
   2 Has his or her eyes open
   3 Is shivering
   4 Is lying with the head of the bed elevated 15 degrees

7. The initial dose of dobutamine for a pharmacologic stress test in an adult is:
   1 1 mcg/kg/min
   2 5 to 10 mcg/kg/min
   3 25 mg oral
   4 50 mg sublingual

Notes

NCLEX C H A P T E R *15* **Answers**—cont'd

5. 1 Ventricular escape beats are the ventricles' attempt to help out a bad situation. If you suppress the only beats you have by administering procainamide or lidocaine or giving cardioversion, you will worsen the situation and cause asystole.

NCLEX C H A P T E R *16* **Answers**

1. 4 An echocardiogram is by definition an acoustic image of the heart and heart valves. An electrocardiogram evaluates the heart's electrical activity, while an electroencephalogram evaluates brain activity. An endoscopic vesselogram is not a real test.

2. 3 TEE evaluates prosthetic heart valves and is particularly useful in seeing the heart in obese persons. An ECG and the Holter monitor evaluate the electrical activity of the heart. A sinoatrial ECG detects low amplitude electrical activity of the heart during diastole.

3. 1 Dizziness (syncope) is a result of a lack of steady oxygen supply to the brain. Diarrhea, fever, headache, and vomiting are not symptoms of pacemaker failure. Shortness of breath is a symptom, but leg cramps are not.

4. 4 Holter monitors monitor the heart. Antidysrhythmic drug therapy is for the heart. Antihypertensives are blood pressure medications. Antidiarrheals are to lessen stool output. Antispasmotics stop muscle spasms.

5. 2 Based on the symptoms cardiac dysrhythmia is suspected. Renal failure, brain tumor, and hypertension would not cause angina.

6. 3 Shivering is movement, and patient movement causes artifact. The patient should be lying still. Having his or her eyes open does not affect the test. Lying with head of the bed elevated 15 degrees has no effect on detecting heart activity during diastole.

7. 2 The correct dose is 5 to 10 mcg/kg/min. A dose of 1 mcg/kg/min is too low to be effective. An oral dose of 25 mg is incorrect because dobutamine is only given intravenously and 25 mg is an incorrect dose. A sublingual dose of 50 mg is also an incorrect dose and route.

CHAPTER *16*—cont'd

8. You have a 42-year-old man scheduled for a stress test. Which of these factors would give you a clue that the test should be canceled?
   1 He had a pulmonary embolism 5 years ago.
   2 He had 30 ml of water this morning.
   3 He denies chest pain.
   4 He is digitalis toxic according to his blood work results.

CHAPTER *17*

1. You are instructing a UAP to perform a 12-lead ECG. You know he or she is learning correct lead placement when he or she says:
   1 "All of the limb leads go across the chest."
   2 "V6 is positioned under the left armpit, just above the last two ribs."
   3 "Accuracy isn't really important when placing the precordial leads."
   4 "V1 is at the left of the sternum in the fourth intercostal space."

2. A patient is said to have had a transmural infarction when he has a:
   1 QRS between 0.10 and 0.12
   2 Prolonged PR interval
   3 High peaked T wave
   4 Q wave one fourth the depth of the R wave

3. The precordial leads are:
   1 I, II, and III
   2 aVR, aVL, aVF
   3 II, III, and aVF
   4 V1 through V6

4. The earliest sign on the ECG that an infarction is occurring is:
   1 A wide Q wave
   2 ST segment depression
   3 T-wave elevation
   4 T-wave depression

CHAPTER *18*

1. Which of the following is not a viral cause of pericarditis?
   1 Liver cancer
   2 Varicella
   3 Influenza
   4 Coxsackie

2. Pericarditis can be caused by what major organ(s) failing?
   1 Gallbladder
   2 Spleen
   3 Kidneys
   4 Brain

Notes

Notes

8.4 As the heart is already stressed because of too much cardiac medication, and overstressing the heart with the stress test could cause death, this patient's stress test should be canceled. Only a recent pulmonary embolism would contraindicate the stress test. Liquids need to be refrained from for 2 hours before the test. If the patient had chest pain the stress test would be canceled, but his denial makes this unnecessary.

NCLEX CHAPTER *17* Answers

1.2 V6 is in the fifth intercostal space at the midaxillary line. Not all 12 leads go across the chest. Lead placement is of the utmost importance because if placed incorrectly they can cause error in readings by the health care provider. V2, not V1, is at the left of the sternum in the fourth intercostal space.

2.4 A transmural infarction causes the loss of the R wave and a deep Q wave that is more than one fourth the height of the patient's R wave. A QRS between .10 and .12 is not long enough for a transmural Q wave. A prolonged PR interval is characteristic of a heart block, not an infarction. T-wave inversion is a characteristic of an infarction.

3.4 The V leads are also called precordial leads and go across the left chest, from the right of the heart to the left. I, II and III are limb leads. aVR, aVL, and aVF are augmented leads. II, III, and aVF look at the inferior surface of the left ventricle.

4.4 T waves flip over, indicating ischemia of myocardial cells. The Q wave is generally the last sign to appear because necrosis takes several hours to evolve. ST depression will occur in the leads opposite of the infarction. T-wave depression is a sign of ischemia, which is the first zone of an infarction.

NCLEX CHAPTER *18* Answers

1.1 Liver cancer is not a virus. Varicella, influenza, and coxsackie are all viruses that can precipitate pericarditis.

2.3 Pericarditis can be caused by renal (kidney) failure. An ECG waveform indicating gallbladder, spleen, or brain failure would be characterized differently.

CHAPTER *18*—cont'd

3. In cardiac tamponade, cardiac output is:
   1   Increased
   2   Decreased
   3   Within normal limits
   4   Only affected if accompanied by hypotension

4. Pleuritic chest pain as a symptom of pericarditis worsens:
   1   During inspiration
   2   During expiration
   3   While sitting up
   4   While leaning forward

5. Your nursing assessment for a patient with probable cardiac tamponade reveals that pulses become weaker during inspiration. This sign is called:
   1   Electrical alternans
   2   Tachycardia
   3   Precordial friction rib
   4   Pulsus paradoxus

6. Electrical alternans in an ECG is assessed in what part of the ECG cycle?
   1   T wave
   2   P wave
   3   PR interval
   4   QRS complex

7. Pericarditis is an inflammatory process that increases what laboratory value?
   1   Hematocrit (HCT)
   2   Total red blood cell (RBC) count
   3   Erythrocyte sedimentation rate (ESR)
   4   Prothrombin time (PT)

8. A pericardial friction rub is best auscultated:
   1   Over the second intercostal space, right midclavicular line (MCL)
   2   Two finger breaths to the right of the xyphoid process at the fourth intercostal space
   3   Over the mid–xyphoid process
   4   Over the left lower sternal border

9. Withdrawal of fluid from the pericardial sac is known as a(n):
   1   Echocardiogram
   2   Pericardiocentesis
   3   Xyphoid endoscopy
   4   Thoracentesis

10. Which of the following is an indication of a successful pericardiocentesis?
   1   Hypotension
   2   Cardiac standstill
   3   Clearer heart sounds to auscultation
   4   Increased temperature

Notes

Notes

NCLEX CHAPTER *18* **Answers**—cont'd

3. 2 Cardiac tamponade decreases cardiac output. Fluid buildup does compress the heart. Cardiac output is not only affected if accompanied by hypotension; it is affected by multiple factors such as decreased stroke volume and increased heart rate.

4. 1 Pleuritic pain worsens on inspiration because this increases pressure within the thoracic cavity and on the heart itself. Pleuritic pain lessens when the patient is sitting or leaning forward.

5. 4 When pulses become weaker during inspiration in a patient with cardiac tamponade, it is known as pulsus paradoxus. Electrical alternans is a phenomenon seen on the ECG strip. Tachycardia would be a fast heart rate and pulse, not a weak one. Precordial friction rub is a high-pitched sound heard on auscultation at the end of inspiration.

6. 4 Electrical alternans can be assessed from the QRS complex on the ECG because the QRS alternates voltage. The T wave, P wave, and PR interval do not help assess electrical alternans.

7. 3 Pericarditis should increase the laboratory values for ESR because this increases with inflammation. HCT is associated with the percentage of red blood cells in volume. Total RBC count is associated with numbers of red blood cells, while PT is associated with clotting.

8. 4 The pericardium lies at the left lower sternal border, so a pericardial friction rub is best auscultated here.

9. 2 Pericardiocentesis. An echocardiogram is a noninvasive ultrasound procedure of the heart. Thoracentesis is the removal of fluid from the lungs, not the pericardial sac. There is no such procedure as a xyphoid endoscopy.

10. 3 Clearer heart sounds on auscultation, increased blood pressure, and distended neck veins are indications of a successful pericardiocentesis. Hypotension could be a sign of cardiac perforation. If cardiac standstill occurs, CPR should be initiated immediately. Increased temperature would be a sign of infection.

CHAPTER *19*

1. ECG changes indicative of hyperkalemia include:
   1 Prolonged QT intervals
   2 ST-segment depression
   3 Tall, peaked T waves
   4 Decreased T-wave amplitude

2. Digitalis may have all of the following effects on the ECG except to:
   1 Shorten the QT interval.
   2 Prolong the PR interval.
   3 Cause scooping of the ST segments.
   4 Increase the heart rate.

3. Calcium channel blockers may be utilized for all of the following except:
   1 Supraventricular tachycardias
   2 Heart blocks
   3 Atrial tachycardias
   4 Hypertension

4. ECG changes indicating hypokalemia may include:
   1 ST-segment depression
   2 Prolonged QT intervals
   3 Development of U waves
   4 Tall, peaked T waves

5. Class IA antidysrhythmics include all of the following except:
   1 Lidocaine
   2 Quinidine
   3 Disopyramide (Norpace)
   4 Procainamide (Pronestyl)

6. Scooping of the ST segment, heart blocks, bradycardia, and prolonged PR intervals are all characteristics of _____ toxicity.
   1 Digitalis (Lanoxin)
   2 Potassium

   3 Procainamide (Pronestyl)
   4 Quinidine (Quinaglute)

7. The patient's potassium level is 3.2 mEq/L. The health care provider knows replacement of potassium is:
   1 Done by administering a 20 mEq potassium bolus
   2 Always done with the potassium diluted
   3 Always done with intramuscular injections
   4 Usually given via rectal suppository

8. The most frequent cause of hypokalemia in a patient is _____ therapy:
   1 Corticosteroid
   2 Diuretic
   3 Calcium
   4 Digoxin

Notes _____

NCLEX CHAPTER *19* Answers

1. 3   Tall, peaked T waves may occur with hyperkalemia. Prolonged QT intervals, ST-segment depression, and decreased T-wave amplitude are all signs of hypokalemia.

2. 4   Digitalis typically decreases the heart rate. Digitalis may also shorten the QT interval and prolong the PR interval. A hallmark sign of digitalis effect is ST-segment scooping

3. 2   Calcium channel blockers should never be given to patients with bradycardia, sick sinus syndrome, or heart blocks. Calcium channel blockers are used to treat supraventricular tachycardias because they slow atrioventricular conduction time and increase the refractoriness of the atrioventricular node. Calcium channel blockers may be used for patients with atrial tachycardias because they slow atrioventricular conduction time. Calcium channel blockers lower blood pressure and can be used in cases of hypertension.

4. 4   Hyperkalemia results in tall, peaked T waves. ST-segment depression, prolonged QT intervals, and the occurrence of U waves indicate hypokalemia.

1. 1   Lidocaine is considered a class IB agent. Quinidine, disopyramide, and procainamide are class IA agents. Class IA agents slow the influx of sodium into the cardiac cell and decrease the rate of depolarization.

6. 1   Scooping of the ST segments, heart blocks, bradycardia, and prolonging of PR intervals are the ECG signs of digitoxicity. Potassium changes depend on whether the patient is hypokalemic or hyperkalemic. ECG changes characteristic of class IA antidysrhythmics include long PR intervals, QRS, and QT. Quinidine and procainamide are class IA antidysrhythmic drugs.

7. 2   No matter the route, potassium is always diluted. Potassium given by rapid IV bolus can result in ventricular fibrillation and death. Potassium is never given by the intramuscular route because it irritates the tissues. Potassium is not readily absorbed as a rectal suppository and is also very irritating to those tissues.

8. 2   Most loop diuretics cause potassium wasting. Corticosteroids cause water retention and hyponatremia. There is no correlation between calcium excess and potassium depletion. Combination therapy of loop diuretic and cardiac glycoside (digoxin) causes hypokalemia.

Notes

CHAPTER **20**

1. A condition that may contribute to rapid heart rates and that is characterized by an accessory pathway called the bundle of Kent is:
   1   Atrial fibrillation
   2   Wolff-Parkinson-White (WPW) syndrome
   3   Lown-Ganong-Levine (LGL) syndrome
   4   Complete heart block

2. Which of the following is not a characteristic of LGL syndrome?
   1   Short PR interval
   2   Normal width QRS complex
   3   Delta wave
   4   Supraventricular tachycardias

3. Which of the following is NOT a characteristic of WPW syndrome?
   1   Short PR interval
   2   Aberrant ventricular conduction
   3   Delta wave
   4   Normal width QRS complex

4. In LGL syndrome, what is the accessory pathway is called?

5. What is premature activation of the ventricular myocardium referred to as?

CHAPTER **21**

1. A patient who is known to have an internal cardioverter-defibrillator (ICD) is admitted to the cardiac care unit with intermittent episodes of dizziness and palpitations. Which of the following should the health care provider do first?
   1   Deactivate the ICD by placing a pacemaker magnet over the pulse generator.
   2   Obtain a 12-lead ECG.

3   Ensure that resuscitation equipment is available and monitor the patient's rhythm continuously.
4   Teach the patient relaxation techniques and deep breathing.

2. A patient who has recently had an ICD implanted is learning about the device. Which of the following statements by the patient demonstrates an understanding of the purpose of this device?
   1   The ICD uses electrical impulses to control dangerous heart rhythms.
   2   The ICD will prevent dangerous heart rhythms from occurring.
   3   The ICD will make my heart stronger.
   4   The ICD will prevent my heart beat from slowing down too much.

3. A patient who has had an ICD implanted expresses anxiety regarding the sensation that will be felt when the device discharges. Appropriate teaching on the part of the health care provider includes which of the following statements?
   1   "When the device discharges, it will make you faint."
   2   "When the device discharges, you will not even feel it."
   3   "Different patients experience the discharging of the device in different ways."
   4   "Different patients have different pain thresholds, but it shouldn't bother you too much."

Notes

NCLEX CHAPTER *20* Answers

1. 2   The accessory pathway in WPW syndrome is the bundle of Kent. Atrial fibrillation does not have an accessory pathway via bundle of Kent, LGL bypasses the AV node through James fibers, and complete heart block is not characterized by tachycardia.

2. 3   In LGL syndrome, there is preexcitation because the impulse bypasses the atrioventricular node by way of James fibers. Because there is no conduction through the atrioventricular node, there is no potential for a delta wave to occur. A short PR interval, a normal width QRS complex, and supraventricular tachycardias are all characteristics of LGL syndrome.

3. 4   Aberrant ventricular contraction occurs because the ventricles are stimulated by the Bundle of Kent and via the atrioventricular node, causing a wide QRS complex. A short PR interval, aberrant ventricular conduction, and a delta wave are characteristics of WPW syndrome.

4.   The accessory pathway in LGL syndrome is James fibers.

5.   Preexcitation is activation of the ventricular myocardium sooner than normal.

NCLEX CHAPTER *21* Answers

1. 3   The patient's symptoms may indicate a malfunctioning ICD. Resuscitation equipment should be immediately available, and the heart rhythm should be continuously monitored. The pulse generator should not be deactivated except during resuscitation. While a 12-lead ECG would be helpful in diagnosis, it is not the first action the provider should take. Relaxation has no effect on internal defibrillation.

2. 1   The ICD controls dangerous heart rhythms. The ICD does not prevent dangerous heart rhythms from occurring or affect the strength or contractility of the heart muscle.

3. 3   Some patients experience collapse, and others are not even aware the device has discharged. Patient response to discharging of the device is an individual phenomenon. Some patients do experience unconsciousness. By telling the patient that it shouldn't "bother" him or her too much, the provider implies that if the discharge of the device is perceived to be uncomfortable, the patient must have a low pain tolerance.

CHAPTER *21*—cont'd

4. A patient is admitted to the hospital unit following a transvenous pacemaker placement. The patient denies pain but is uncomfortable because of unrelenting hiccups. Vital signs are within normal limits and respirations are unlabored. An appropriate action on the part of the health care provider is to:

   1 Ascertain that the patient has an intact gag reflex, then offer clear liquids.
   2 Determine how the patient treats hiccups at home and assist in carrying out the treatment.
   3 Call the physician to report the hiccups and place the patient on continuous cardiac monitoring.
   4 Position the patient on the right side and contact the physician for a chlorpromazine (Thorazine) order.

5. Which of the following patient statements indicates an understanding of pacemaker precautions?

   1 "I should avoid microwave ovens."
   2 "I should avoid high frequency sounds."
   3 "I should avoid cordless telephones."
   4 "I should avoid powerful magnetic sources."

6. Reprogramming of implanted permanent pacemakers is accomplished by:

   1 A simple outpatient surgical procedure
   2 Radio frequencies transmitted through the skin
   3 A pacemaker magnet
   4 A telephone call to the health care provider's office

7. Mrs. Flanceski is a patient admitted to the ambulatory surgery unit for a minor orthopedic procedure. The patient states she is feeling well this morning. Her chart indicates that she has an implanted dual-chamber pacemaker. When the nurse initiates ECG monitoring per unit procedure, the patient's heart rate is 80 bpm but no pacemaker spikes are visible. This situation indicates:

   1 Mrs. Flanceski needs a battery replacement for her pacemaker.
   2 Mrs. Flanceski needs her pacemaker reprogrammed.
   3 The physician should be notified and resuscitation equipment taken to the bedside.
   4 The pacemaker is sensing Mrs. Flanceski's naturally occurring heart rate.

8. Cardiomyopathy is a common cardiac problem for individuals who chronically abuse drugs. Which of the following drugs would not cause this problem?

   1 Cocaine
   2 Marijuana
   3 Amphetamines
   4 Alcohol

9. Myocardial infarction can occur with use of which of the following illicit drugs?

   1 Alcohol
   2 Crack
   3 Angel dust
   4 Inhalants

Notes

4.3 The pacemaker leads can become dislodged, irritate the diaphragm, and cause the patient to have hiccups. When pacemaker malfunction is suspected, the patient should be monitored continuously. Home remedies will not stop hiccups that are the result of a pacemaker malfunction. Putting the patient on continuous cardiac monitoring could cause more damage to the pacemaker. Although Thorazine is sometimes used to stop hiccups, in this case it can cause more cardiac problems.

5.4 Powerful magnetic sources may affect pacemaker function. Pacemakers are not affected by the microwave ovens in use today. While pacemakers can be reprogrammed by radiofrequency through the skin, hearing high frequency sounds has no effect. Cordless telephones do not affect pacemaker function.

6.2 Reprogramming of implanted permanent pacemakers is accomplished by radio frequencies transmitted through the skin. A simple surgical procedure is sometimes necessary to change the battery. A pacemaker magnet will deactivate the device. While pacemaker function can be monitored via telephone, reprogramming cannot currently be accomplished in this way.

7.4 Because the rate is 80 bpm and the patient is asymptomatic, the absence of pacemaker spikes is an indication that the pacemaker is not in control of the patient's heart rhythm. Since the patient's heart rate is 80 bpm without pacing and she is asymptomatic, it is likely that the device senses the adequacy of the patient's naturally occurring rhythm. There is no "demand" for pacing in this situation.

8.2 Marijuana does not cause cardiomyopathy. Cocaine, amphetamines, and alcohol increase heart rate.

9.2 Cocaine and crack use stimulates the sympathetic nervous system, increasing production of epinephrine and norepinephrine; this may cause coronary vasospasm and vasoconstriction. Local damage to the endothelial lining of the coronary vessels can cause platelet aggregation and thrombus formation. A myocardial infarction can occur with no history of heart disease. The three remaining drugs do not affect the heart in the same way. With alcohol, angel dust, and inhalants, no myocardial infarction occurs.

CHAPTER **21**—cont'd

10. Mr. Smith underwent a cardiac transplantation 24 hours ago. The health care provider observed a change in his ECG strip indicating a supraventricular tachycardia. The treatment of choice is:

    1 Digitalis

    2 Carotid sinus pressure

    3 Cardioversion

    4 Valsalva maneuver

11. As an emergency nurse, you have just received a patient who had been in a motorcycle accident. It was reported that the motorcycle had landed on his chest. Ecchymotic lesions were evident on the chest, a pericardial friction rub was heard, and retrosternal pain was present. Your first priority as an emergency room nurse would be to:

    1 Obtain a complete medical history.

    2 Administer oxygen.

    3 Monitor the ECG.

    4 Assess airway, breathing, and circulation.

12. ECG changes with cardiac trauma include:

    1 Bradycardia

    2 Tachycardia

    3 Normal sinus rhythm

    4 Right bundle branch block

10. 3 Treatment of supraventricular tachycardia is limited because of denervation of the heart; therefore cardioversion may be required. Because of the denervation (absence of autonomic innervation) effect on the transplanted heart's responses to digitalis, carotid sinus pressure will not be effective. The Valsalva maneuver stimulates the vagus nerve, causing a slowing of the heart in a normal autonomic innervation. Since the transplanted heart is denervated, the heart is dependent upon circulating catecholamines and an increased venous return to manage heart rate and contractility.

11. 4 Maintaining the airway, breathing, and circulation is obviously essential to the life of the patient. Obtaining a complete medical history is not the first priority, and assessment is needed before treating the patient by administering oxygen. An ECG cannot provide all necessary data on the airway, breathing, and circulation.

12. 2 Tachycardia acts to increase the amount of oxygen delivered to cells of the body by increasing the amount of blood circulated through the vessels. Tachycardia accompanies anoxia, such as that caused by cardiac trauma. Only tachycardia has an increased heart rate over 100 bpm. A normal sinus rhythm is not a threat, and right bundle branch block is not associated with cardiac trauma.

Index

Page numbers followed by *f* indicate figures; *t*, tables.